HANDBOOK OF PHYSICAL MEASUREMENTS

HANDBOOK OF PHYSICAL MEASUREMENTS

Karen W. Gripp

CHIEF OF THE DIVISION OF MEDICAL GENETICS
A. I. DU PONT HOSPITAL FOR CHILDREN
PROFESSOR OF PEDIATRICS
THOMAS JEFFERSON MEDICAL COLLEGE

Anne M. Slavotinek

PROFESSOR OF CLINICAL PEDIATRICS
UNIVERSITY OF CALIFORNIA, SAN FRANCISCO

Judith E. Allanson

PROFESSOR OF PEDIATRICS
UNIVERSITY OF OTTAWA

Judith G. Hall

PROFESSOR EMERITA
UNIVERSITY OF BRITISH COLUMBIA

OXFORD
UNIVERSITY PRESS

OXFORD
UNIVERSITY PRESS

Oxford University Press is a department of the University of Oxford.
It furthers the University's objective of excellence in research, scholarship,
and education by publishing worldwide.

Oxford New York
Auckland Cape Town Dar es Salaam Hong Kong Karachi
Kuala Lumpur Madrid Melbourne Mexico City Nairobi
New Delhi Shanghai Taipei Toronto

With offices in
Argentina Austria Brazil Chile Czech Republic France Greece
Guatemala Hungary Italy Japan Poland Portugal Singapore
South Korea Switzerland Thailand Turkey Ukraine Vietnam

Published in the United States of America by
Oxford University Press
198 Madison Avenue, New York, NY 10016

Library of Congress Cataloging in Publication Data
Handbook of physical measurements / edited by Karen W. Gripp ... [et al.].—3rd ed.
p. ; cm.
Includes bibliographical references and index.
ISBN 978-0-19-993571-0 (pbk. : alk. paper)—ISBN 978-0-19-998979-9
(uPDF ebook)—ISBN 978-0-19-932563-4 (epub ebook)
I. Gripp, Karen W.
[DNLM: 1. Body Weights and Measures—methods—Handbooks. 2. Infant. 3. Child.
4. Growth—Handbooks. 5. Growth Disorders—diagnosis—Handbooks. 6. Reference
Values—Handbooks. WS 39]
QM28
573.6—dc23
2013003366

1 3 5 7 9 8 6 4 2
Printed in the United States of America
on acid-free paper

CONTENTS

1. Introduction 1
2. Measurement 4
3. Proportional Growth and Normal Variants 14
4. Height and Length 16
5. Weight 50
6. Head Circumference (Occipitofrontal Circumference, OFC) 77
7. Craniofacies 86
8. Limbs 197
9. Chest and Trunk 262
10. Genitalia 285
11. Skin and Hair 309
12. Dermatoglyphics and Trichoglyphics 330
13. Use of Radiographs for Measurement 345
14. Developmental Data 365
15. Prenatal Ultrasound Measurements 376
16. Postmortem Organ Weights 394

17. Measurements for Specific Syndromes 408
18. An Approach to the Child with Dysmorphic Features 544

Glossary *549*
Index *563*

HANDBOOK OF PHYSICAL MEASUREMENTS

Chapter 1

Introduction

The purpose of this handbook is to provide a practical collection of reference data on a variety of physical measurements for use in the evaluation of children and adults with dysmorphic features and/or structural anomalies. It has been prepared as a small pocket book so that it can easily be carried by the physician to the ward or "the field" and a companion digital application is available for handheld devices. This book and the application are intended for use by health professionals evaluating the size of various physical features. It is an attempt to provide standards both for comparison and for improved definition of normal patterns of human development and growth.

There is a need for a standardized approach to physical measurement in patients with congenital anomalies and syndromes. Until recently, the study of children with dysmorphic features has primarily involved qualitative descriptions. Descriptive terms have since been standardized and this edition of the handbook uses the preferred terminology. The descriptive terminology is accurate and should be used consistently, as the definition and delineation of new clinical entities require precise and reproducible methods. Careful documentation by measurement, in well-known conditions, will allow one to distinguish heterogeneity, learn more about natural history, and provide a basis for the future application of techniques and concepts from developmental biology and molecular genetics.

The real value of a single measurement lies in comparison with a standard. The standard can be an age-related norm, or it can be the individual patient at another point in time. Comparisons can also be made for the growth of different parts of the body; for example, to see whether head circumference, height, and weight are at the same percentile or at different percentiles. While graphs or tables of standard growth parameters—length, weight, and head circumference —are easy to find, it is often difficult to obtain comparable standards for other body structures. For this reason, we have compiled a comprehensive set of normal curves for ocular measurements and other craniofacial features, such as the ear. For the measurement graphs we have chosen to illustrate percentiles, if available, rather than standard deviations, in order to be consistent. Standard deviations do allow comparison of the individual patient to an age-related normal population, but percentiles have the additional advantage of allowing serial growth measurements in the same person and comparison of the growth of different body parts in one individual in a more easily interpretable form (unless, of course, the measurements are substantially below the 3rd or substantially above the 97th percentile).

We recognize that obtaining precise physical measurements is, in fact, a complex and specialized field in itself. However, for routine clinical use, the method must be simple enough to "get the job done." Therefore, we have outlined and illustrated practical and simple methods and have chosen those graphs and tables that, in our experience as practicing clinical geneticists, are the most useful.

STRUCTURE OF THE BOOK

We have chosen charts and graphs that are in common use and, as often as possible, have combined sources. Body proportions and norms for one ethnic group may not be appropriate for individuals from other ethnic backgrounds; however, little ethnic data are available. Each chapter concentrates on a specific body area and includes:

1. an introduction with embryology, the landmarks from which the measurements were taken, the necessary instruments, and the ways in which the measurements can be obtained;
2. growth charts;

3. references to which the reader should refer for an in-depth understanding of statistics, methodology, anthropometrics, and anthropologic approach.

There is a chapter on the approach to the patient with structural anomalies. A glossary at the end of the book defines many of the terms that have been used.

This book and application are an attempt to provide an "easy to use" collection of data on physical measurements aimed at better defining congenital anomalies and syndromes. The authors are aware that this collection is incomplete and will need revision, additions, and updating; therefore, suggestions to improve the quality and usability of the book are welcomed.

Chapter 2

Measurement

WHY MEASUREMENTS ARE USEFUL

Growth is the essence of the developing organism. Physical growth starts shortly after fertilization and continues throughout gestation, childhood, and adolescence. It may even occur in the adult. Growth of different parts of the body follows a predictable schedule during normal development and maturation. This timetable of development is influenced and controlled by many genetic and environmental factors. Any disturbance in the "normal" sequence of development and growth may lead to disproportion of physical features. These imbalances may be transient and can sometimes be compensated for by subsequent catch-up growth. Most syndromes with dysmorphic features, however, display more or less recognizable patterns of disproportionate growth.

The growth of different parts of the body can be observed and measured at one point in time or at specific time intervals. It can be expressed as a number, a comparison, a percentile, or a standard deviation from the norm. The comparison may be with the growing individual at different ages (so that one can observe changes over time) or with standardized normal values (obtained from either cross-sectional or longitudinal studies of a specific group of individuals). One can assess and compare differential growth of various parts of the body.

Longitudinal studies follow a group of individuals or cohort over time, with standardized measurements obtained at precise intervals. Longitudinal studies are difficult because they include a large number of individuals who must be measured at set intervals, using the same techniques, and, ideally, by the same person(s). Longitudinal studies provide data on patterns of growth and growth velocity. Velocity curves are valuable in demonstrating the rate of change of a specific dimension with time. However, the work involved and the time span can prevent the collection of longitudinal data.

Cross-sectional studies utilize data obtained from a large number of individuals of the same age, usually collected at one time. Cross-sectional studies are technically less difficult to do because they do not rely on the long-term cooperation of many individuals. Cross-sectional studies are used mainly as standards of physical measurement and provide less information about variability, velocity, or patterns of growth over time.

Statistical and data collection methods involved in the construction of normal growth curves will not be discussed further. Details are available in the literature references listed. It is important for the reader to be aware that the various standards provided in this book often come from different populations using different methodologies and so are not really comparable. Nevertheless, they are the only measurements presently available.

Most syndromes with dysmorphic features show disturbances of growth either of the entire body or of certain body parts. In the past, various atypical features have been expressed in qualitative terms, such as short stature, long fingers, or other terms that imply a comparison with other body proportions. An impression of the patient or a "gestalt" is formed in the reader's mind. The terminology used to describe physical findings and their variation among people has been standardized. A more objective way to assess body proportions is by quantitative measurement. This is especially important when the disturbance in growth involves only a specific body area or can be related to a disease process, because it may give insight into the basic mechanisms underlying the growth disturbance and thus to the pathogenesis of the disease.

Comparison of the dimensions obtained for a specific individual or patient with a normal standard curve requires three things:

1. standardized landmarks on the body from which and to which measurements can be taken;
2. standardized methods of taking measurements;
3. standard equipment.

The landmarks that we will use are shown in Figure 2.1 and will be referred to at the beginning of each measurement section. In general, they represent surface landmarks of underlying bony structures that can be palpated easily through the skin. To obtain a minimum degree of accuracy in physical measurement, the examiner should be aware of these landmarks. There are individual anatomical variations, especially in patients with congenital anomalies or syndromes

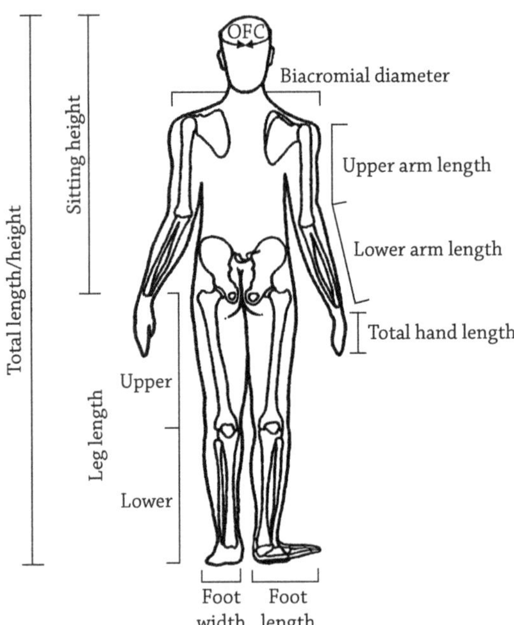

Figure 2.1. Body landmarks to and from which measurements can be taken.

with dysmorphic features. Landmarks for measurements of the head and facial structures will be discussed in detail in Chapter 7.

SUMMARY

By taking accurate physical measurements, we can express and communicate observations on growth, proportion, and disturbances of the developmental process in quantitative terms. Single measurements are meaningless in isolation. They are valuable only in relation to other parameters and in comparison with normal values.

ANTHROPOMETRY

Anthropometry is the study of comparative measurement of the human body. A number of precision instruments are available for accurate anthropometric studies. A decision to use these instruments will depend upon the degree of precision that is desired or required.

The pediatrician, physician, medical geneticist, dysmorphologist, or clinician interested in taking precise physical measurements may want to use anthropometric instruments. However, adequate training is necessary to use these devices properly (Fig. 2.2). Most clinics will have an upright measuring device (stadiometer), a supine measuring table, and an infant scale as well as a regular scale. In clinics in which growth is frequently measured, skinfold calipers, orchidometers, and other types of calipers will probably be available. In research centers, such as those dealing with reconstructive surgery of the face, precision instruments for technical measurements are used. Digital technology including three-dimensional photography and computerized data analysis may also be available.

In general, the accuracy required to create standard curves in anthropological research under laboratory circumstances will be much greater than the precision that can be expected from the physician who is measuring an unwilling, screaming child. Use of precision

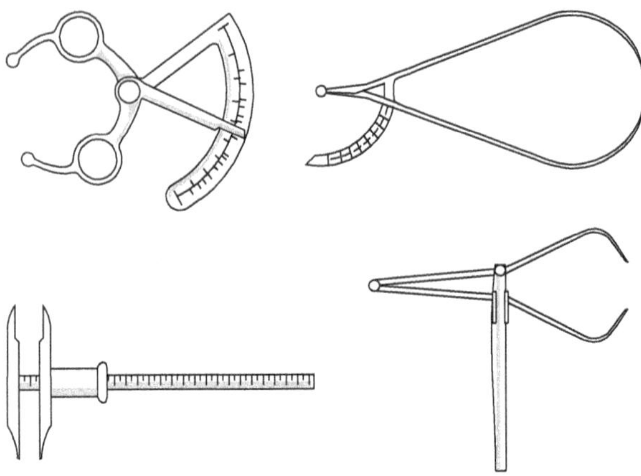

Figure 2.2. Anthropometric instruments: calipers.

instruments usually demands a great deal of cooperation from the patient.

Alternatively, precise physical measurements can be extrapolated from a standardized photograph in a technique called *photogrammetric anthropometry*. This method is costly, requiring standardized cameras and computational technology, and again it is not an everyday, practical approach. Clinical geneticists frequently take photographs to document clinical features. A standard set includes face, front, and side; total body, front, back, and side with palms forward; close-up of hands and feet, and any other atypical features. However, without a reference standard of size in the photograph, they cannot be used for accurate measurements.

For the clinic or ward examination, ordinary tape measures will be most frequently used. It is important to note that metallic or disposable paper tapes are more reliable for long-term use than cloth tapes. Cloth tapes tend to wear out and become stretched over a period of time. If a cloth tape is used, it should be checked from time to time against a metal or wooden standard.

For a long time, there has been a dual measurement system—most European countries used metric units (meters and grams), whereas many physicians in the United States used Imperial units (inches and

millimeter (mm) ÷ 25.4 = inch (in)	inch (in) ÷ 0.039 = millimeter (mm)
centimeter (cm) ÷ 2.54 = inch (in)	inch (in) ÷ 0.394 = centimeter (cm)
centimeter (cm) ÷ 30.5 = foot (ft)	foot (ft) ÷ 0.033 = centimeter (cm)
meter (m) ÷ 0.305 = foot (ft)	foot (ft) ÷ 3.279 = meter (m)
meter (m) ÷ 0.915 = yard (yd)	yard (yd) ÷ 1.093 = meter (m)
1 foot (ft) = 12 inches (in);	1 yard (yd) = 3 feet (ft); 1 yard (yd) = 36 inches (in)

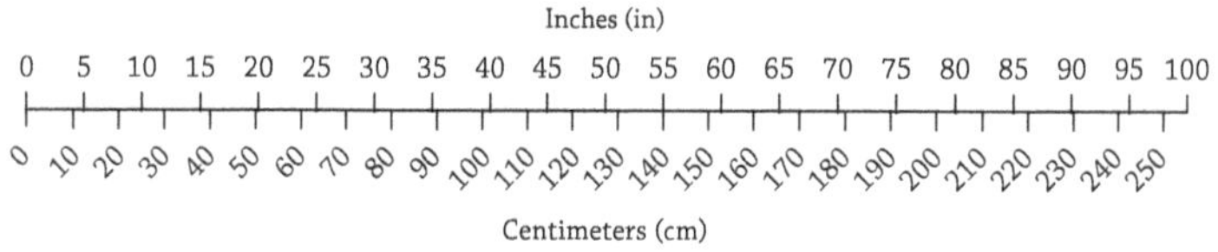

Inches (in)
0 5 10 15 20 25 30 35 40 45 50 55 60 65 70 75 80 85 90 95 100
0 10 20 30 40 50 60 70 80 90 100 110 120 130 140 150 160 170 180 190 200 210 220 230 240 250
Centimeters (cm)

Figure 2.3. Linear conversions of metric to imperial units.

pounds). However, the metric system has become internationally accepted in medicine. In this book, to avoid confusion, most graphs will have both systems of units. Figure 2.3 provides the methods to convert centimeters and inches, and Figure 2.4 gives pounds and kilograms.

Any documentation of measurement(s) should be given together with the age of the individual, the date on which the measurement was obtained, the method used to obtain that measurement, and the name of the person doing the measuring. This makes it easier to compare the values obtained and enables one to anticipate the possible failures of the method employed. In addition, reports or descriptions should include percentiles (or standard deviations) for easy reference and comparison.

gram (g) ÷ 28.4 = ounce (oz)	ounce (oz) ÷ 0.035 = gram (g)
kilogram (kg) ÷ 0.455 = pound (lb)	pound (lb) ÷ 2.20 = kilogram (kg)

Ounces (oz)
0 5 10 15 20 25 30 35 40 45 50 55 60 65 70 75 80 85 90 95 100
0 200 400 600 800 1000 1200 1400 1600 1800 2000 2200 2400 2600 2800
Grams (g)

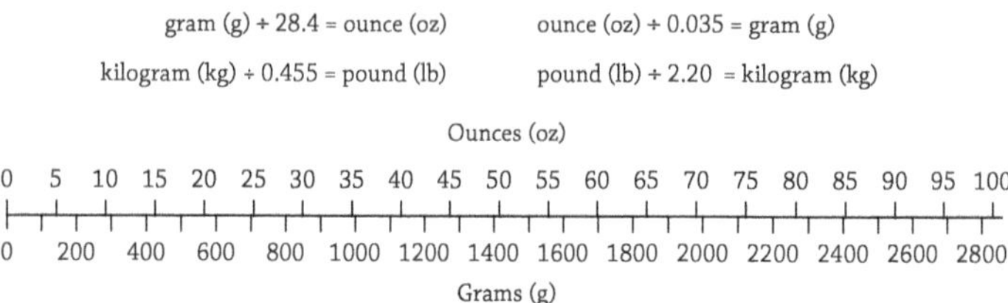

Figure 2.4. Weight conversions of metric to imperial units.

USEFUL PARAMETERS AND LANDMARKS

Measurements of length, weight, and head circumference are standard measurements of a physical examination. These three measurements are the parameters against which all others are compared. They document growth and body proportions. They should be obtained routinely at every visit to a physician in order to be able to assess longitudinal growth and growth relative to an age- and sex-matched standard. Curves of normal standards of growth, weight, and head circumference are included in every text on pediatrics. They usually start from the late stages of pregnancy, include birth parameters, and continue until 18 or 20 years of age. In this book, we have chosen the most commonly used standards and taken the liberty, for practicality, of combining some curves. Although the purist may question this process, we do not think it will markedly affect accuracy in most cases, and we hope the easy utilization of having only one curve will encourage regular and complete measurement. We have included geographic data when available, or when markedly different measurements can be observed (e.g., North America and North European heights). Unfortunately, ethnic comparisons of most areas of the body are not available.

Ultrasound examination permits monitoring of fetal development (Chapter 15). Routine measurements include biparietal diameter (BPD), crown–rump length (CRL), chest circumference, and femur length. These are useful standards with which to observe the growth of the fetus prior to birth.

Head circumference (OFC) is regarded as one of the most important measurements in infancy and early childhood, since it reflects intracranial volume and brain growth. The head circumference charts chosen for this book are the ones most widely used. Often centers will have their own OFC charts, related to the population and ethnic groups that they serve (Chapter 6).

When length, weight, or head circumference deviate from the normal growth curve, further investigation may be warranted. Many different pathological processes, some of which may be treatable, can lead to growth failure. Discrepancies in growth proportions may provide clues to the pathological process; for instance, chronic infection and renal failure lead to relative loss in weight, while growth hormone deficiency and Cushing syndrome produce relative increase in weight. By two years of age, a child will usually have established a pattern of growth that will predictably follow percentile growth curves. These growth curves, on average, are similar for OFC, height, and weight. During the first year of life, a child may change percentile growth curves as he or she establishes an extrauterine pattern of growth.

Bone age is an additional parameter of growth that reflects physiological growth. Bone age is determined from radiographs of the hand or other epiphyseal centers (different ones for different ages). If a disturbance of normal growth is suggested, additional X-rays may be necessary (Chapter 13).

Weight and skinfold thickness will be of special value in nutritional problems (Chapter 5).

During adulthood, particular measurements may also reflect an underlying pathological process. Routinely, weight and total body length are measured in the adult, but head size is often excluded because the head usually does not grow in the normal adult. Familial patterns of growth ("latebloomers") and disproportion (large heads or "short waisted") may identify genetically determined influences on growth.

One should always include the measurements of the parents of the child under assessment so that mid-parental parameters can be established for comparison. This is particularly important and appropriate when evaluating deviations from normal of head size and height.

Growth velocity is most rapid immediately after birth and up to 3 years of age, after which there is a continued deceleration of growth until puberty. The adolescent growth peak in girls is at approximately 12 years, and in boys at approximately 14 years. It is useful to compare growth at yearly intervals, although in infancy shorter time intervals will be used because the velocity is greater.

MEASUREMENTS IN DYSMORPHOLOGY AND CLINICAL GENETICS

The human body is expected to grow predictably and proportionately. The relationship between individual measurements is expected to be constant at specific ages. These relationships can be expressed as ratios, as an index, or by the use of regression techniques. Those in common use are the relationship between height and weight. They are mainly correlated with the chronological age or the bone age of the patient. These proportions and relationships can change dramatically from the fetal period through childhood to adolescence because of various interactions among genetic, hormonal, and environmental factors.

In the study of syndromes with dysmorphic features, we are looking for recognizable signs that help to define and delineate the specific condition. Those recognizable features may be quite different during different life periods. Using Down syndrome as an example, from embryofetal pathology, we have learned that manifestation of the Down syndrome phenotype in a fetus depends on the gestational week, and often very few features are present until close to birth. Similarly, there is a changing phenotype during childhood and into adulthood, with the typical phenotype of Down syndrome sometimes becoming more difficult to recognize in the adult. Because of the change in physical appearance and therefore in the pattern of measurements with time, we can expect that some diseases or disorders will be more obvious and more easily recognized during certain stages of development. The patterns of relative measurements may partly relate to the growth spurts that occur in different organ systems at different times.

Measurements of individual body parts can never be separated from a general clinical impression or "gestalt." This type of general impression of the patient will usually be obtained by observing the patient for a while before taking specific measurements. The specific measurements and general clinical impression should be integrated with additional factors such as the presence of anomalies, movement pattern, mode of communication, and type of developmental disability into an overall description and impression.

There is a tendency to neglect the observation and description of the adult patient with malformations, for those with specific syndromes or even with isolated intellectual disability. As a consequence, we have limited knowledge of physical changes in syndromes with dysmorphic features as related to the aging process. Studying the natural history of the growth relationships may lead to a better understanding of the underlying pathophysiology and natural history of these disorders.

Chapter 3

Proportional Growth and Normal Variants

BODY PROPORTIONS

Body proportions change considerably during fetal and postnatal life. For example, during fetal life the head appears disproportionately large compared with the body. Late in gestation, subcutaneous fat begins to accumulate, and from then until birth, the major changes in proportions are due to the accumulation of fat (Fig. 3.1).

The alteration of body configuration is the result of selective regional growth. In infancy the head grows most rapidly, so that during the first year of life, occipito-frontal circumference (OFC) is greater than chest circumference. After the first year, head growth

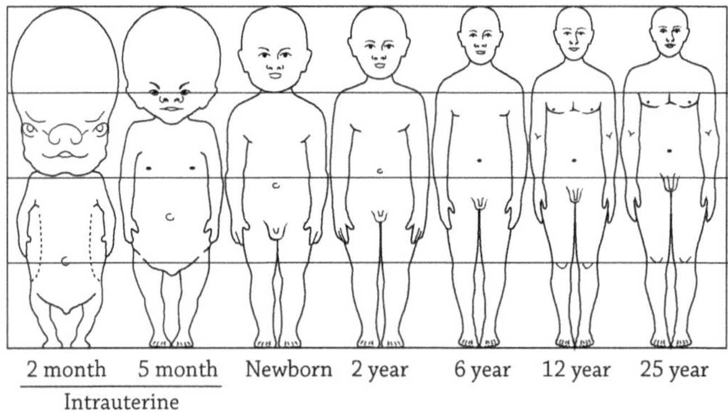

Figure 3.1. Body proportions during human development.

slows down. At birth the limbs are shorter than the trunk; they grow more rapidly and proportions become reversed. Leg growth ceases earlier than growth of the arms.

The changing proportions are mainly reflected in two ratios. First, the upper/lower segment ratio is the ratio of the distance from the top of the head to the symphysis pubis and the distance from the symphysis pubis to the sole of the foot. At birth, this ratio is about 1.7; at 10 years of age, it is about 1.0; after 10 years of age, the ratio is normally less than 1.0. The second ratio is the comparison of arm span with height. At birth, the span is over an inch less than height. Normally in boys, the arm span exceeds standing height by about 10 years of age; in girls normally, arm span exceeds height at about 12 years of age.

Chapter 4

Height and Length

INTRODUCTION

There are two different ways of evaluating height and length. Total body length is the distance between the top of the head and the sole of the foot when the individual is in a recumbent position (lying down) with the foot dorsiflexed (Fig. 4.1). Total standing height is the distance from the highest point of the head to the sole of the foot in the midsagittal plane with the individual standing in an upright position (Fig. 4.5). The head should be held erect with the eyes looking straight forward, so that the lower margin of the bony orbit and upper margin of the external auditory canal opening are in the same horizontal plane (Frankfort plane).

The charts for standard measurement of length or height are ordered in three age groups:

1. length by gestational age at birth (Figs. 4.2, 4.3, 4.4), including twins;
2. birth to 4 years (infants are measured in a recumbent position, typically to age 2 years) (Figs. 4.7, 4.9, 4.12, 4.14);
3. 2 to 18 years (children are measured standing upright) (Figs. 4.8, 4.10, 4.13, 4.16).

TOTAL BODY LENGTH

Definition Length of the supine body.

Landmarks Measure from the top of the head to the sole of the foot with the patient lying on the back with hips and knees extended (Fig. 4.1a, b).

Instruments Ideally, measuring table with engraved measurements, a firm headblock, and a moveable footblock (Fig. 4.1a).

Position For this measurement, ideally, two persons work together. One holds the head of the child, while the other straightens the legs of the child with one hand and moves the footblock toward the heel

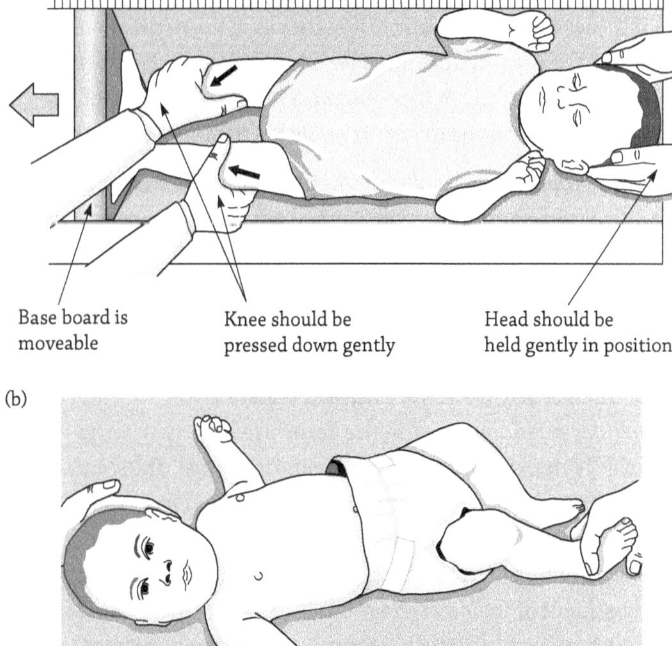

Figure 4.1. Measuring a child less than 2 years old with a measuring table (a) or a tape measure (b).

of the child with the other hand. The top of the head of the patient should be placed against the headboard, eyes looking upward. The ideal head position is with the Frankfort horizontal position held in a vertical plane (i.e., the lower edge of the bony orbit and the upper margin of the external opening of the auditory canal of the ear are in the same vertical plane). The legs, or at least one leg, should be straightened, the ankle at a right angle to the leg with the toes pointing upward. The moveable footboard should be brought in direct contact with the sole of the foot and the measurement read.

Alternatives When a measuring table is not available, a less accurate way is to mark the sheet or the paper on which the child is lying above the child's head and at the foot, after stretching the patient out. Remove the patient and measure the distance on the paper or sheet between the markings. Alternatively, a tape measure can be placed under the child who is positioned supine on top of or beside the tape (Fig. 4.1b).

Remarks Ideally, each measurement should be taken at least twice and the patient should be repositioned between measurements. The experience in clinics dealing with growth problems has shown this to be necessary to obtain accurate measurements of height and length. Measurements in the age group birth to 2 years are difficult to obtain because the children are sometimes not very cooperative. Thus, the measurements may be less accurate in general.

Small for gestational age is the term used for newborns who are below the 10th percentile for their gestational age. Thus, infants less than the 10th percentile in length, even if normal in weight, must be considered small for gestational age.

To determine whether babies born prematurely are small for their age, adjustment of their stated age has to be made (the number of weeks they were born prematurely is subtracted from their postnatal age, and the measurement is compared to the corrected age). Premature babies, by definition, are those born before 37 weeks of gestation. Such individuals catch up to normal at about 2 years of age.

Pitfalls When the head is tipped forward or up, the measurement may be increased. Lack of full extension of the legs or mild contractures

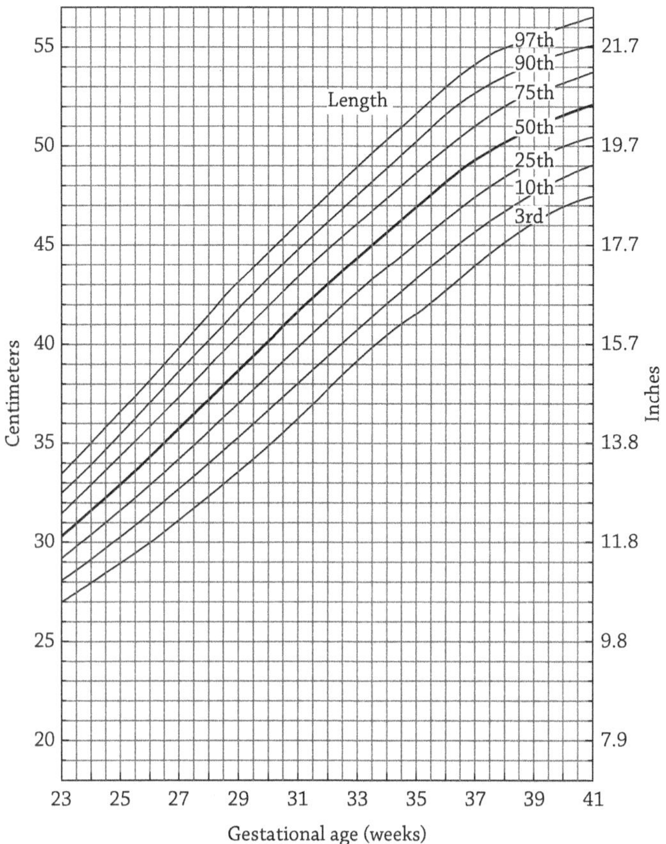

Figure 4.2. Length by gestational age for males. Adapted from Olsen et al. (2010).

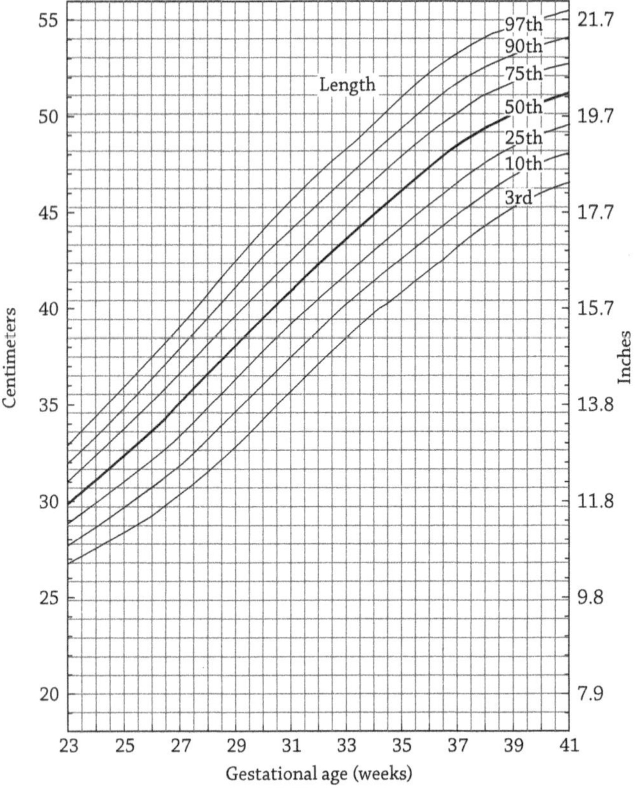

Figure 4.3. Length by gestational age for females. Adapted from Olsen et al. (2010).

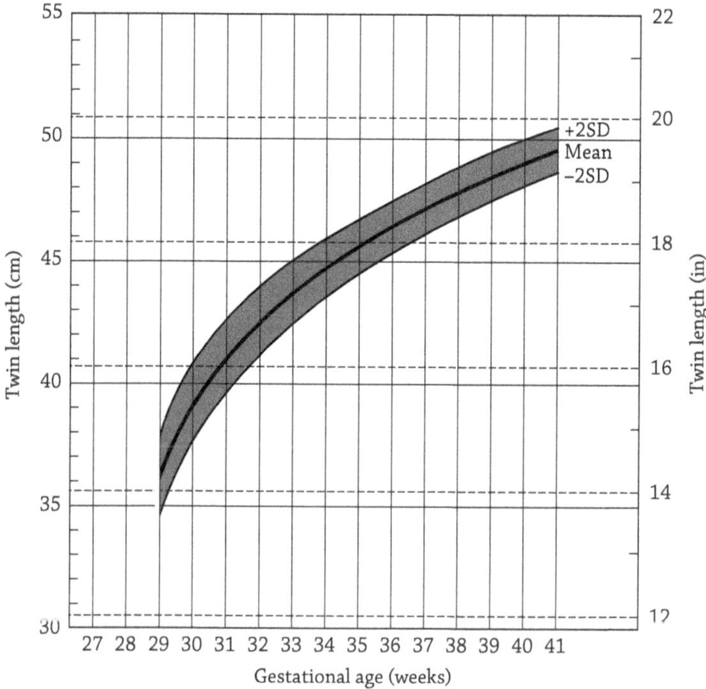

Figure 4.4. Twin-length at birth, both sexes. From Waelli et al. (1980), by permission.

of knees or hips, particularly in newborns, will give artificially shortened measurements.

STANDING HEIGHT

Definition Total height in the standing position.

Landmarks Top of the head to the soles of the feet (Fig. 4.5a, b).

Instruments Ideally, a stadiometer (stable, accurate measuring device) with a moveable headboard is used. Alternatively, a tape measure may be fixed to the wall from the floor upward to at least 6 feet and a right-angle board used to mark the point of greatest height (Fig. 4.5b).

Position The patient should stand upright, with the back against the wall and the head erect (Frankfort horizontal plane), facing forward, and looking straight ahead. The patient should be gently straightened

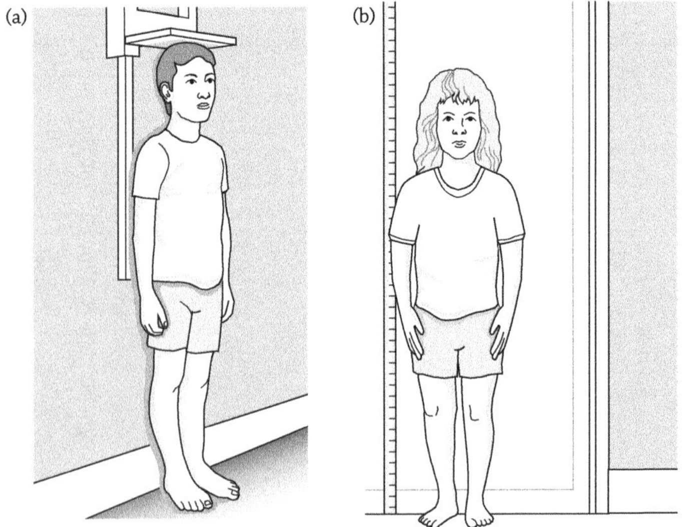

Figure 4.5. Measuring standard height with (a) a stadiometer or (b) a tape measure.

upright; the heels placed together; buttocks and shoulders should be in contact with the wall or measuring device. The moveable headboard is lowered gently until it touches the top of the head. Appropriate clothing should be worn: no socks or shoes (Fig. 4.5).

Alternative A door jamb or the wall and a tape measure can be used if a stadiometer is not available (Fig. 4.5b). The patient stands straight in the position described earlier, with heels together against the door jamb. Heels, buttocks, and shoulders should be in contact with the vertical door jamb. A book or a ruler can be used to replace the headboard, and the point of greatest height is marked on the door jamb. The total standing height is measured from the floor to the marking on the door jamb or wall.

Remarks Repeat the measurement. The patient has to step off after the first measurement and take the position again in between measurements.

The total standing height (upright position) in the 2- to 18-year-old is 1–2 cm less than the total body length (recumbent position). The growth of a normal child usually follows one particular percentile. Any rapid change in measurements to above or below this percentile should be a reason for close follow-up and, if necessary, for further diagnostic procedures.

There are significant differences between the growth charts used in North America and those used for some European countries. The data widely used in North Europe show, for example, that the 50th percentile at 1 year of age equals the 75th percentile in the North American growth charts. Thus, we provided two sets of growth charts, one with North American standards (Figs. 4.7, 4.8, 4.12, 4.13) and one for European standards (Figs. 4.9, 4.10, 4.14, 4.16). It is important to use one or the other standard consistently when making comparisons over time. To develop universal growth charts, the World Health Organization (WHO) systematically studied growth in breastfed infants from several countries (Brazil, Ghana, India, Norway, Oman, and the United States), and these charts are provided here (Figs. 4.11, 4.15).

Pitfalls If the patient is unable to stand, the recumbent length should be measured, recognizing that it will be slightly greater than total standing height.

In individuals with contractures of the legs, the tape is worked along the middle of the patient's leg along the angle of the contracture as in the illustration (Fig. 4.6) to estimate total length.

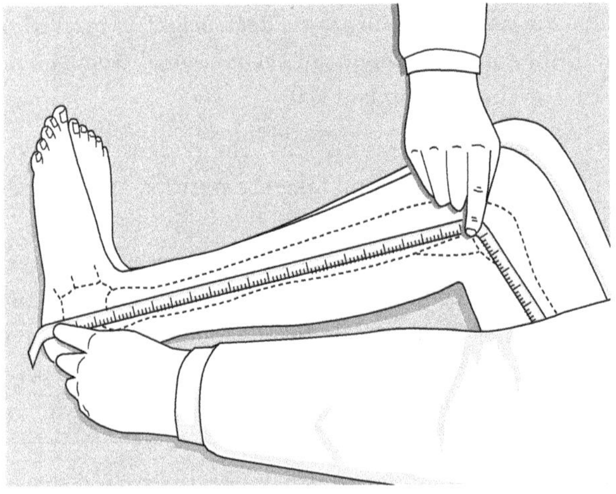

Figure 4.6. Measuring an individual with contractures by "walking the tape."

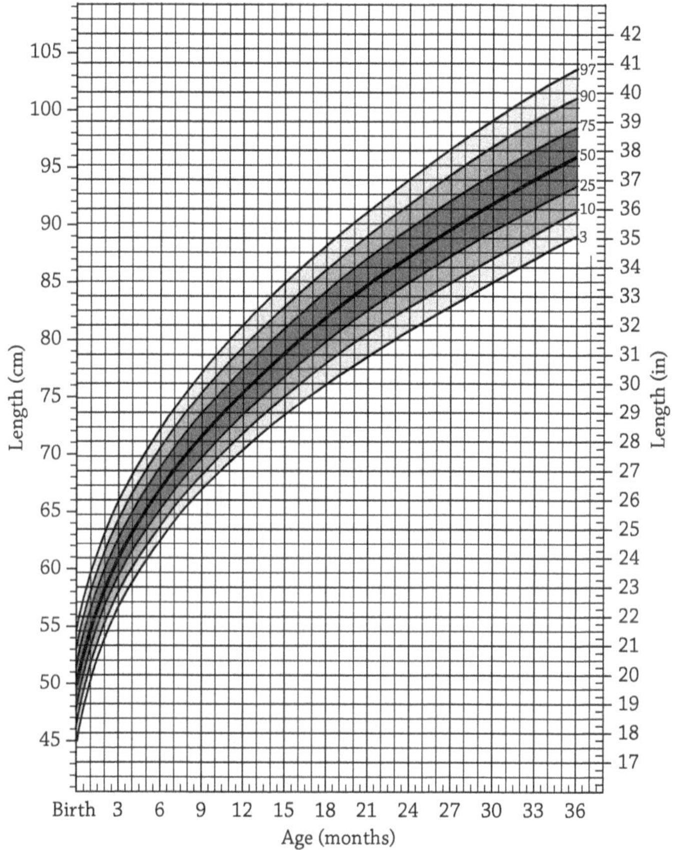

Figure 4.7. Length, North American males, birth to 3 years. Adapted from Centers for Disease Control and Prevention (CDC); available at http://www.cdc.gov/growthcharts

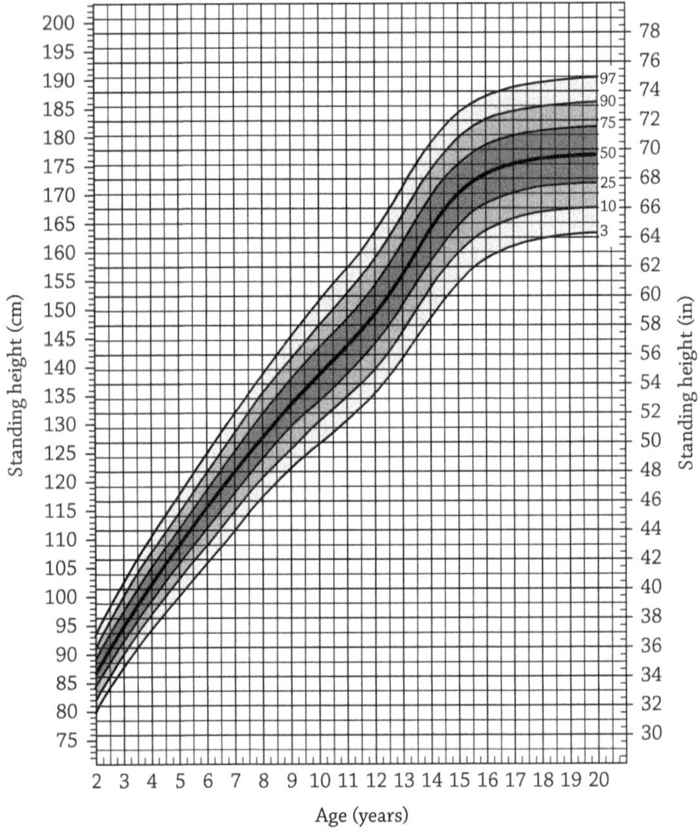

Figure 4.8. Standing height, North American males, 2 to 20 years. Adapted from Centers for Disease Control and Prevention (CDC); available at http://www.cdc.gov/growthcharts

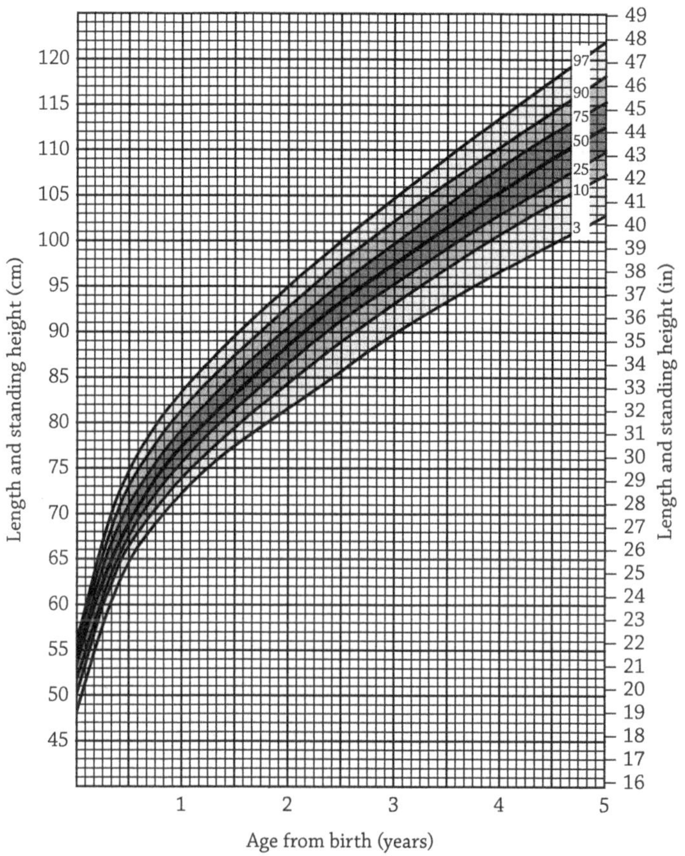

Figure 4.9. Recumbent length and standing height, North European males, birth to 5 years. Adapted from Brandt (1986); available at http://www.wachstum-ipep.de/WTK/WTK.html

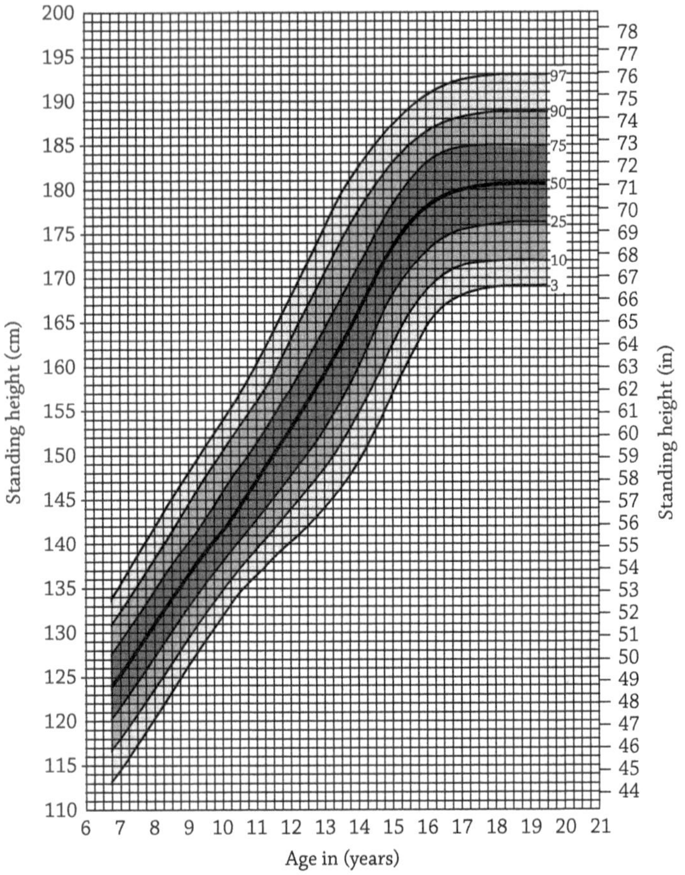

Figure 4.10. Standing height, North European males, 6 to 19 years. Adapted from Georgi et al. (1996); available at http://www.wachstum-ipep.de/WTK/WTK.html

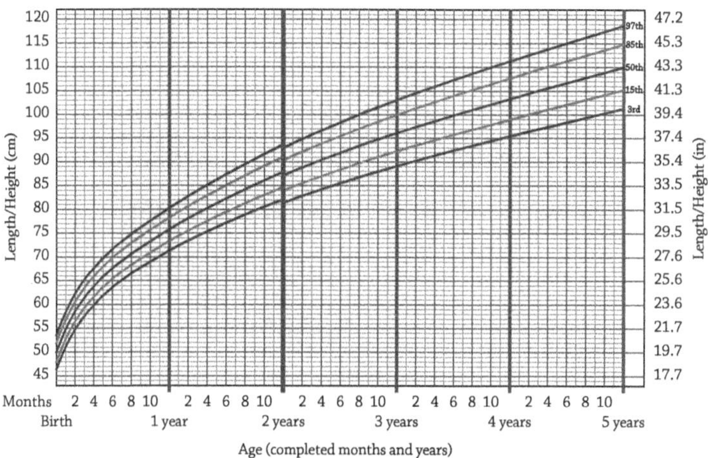

Figure 4.11. Length/height for age in males. Adapted from http://www.who.int/child-growth/standards/en/

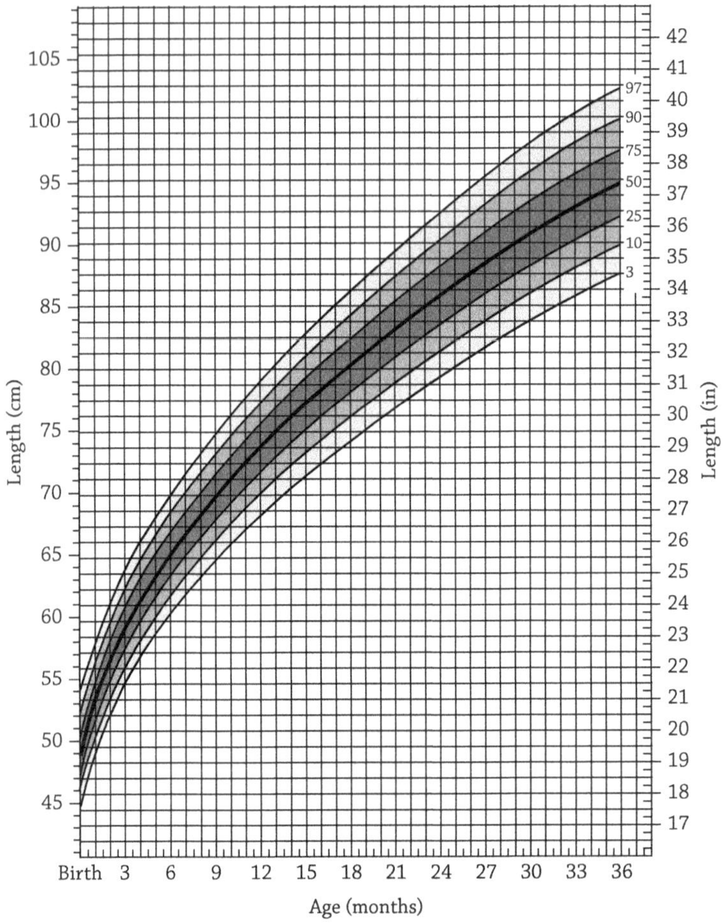

Figure 4.12. Length, North American females, birth to 3 years. Adapted from Centers for Disease Control and Prevention (CDC); available at http://www.cdc.gov/growthcharts

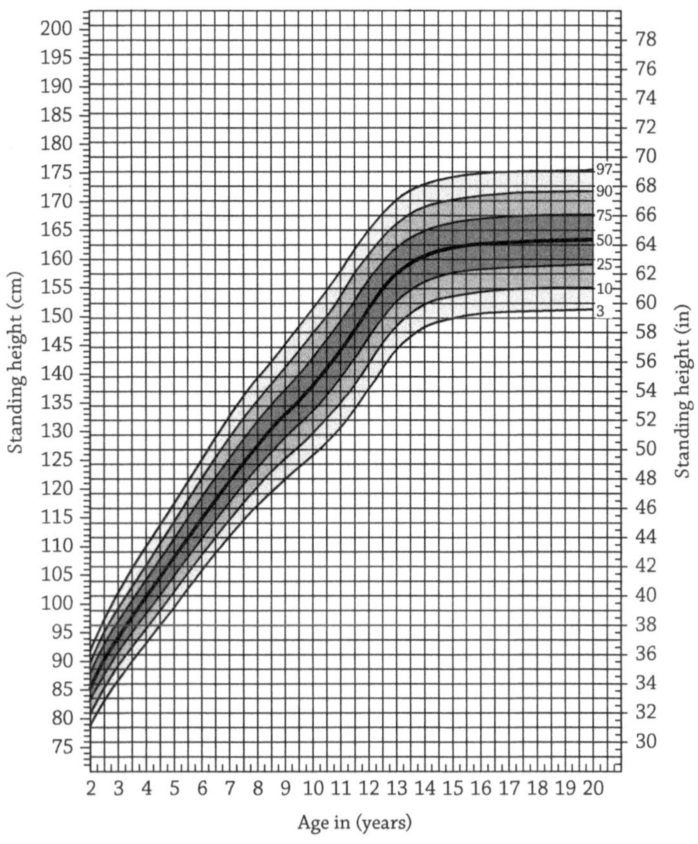

Figure 4.13. Standing height, North American females, 2 to 20 years. Adapted from Centers for Disease Control and Prevention (CDC); available at http://www.gov/growthcharts

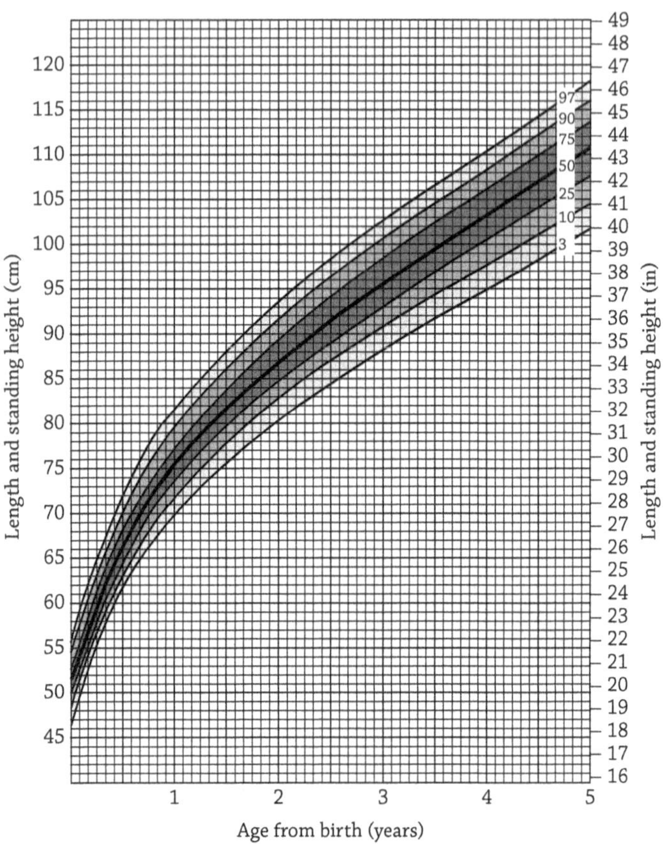

Figure 4.14. Recumbent length and standing height, North European females, birth to 5 years. Adapted from Brandt (1986); available at http:www.wachstum-ipep.de/WTK/WTK.html

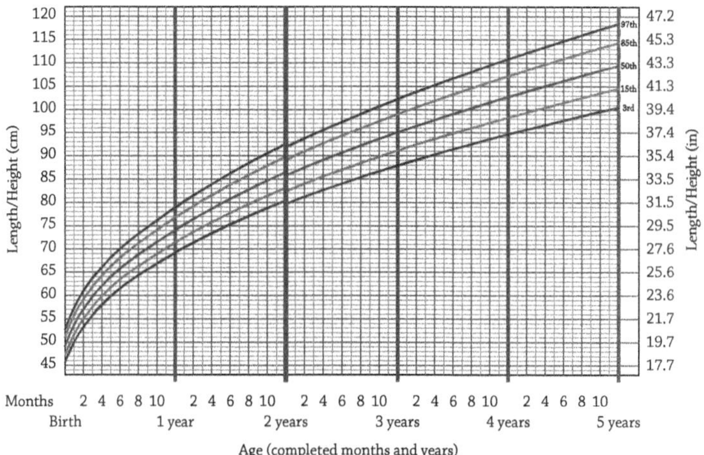

Figure 4.15. Length/height for females. Adapted from http://www.who.int/childgrowth/standards/en/

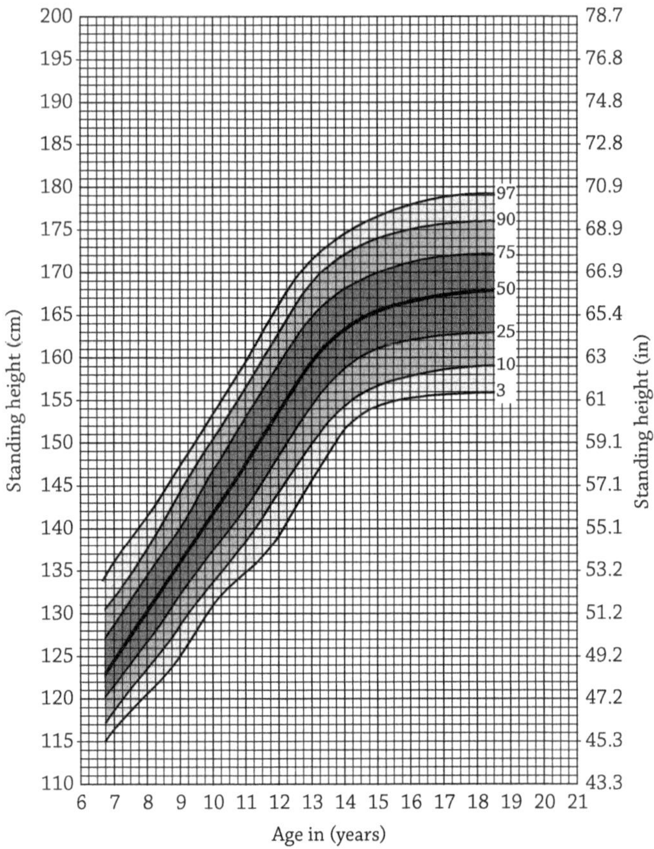

Figure 4.16. Standing height, North European females, 6 to 19 years. Adapted from Georgi et al. (1996); available at http://www.wachstum-ipep.de/WTK/WTK.html

CROWN–RUMP LENGTH

Definition Crown–rump length is the distance from the top of the head to the bottom of the buttocks.

Landmarks Measure from the top of the head to the posterior distal part of the thighs with legs extended at right angles at the hips (Fig. 4.17a).

Instruments A recumbent measurement table or tape and table.

Position The patient is lying on the side with the hips flexed to 90 degrees.

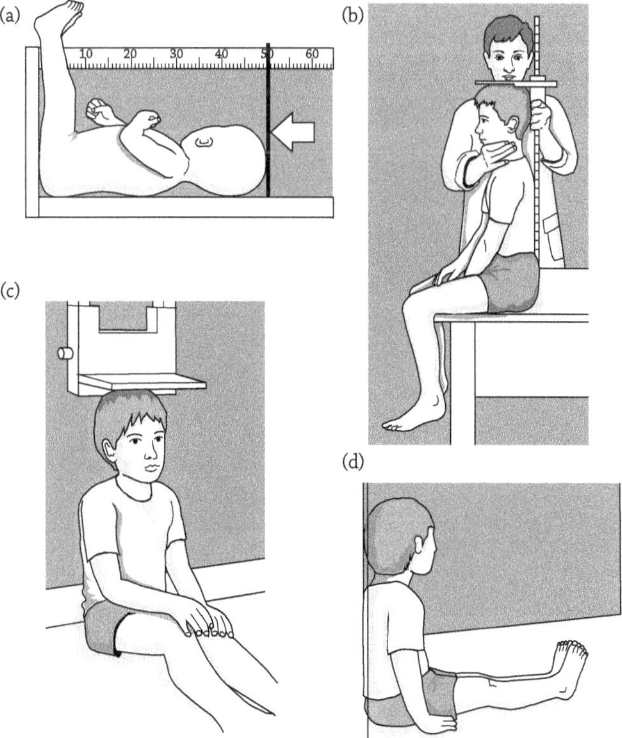

Figure 4.17. Measuring (a) crown–rump length and (b–d) sitting height.

Remarks Crown–rump length is a standard measurement to define fetal size (Chapter 15) and can be a useful measurement in the first few years of life. It can give valuable information to define disproportionate growth, especially in patients with reduction defects of the limbs or contractures (Figs. 4.18–4.20).

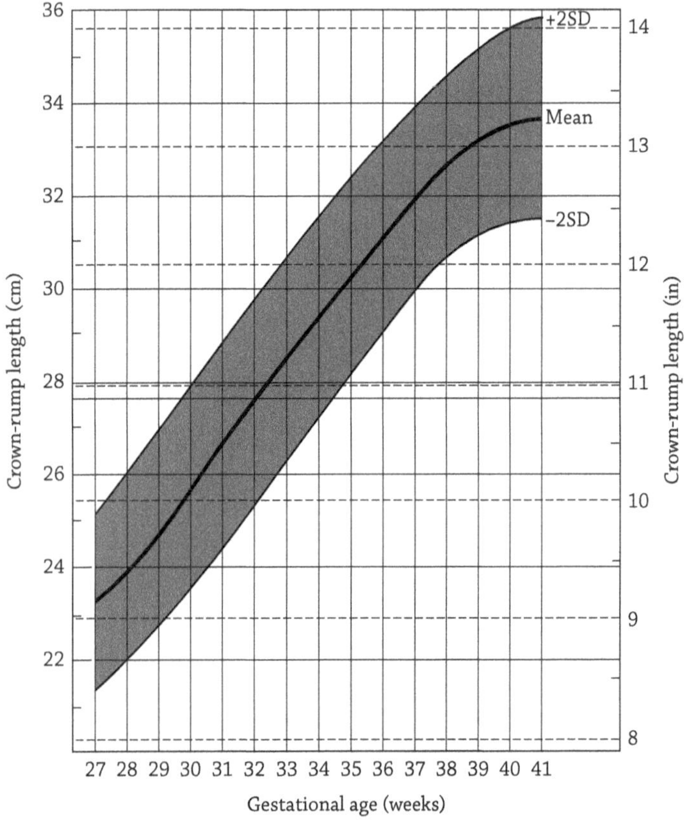

Figure 4.18. Crown–rump length at birth, both sexes. From Merlob et al. (1986), by permission.

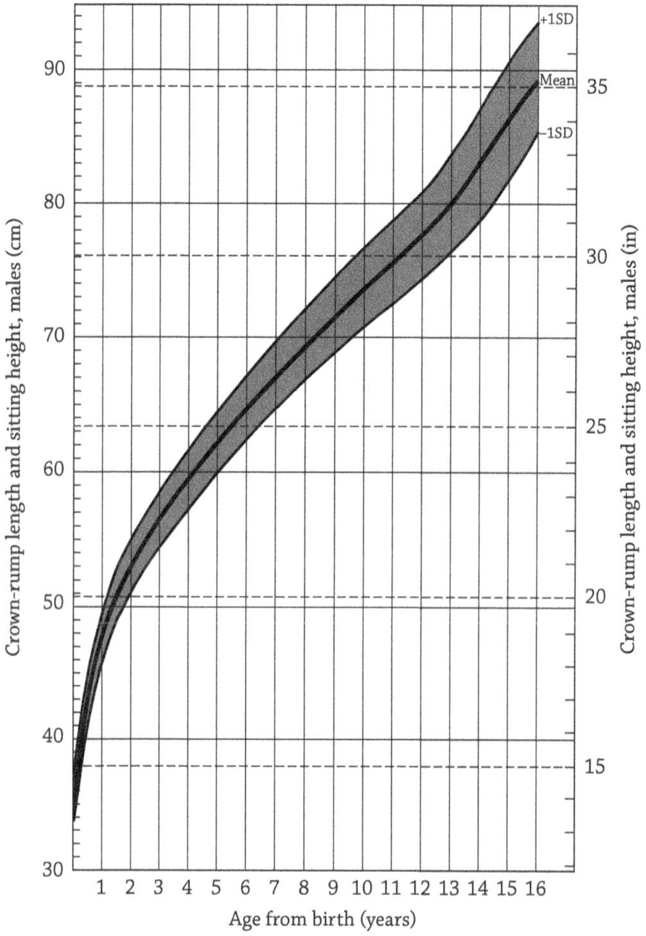

Figure 4.19. Crown–rump length and sitting height, males, birth to 16 years. From Tanner (1978), by permission.

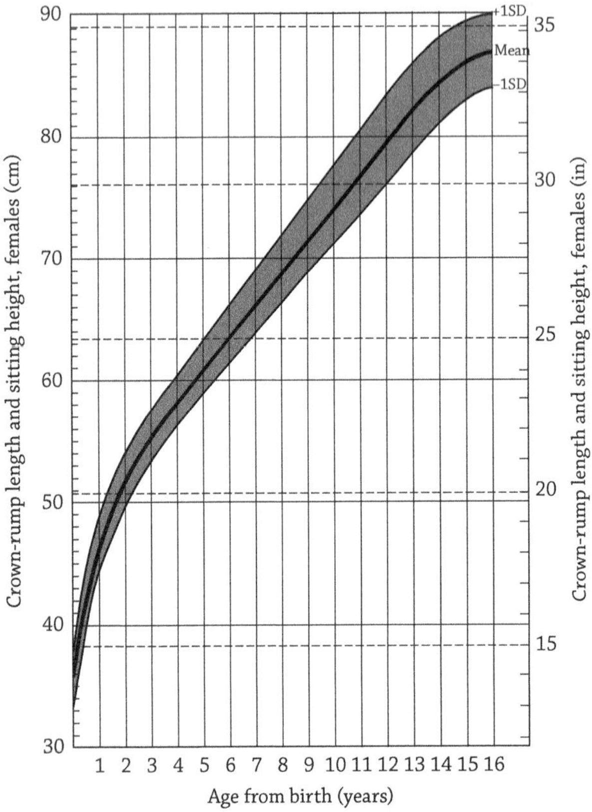

Figure 4.20. Crown–rump length and sitting height, females, birth to 16 years. From Tanner (1978), by permission.

SITTING HEIGHT

Definition Sitting height is the distance from the top of the head to the buttocks when a sitting position.

Landmarks Measure from the top of the head to the bottom of the thighs (surface on which the patient is sitting) (Fig. 4.17b and c).

Instruments Sitting height table or stadiometer.

Position The patient sits straight, eyes looking straight ahead (Frankfort horizontal plane). The back of the head, back, buttocks, and the shoulders are in contact with the vertical board. A moveable headboard is used to adjust the measurement (Fig. 4.17b and c).

Alternatives The patient sits at the door jamb with legs straight out in front; the back of the head, shoulders, and buttocks are in contact with the wall. A ruler or book can be used instead of a headboard. Measurements are taken with a tape from the floor to a marking on the door jamb (Fig. 4.17d).

Remarks The charts from birth to 16 years are provided in Figures 4.18–4.20.

MID-PARENTAL HEIGHT (USED TO ASSESS CHILD'S GROWTH PATTERN)

Definition Sum of parental heights divided by 2.

Remarks Mid-parental height is an important parameter for children who appear to be smaller or taller than average. There is an almost linear correlation between the height of children 2–9 years and the heights of their biological parents. Using mid-parental height, projections can be made of the child's growth centile using the combination curve of Tanner (Figs. 4.21 and 4.22).

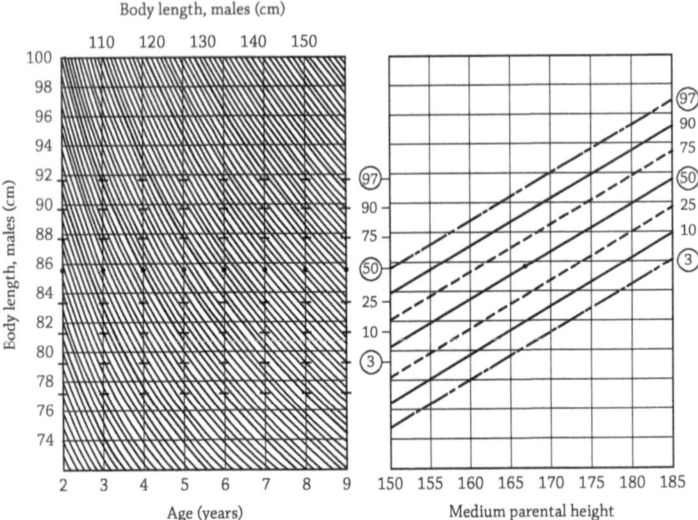

Figure 4.21. Mid-parental height, males, combination curve. From Tanner et al. (1970), by permission.

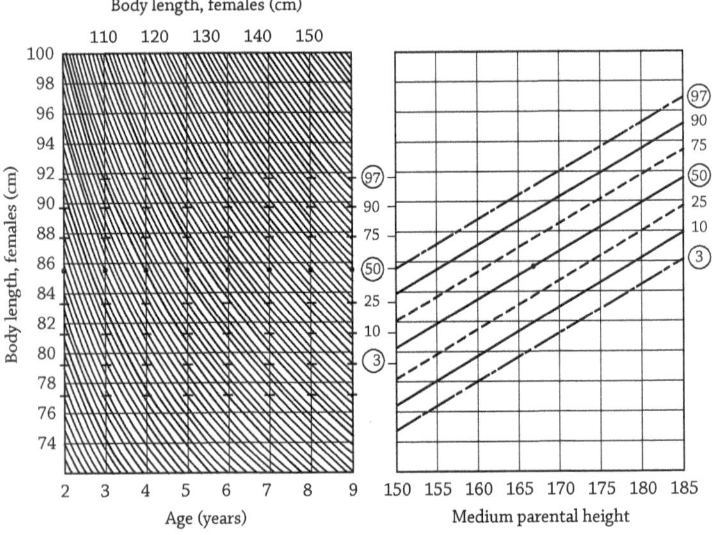

Figure 4.22. Mid-parental height, females, combination curve. From Tanner et al. (1970), by permission.

HOW TO USE THE COMBINATION CURVE

Look up the child's height at the left margin (73–100 cm) or at the upper margin (101–150 cm).

- Follow the curved line from the left border of the chart until you cross the line for the child's age.
- Then draw a horizontal line to the second chart until you meet the vertical line coming from mid-parental height.
- Find the percentile of the child's height along the right-hand margin in relation to the parents' mid-parental height.

Example A 6-year-old boy has a height of 110 cm, his parents (mother, 165 cm; father, 175 cm) have a mid-parental height of 170 cm. He is on the 10th percentile for expected height in view of his mid-parental height.

PREDICTION OF HEIGHT

In normal children, one can predict height with some accuracy after 4 years of age using height and an assessment of bone age. Elaborate tables have been developed by Bayley and Pinneau (1952) that are said to be accurate within 2 inches of adult height. However, the tables do not take into account parental height and velocity of puberty (although delayed and precocious puberty are taken into account by using the tables for delayed and advanced bone age). Many other methods to predict final adult height have been developed.

Garn has developed a "multiplier" for each age that can be used with the present height to predict ultimate height if bone age is normal. The tradition of doubling the height at 2 years to give predicted height was derived from this source (Fig. 4.23).

Multiplier (boys)	*Age*	*Multiplier (girls)*
2.46	1	2.30
2.06	2	2.01
1.86	3	1.76
1.73	4	1.62
1.62	5	1.51
1.54	6	1.43
1.47	7	1.35
1.40	8	1.29
1.35	9	1.23
1.29	10	1.17
1.24	11	1.12
1.19	12	1.07
1.14	13	1.03
1.09	14	1.01
1.04	15	1.002
1.02	16	1.001
1.01	17	1.001
1.00	18	1.00

Figure 4.23. Multipliers for prediction of height of boys and girls of average parental stature. From Garn (1966), by permission.

PROSPECTIVE HEIGHT

When parents or children are at the lower or upper ends of the growth curve, prospective adult height may be of concern. There is a correlation between parental height and the final height of children. Formulas to calculate final height taking parental height into account are as follows.

Height at maturity

Boys = 0.545 height at 2 years + 0.544 parental height + 14.85 inches
Girls = 0.545 height at 2 years + 0.544 parental height + 10.09 inches

PREDICTION OF ADULT HEIGHT FOR FEMALES FROM HEIGHT AT THE AGE OF MENARCHE

An alternative method for predicting height in females is the use of height at age of menarche. The data for females related to age of menarche are provided in Figure 4.24.

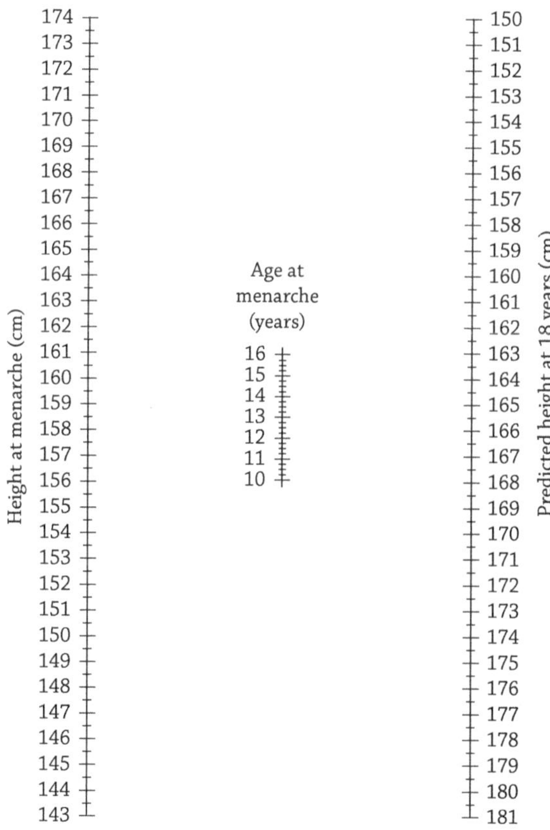

Figure 4.24. Nomogram for the prediction of adult height from the height and age at menarche. From Headings (1975), by permission.

HEIGHT VELOCITY

Growth velocity is the rate of growth over a period of time (Figs. 4.25–4.27). It is most rapid immediately after birth and then, between the ages of 2 and 12 years in boys, or 2 and 10 years in girls, growth velocity slowly but continuously decelerates. During adolescence, it increases again. The adolescence peak for girls is approximately 12 years and boys, at approximately 14 years of age.

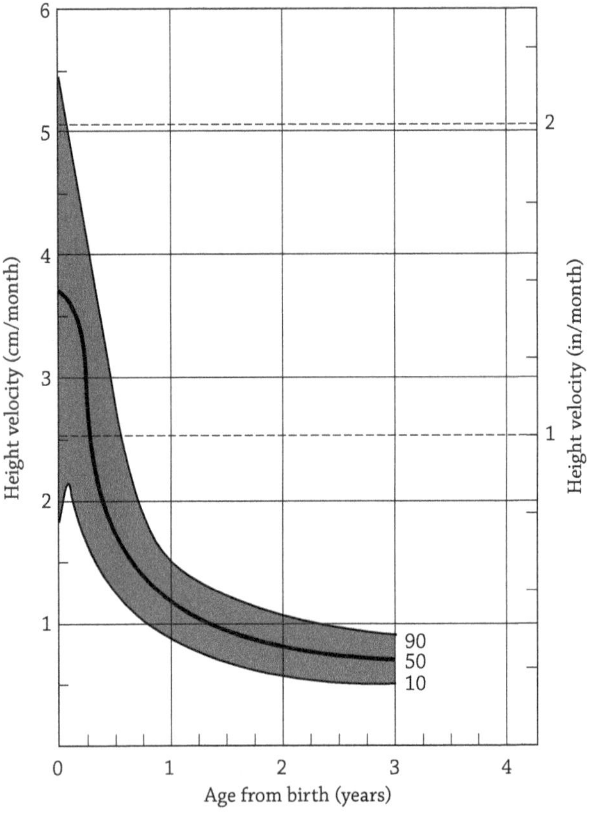

Figure 4.25. Height velocity, both sexes, birth to 4 years. From Brandt (1986), by permission.

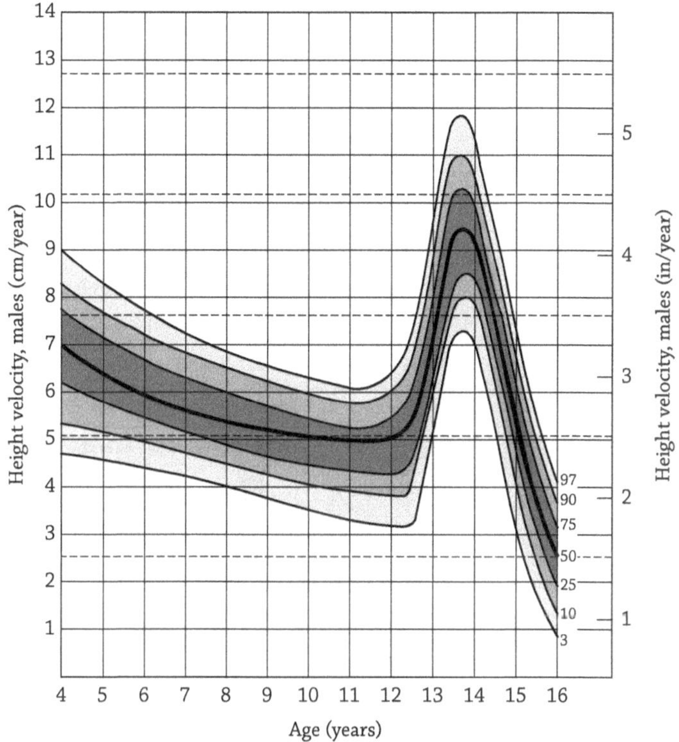

Figure 4.26. Height velocity, males. From Tanner and Whitehouse (1976), by permission.

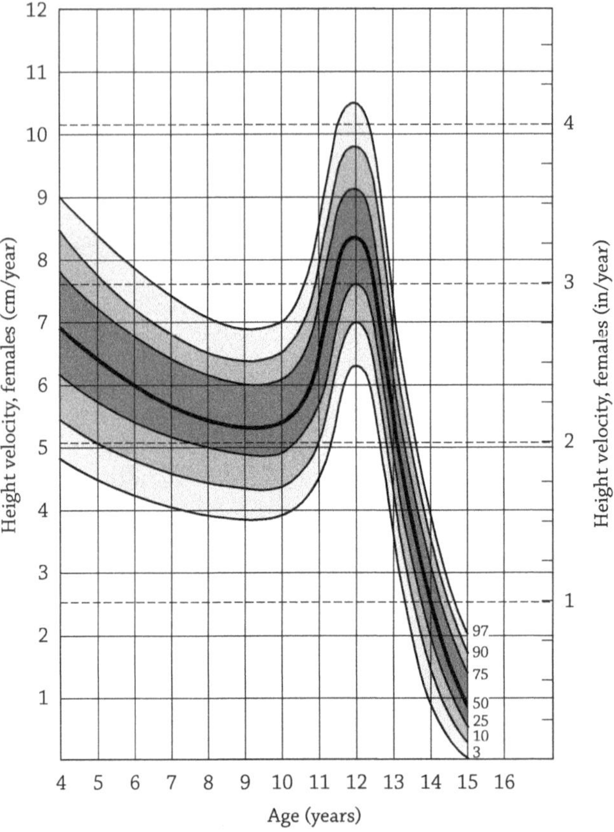

Figure 4.27. Height velocity, females. From Tanner and Whitehouse (1976), by permission.

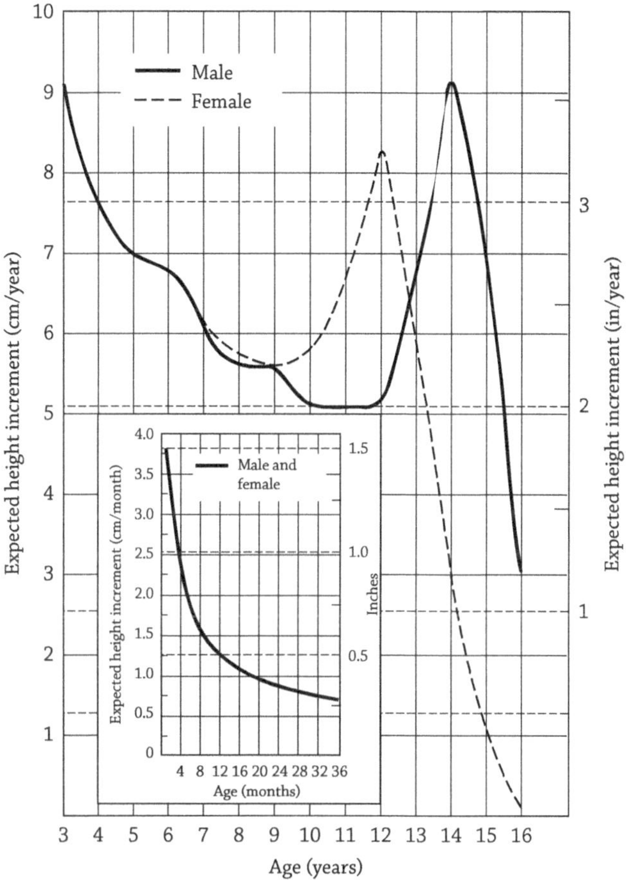

Figure 4.28. Expected increments in height, both sexes, birth to 16 years. From Lowrey (1986), by permission.

It is useful to compare growth velocity with the normal yearly intervals: If a girl was 99 cm at 3 years 6 months and measured 106 cm at 4 years 4 months, she has grown 7 cm in 10 months (or presumably 6 cm per year). This rate is compared to her age at the middle of this time interval (3 years, 11 months) and gives the growth velocity for her at that age. In infancy, shorter time intervals are used to evaluate growth velocity.

EXPECTED INCREMENTS

There is a predictable height increase for each specific time interval. This increment changes with age. Males and females have the same incremental height increases for the first 48 months of life, then sex differences are noted. Expected height increase increment charts can be found in Figure 4.28.

BIBLIOGRAPHY

Bayley, N., and Pinneau, S. R. (1952). Tables for predicting adult height from skeletal age: revised for use with the Greulich–Pyle hand standards. *Journal of Pediatrics*, 40, 423–444.

Brandt, I. (1986). Growth dynamics of low-birth-weight infants with emphasis on the prenatal period. In *Human growth: A comprehensive treatise, Vol. 1* (eds. F. Falkner and J. M. Tanner), pp. 415–475. New York: Plenum.

Brooke, O. G., Butters, F., Wood, C., Bailay, P., and Tudkmachi, F. (1981). Size at birth from 31–41 weeks gestation: Ethnic standards for British infants of both sexes. *Journal of Human Nutrition*, 35, 415–443

Garn, S. M. (1966). Body size and its implications. In *Review of child development research* (eds. L. W. Hoffman and M. L. Hoffman), Vol. 2, pp. 529– 561. New York: Russell Sage Foundation.

Garn, S. M., and Rohmann, C. G. (1966). Interaction of nutrition and genetics in the timing of growth and development. *Pediatric Clinics of North America*, 13, 353–379.

Georgi, M., Schaefer, F., Wuehl, E., Schaerer, K. (1996). Heidelberger Wachstumskurven. *Monatsschrift Kinderheilkunde*, 144, 813–824.

Hamill, P. V., Drizd, T. A., Johnson, C. L., Reed, R. B., Roche, A. F., and Moore, W. M. (1979). Physical growth: National Center for Health Statistics percentile. *American Journal of Clinical Nutrition*, 32, 607–629.

Headings, D. L. (ed.) (1975). *The Harriet Lane handbook* (7th ed.). Chicago: Year Book Medical Publishers.

Hohenauer, L. (1980). Intrauterine Wachtumskurven fuer den Deutschen Sprachraum. *Zeitschrift fuer Geburtshilfe und Frauenheilkunde*, 184, 167–179.

Largo, R. H., Waelli, R., Duc, G., Fanconi, A., and Prader, A. (1980). Evaluation of perinatal growth. *Helvetia Paediatrica Acta*, 35, 419–436.

Lowrey, G. H. (1986). *Growth and development of children* (8th ed). Chicago: Year Book Medical Publishers.

Merlob, P., Sivan, Y., and Reisner, S. H. (1986). Ratio of crown–rump distance to total length in preterm and term infants. *Journal of Medical Genetics*, 23, 338–340.

Naeye, R. L., Benirschke, K., Hagstrom, J. W. C., and Marcus, C. C. (1966). Intrauterine growth of twins as estimated from liveborn birth-weight data. *Pediatrics*, 37, 409–416.

Olsen, I. E., Groveman, S. A., Lawson, M. L., Clark, R. H., and Zemel, B. S. (2010). New intrauterine growth curves based on United States Data. *Pediatrics*, 125, e214.

Tanner, J. M. (1978). Physical growth and development. In *Textbook of pediatrics* (eds. J. O. Forfar and G. C. Arneil), pp. 253–303. Edinburgh: Churchill Livingstone.

Tanner, J. M., and Whitehouse, R. H. (1973). Height and weight charts from birth to 5 years allowing for length of gestation. *Archives of Disease in Childhood*, 48, 786–789.

Tanner, J. M., and Whitehouse, R. H. (1976). Clinical longitudinal standards for height, weight, height velocity, weight velocity, and stages of puberty. *Archives of Disease in Childhood*, 51, 170–179.

Tanner, J. M., Goldstein, H., and Whitehouse, R. H. (1970) Standards for children's height at ages 2–9 years allowing for height of parents. *Archives of Disease in Childhood*, 45, 755–762.

Waelli, R., Stettler, T., Largo, R. H., Fanconi, A., and Prader, A. (1980). Gewicht, Laenge und Kopfumfang neugeborener Kinder and ihre Abhaengigkeit von muetterlichen und kindlichen Faktoren. *Helvetia Paediatrica Acta*, 35, 397–418.

WHO standard growth curves. Available at http://www.who.int/childgrowth/standards/en/

Chapter 5

Weight

WEIGHT

Definition Weight or heaviness of the individual.

Instruments For infants and younger children, a scale in which the individual can lie or sit is used. For older children and adults, a standing scale is used.

Position In a newborn infant or young child, weight is taken by laying the baby on the weighing table or infant scale (Fig. 5.1a); in older children and adults able to stand, a standing scale is used (Fig. 5.1b).

The individual should not be touching anything except the scale (wall, floor, scale upright, etc.) because that will affect the weight measurement. Most clothing is removed since it will affect the weight measurement.

Alternative If no infant scales are available, a normal scale can be used, weighing an adult and child together, transferring the child to an assistant, and taking the adult's weight alone. The baby's weight will be calculated by the difference between the weight of the adult plus the child and the weight of the adult alone. In older individuals unable to stand, the weight of the bed or wheelchair is taken and subtracted.

Remarks Weight measurement should be performed at least twice, preferably three times, to ensure accuracy. The patient should step on and off the scale between measurements.

As little clothing as possible should be worn for the weighing. In newborns and infants, the diaper is removed. A blanket may be used if the scale is cold, but its weight should be subtracted from the total. If weight is taken with the diaper on, the weight of the diaper should

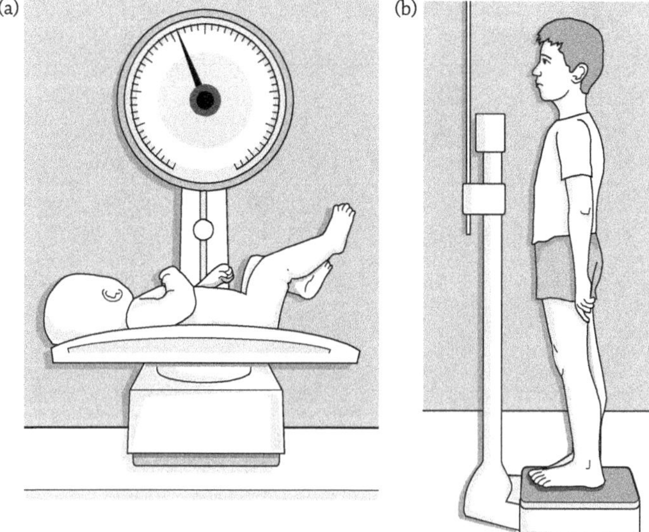

Figure 5.1. Measuring weight with (a) an infant scale and (b) a standing scale.

be subtracted from the baby's weight. In older patients, light underwear is usually worn (Fig. 5.1b). However, shoes, belts, regular clothing, and any jewelry should be removed.

In the absence of a limb, one has to adjust the expected weight in relationship to height. It is estimated that the upper limbs together account for approximately 11% of the total weight and the lower limbs together for approximately 20% of the total weight.

During the first days of life, a natural weight loss occurs. It usually is greatest at the third day of life, when it equals approximately 7% of the birthweight.

Weight for North European and North American children are shown in Figs. 5.2–5.13.

Pitfalls In infants the effects of feeding and bowel movement can alter weight.

The weight should be recorded when the individual is quiet and still. Shifting weight and movement can change the measurement by several pounds.

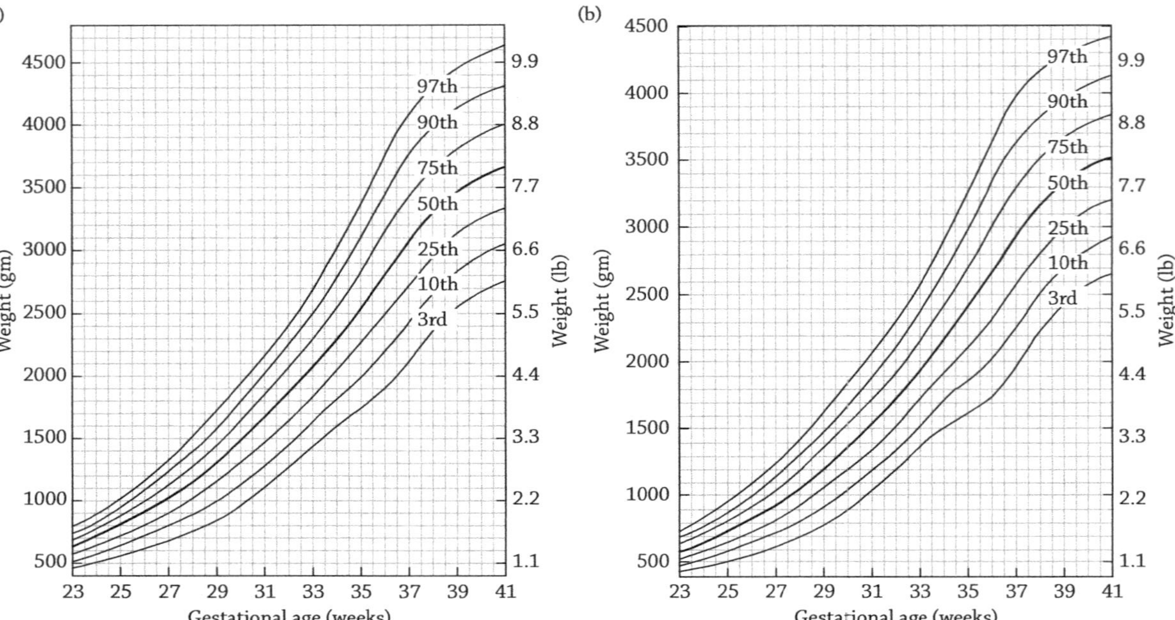

Figure 5.2. Weight at birth by gestational age for (a) males and (b) females. Adapted from Olsen et al. (2010).

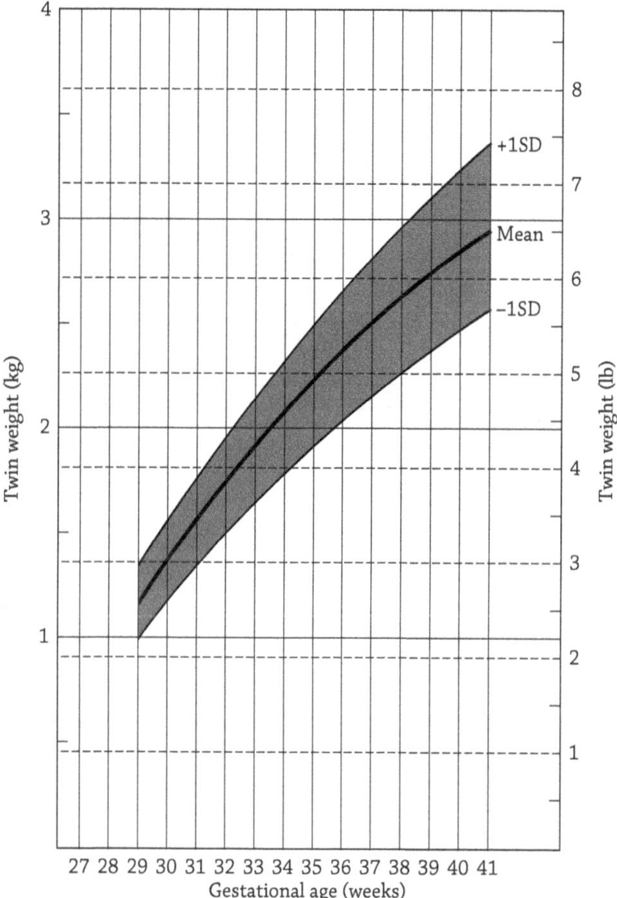

Figure 5.3. Twin weight, both sexes at birth. From Waelli et al. (1980), by permission.

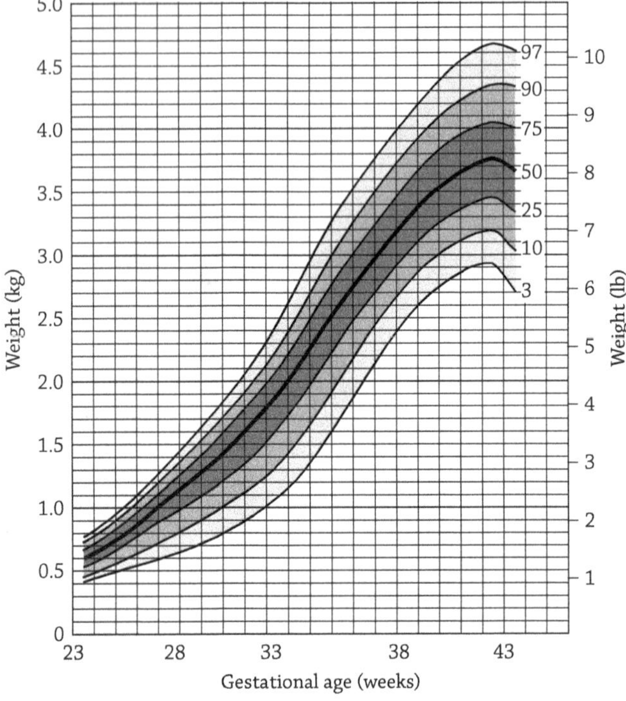

Figure 5.4. Weight, North European males at birth. Adapted from Voigt et al. (1996).

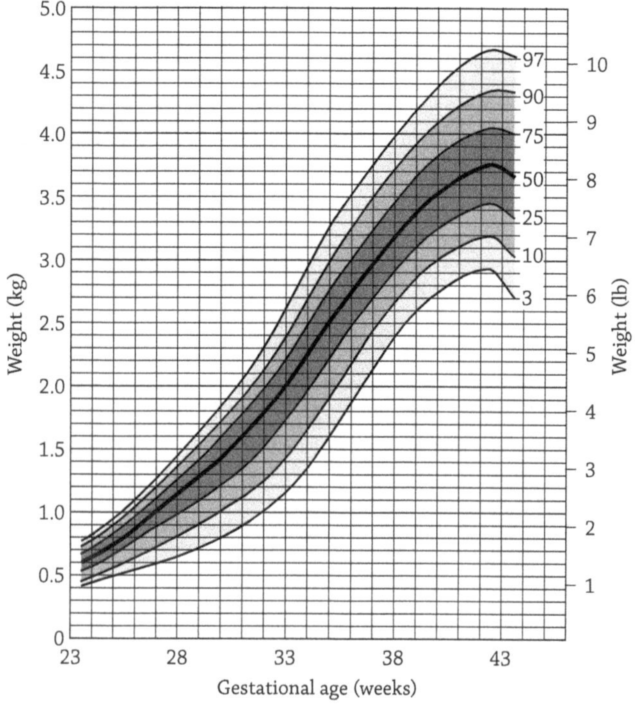

Figure 5.5. Weight, North European females at birth. Adapted from Voigt et al. (1996).

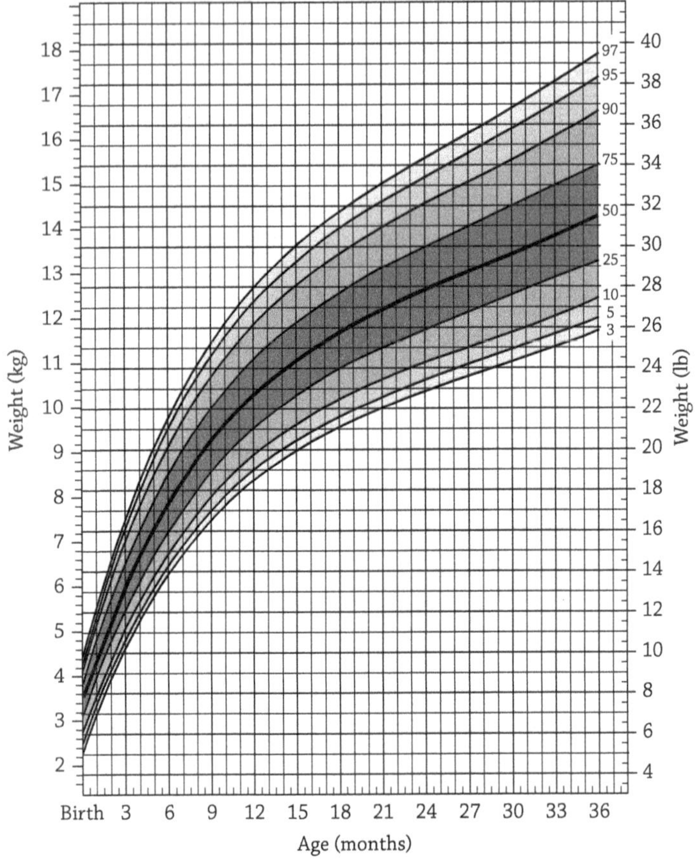

Figure 5.6. Weight, males, birth to 3 years. Adapted from the Centers for Disease Control and Prevention (CDC); available at http://www.gov/growthcharts

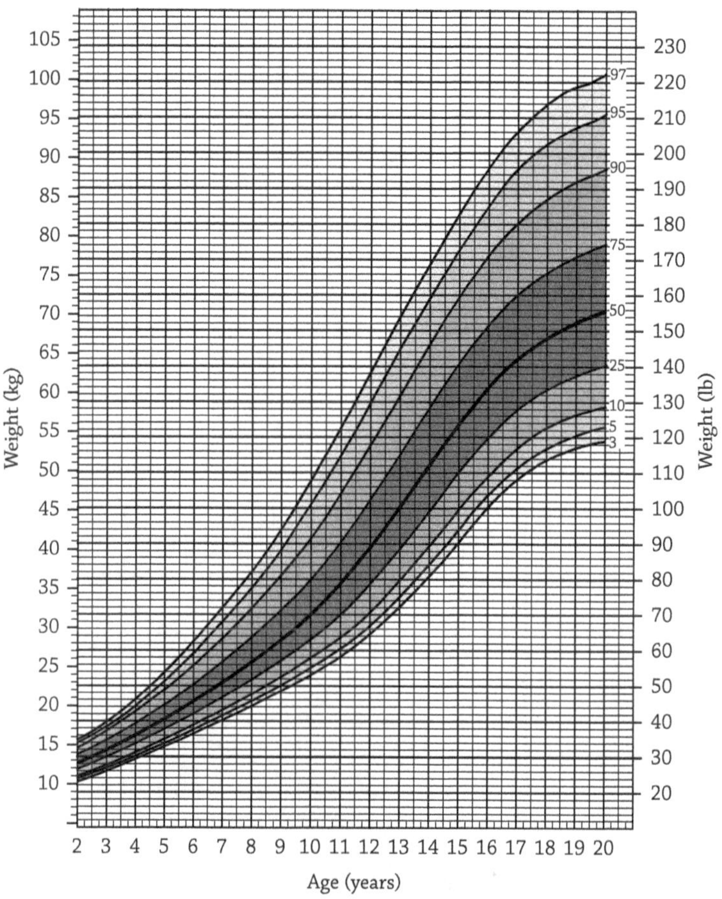

Figure 5.7. Weight, males, 2 to 20 years. Adapted from the Centers for Disease Control and Prevention (CDC); available at http://www.gov/growthcharts

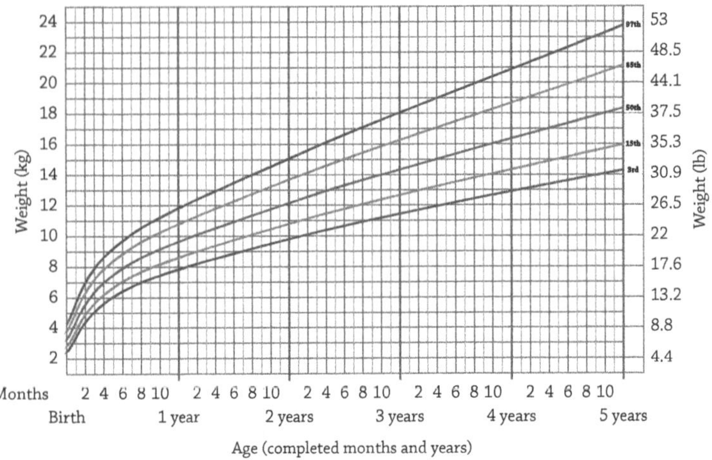

Figure 5.8. Weight for age in males. Adapted from http://www.who.int/childgrowth/standards/en/

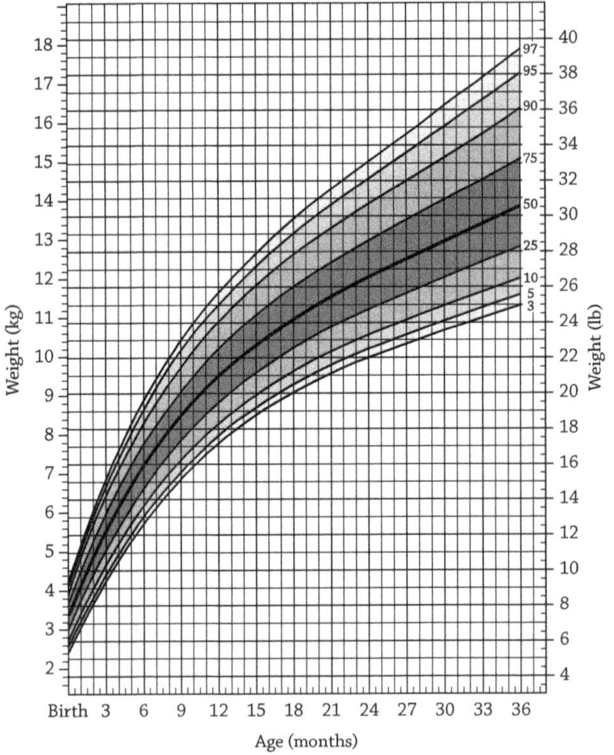

Figure 5.9. Weight, females, birth to 3 years. Adapted from the Centers for Disease Control and Prevention (CDC); available at http://www.gov/growthcharts

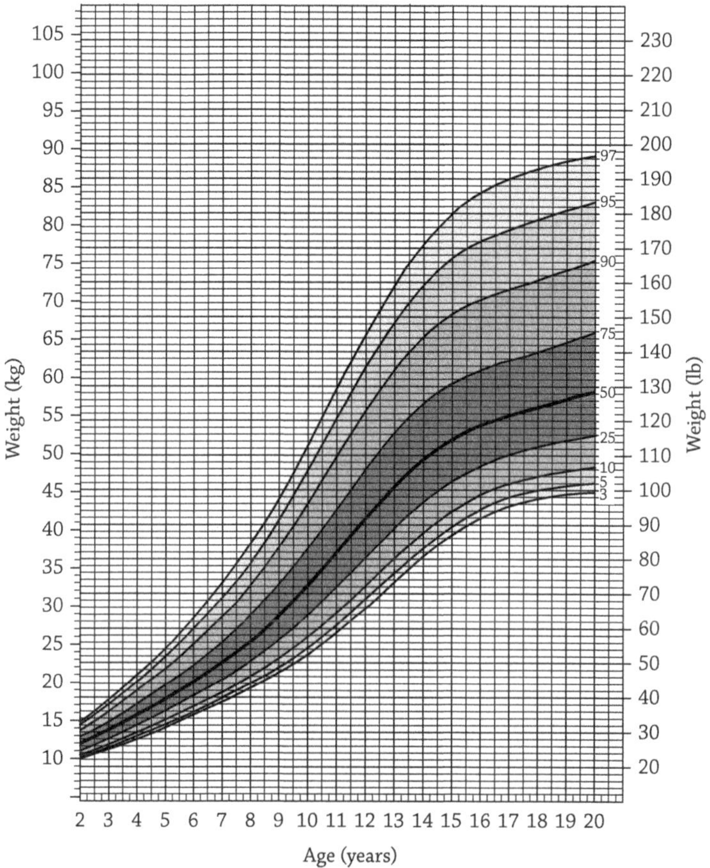

Figure 5.10. Weight, females, 2 to 20 years. Adapted from the Centers for Disease Control and Prevention (CDC); available at http://www.gov/growthcharts

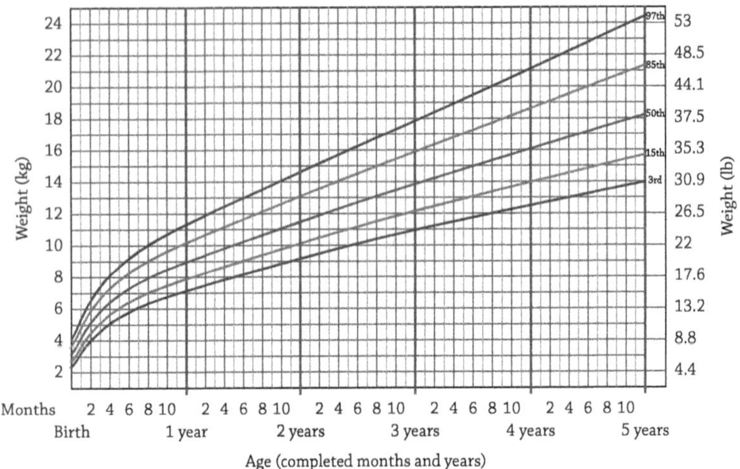

Figure 5.11. Weight for age in females. Adapted from http://www.who.int/childgrowth/standards/en/

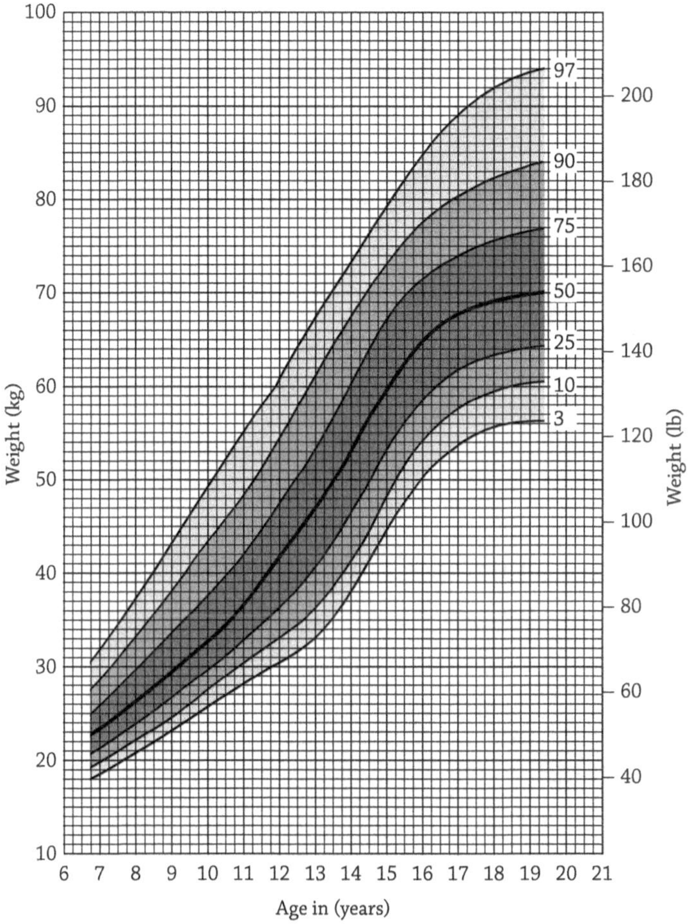

Figure 5.12. Weight, North European males, 7 to 19 years. Adapted from Georgi et al. (1996).

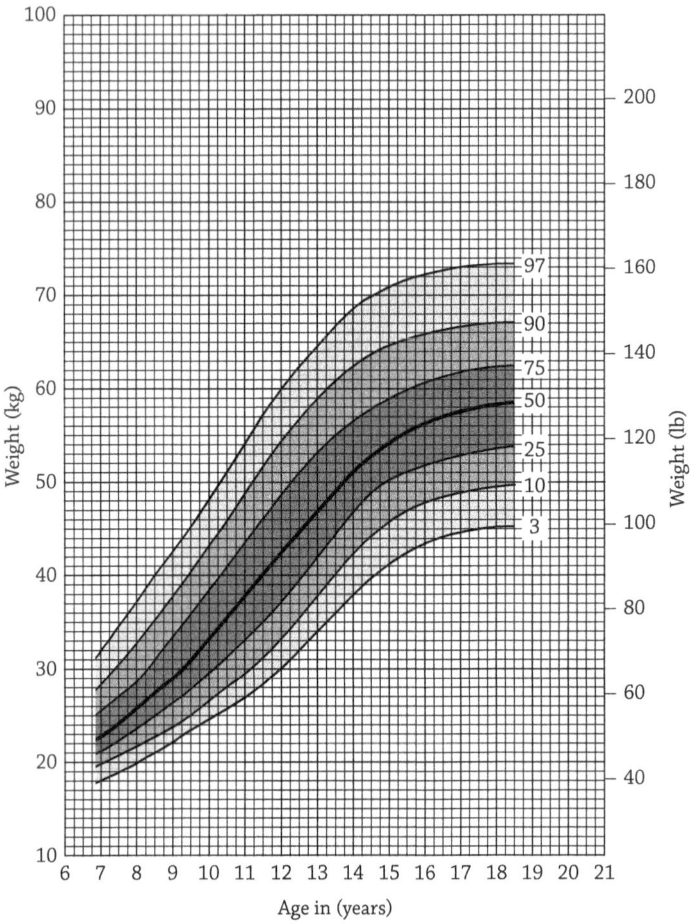

Figure 5.13. Weight, North European females, 7 to 19 years. Adapted from Georgi et al. (1996).

BODY MASS INDEX

Definition Body mass index (BMI) is defined as

$$\text{BMI} = \frac{\text{Weight in kg}}{(\text{Height in m})^2}$$

By definition, a person with a BMI greater than 25 is considered overweight; a BMI greater than 30 indicates obesity (Figs. 5.14–5.17).

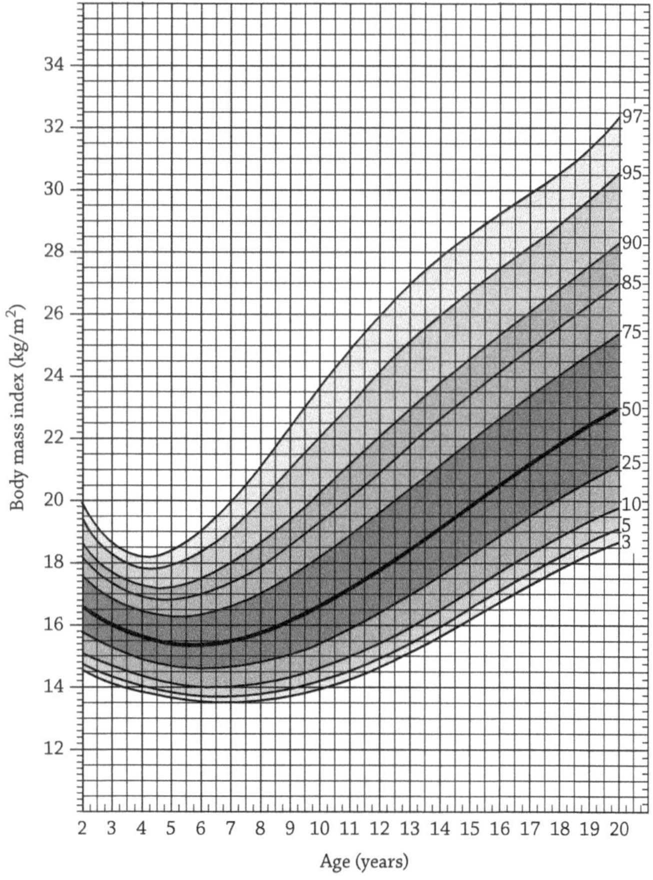

Figure 5.14. Body mass index for North American males, ages 2 to 20 years. Adapted from the Centers for Disease Control and Prevention (CDC); available at http://www.gov/growthcharts

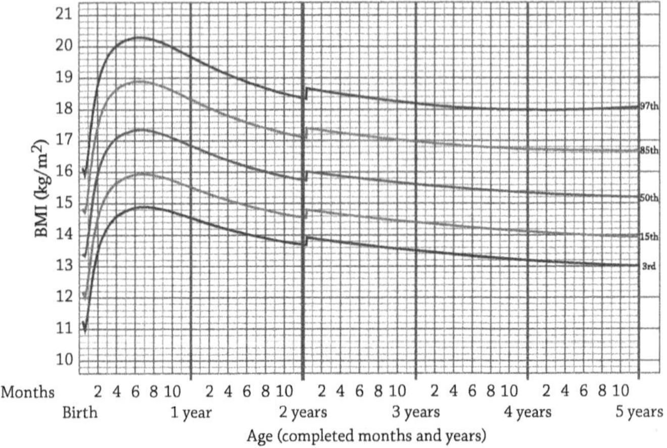

Figure 5.15. Body mass index (BMI) for age in males. Adapted from http://www.who.int/childgrowth/standards/en/

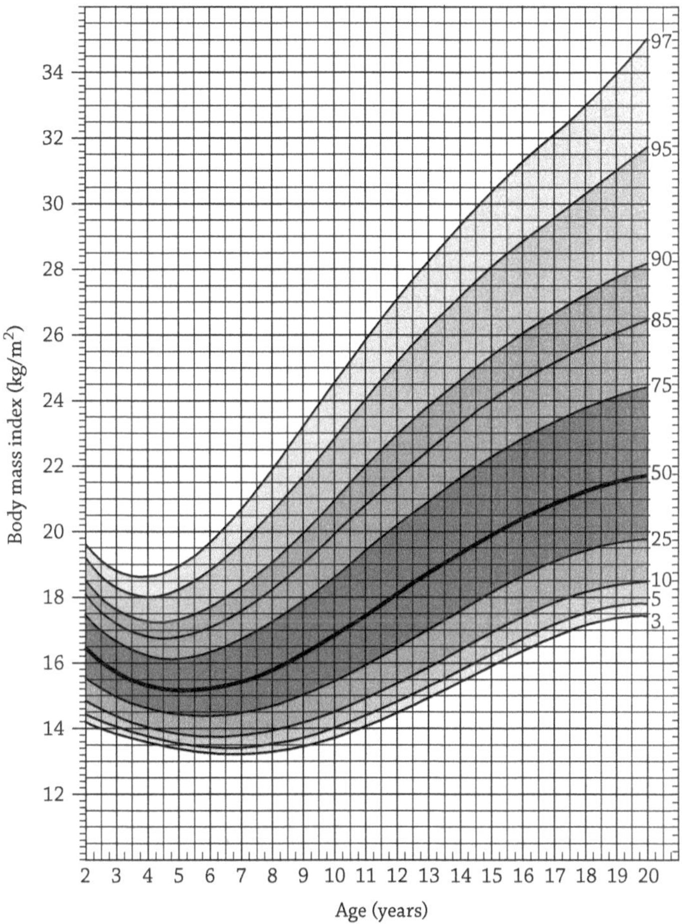

Figure 5.16. Body mass index (BMI) for North American females, ages 2 to 20 years. Adapted from the Centers for Disease Control and Prevention (CDC); available at http://www.gov/growthcharts

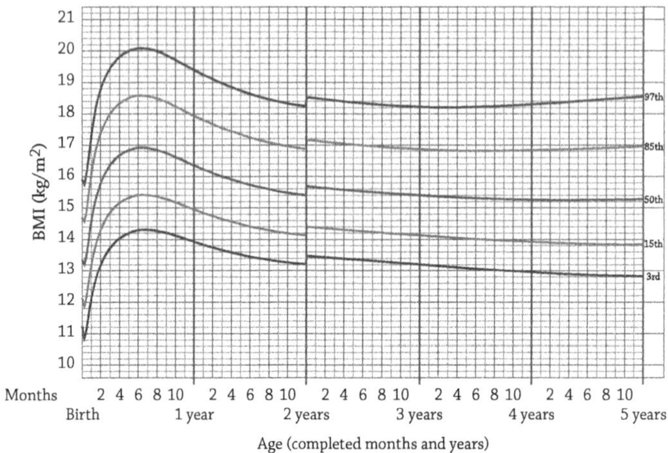

Figure 5.17. Body mass index (BMI) for age in females. Adapted from http://www.who.int/childgrowth/standards/en/

WEIGHT VELOCITY

Definition Weight velocity is the rate of weight gain or loss over a period of time (Figs. 5.18–5.20).

Remarks As with other parameters of growth, weight gain is most rapid in the first months of life, and again between 12–16 years.

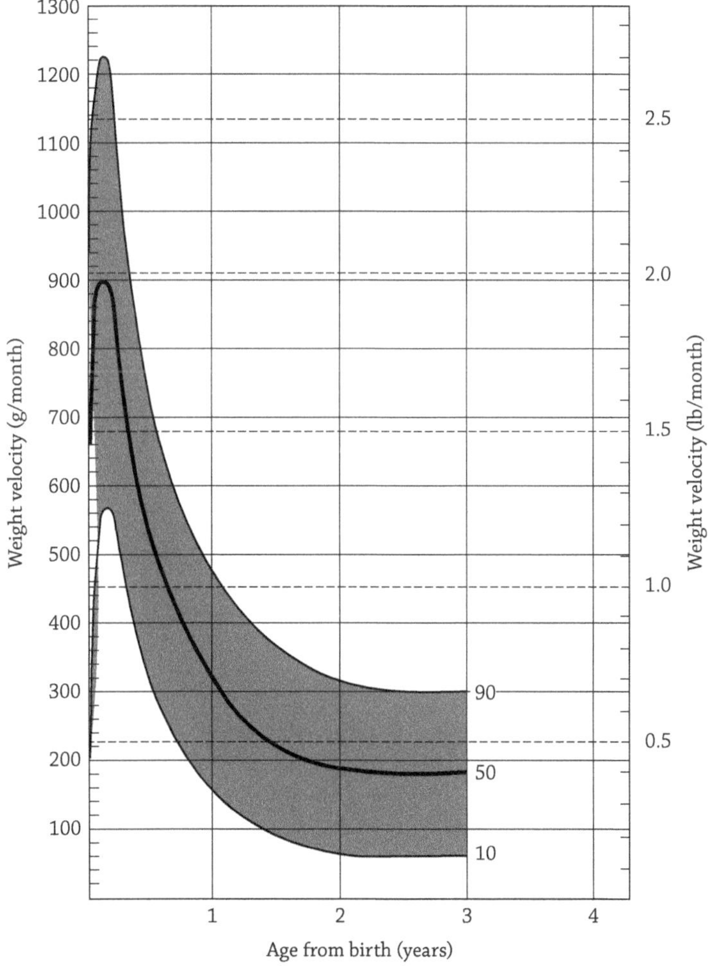

Figure 5.18. Weight velocity, both sexes, birth to 4 years. From Brandt (1986), by permission.

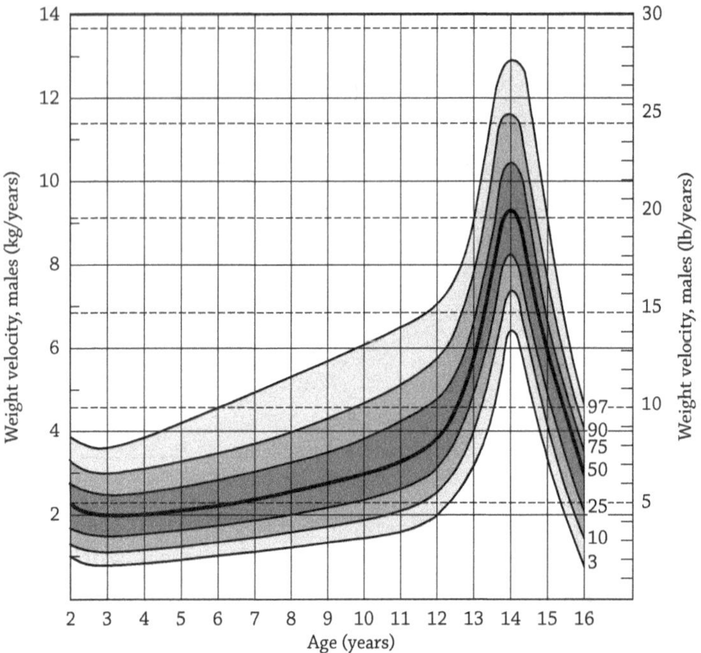

Figure 5.19. Weight velocity, males, 2 to 16 years. From Tanner and Whitehouse (1976), by permission.

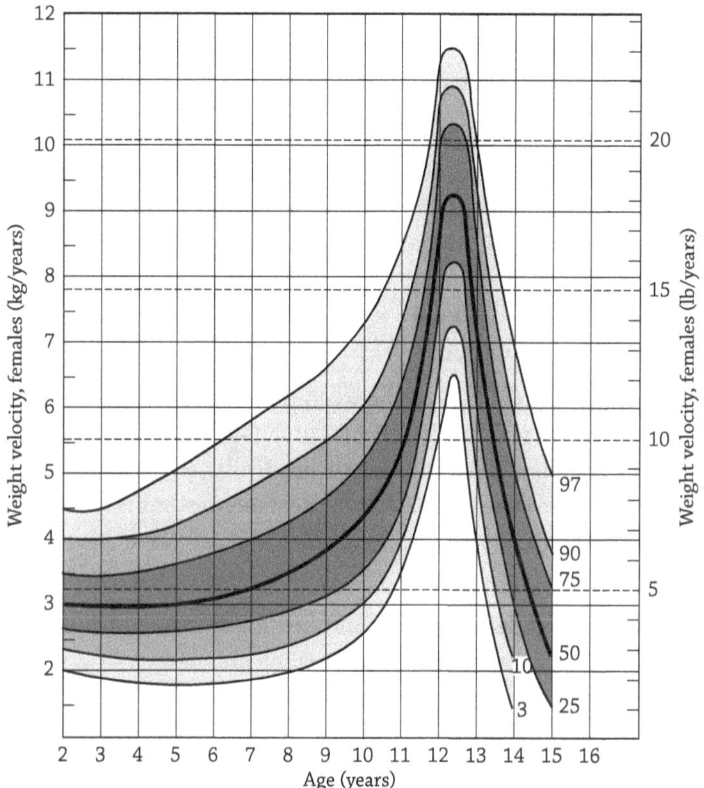

Figure 5.20. Weight velocity, females, 2 to 16 years. From Tanner and Whitehouse (1976), by permission.

SKINFOLD THICKNESS

Definition Thickness of the skinfold.

Landmarks Triceps and subscapular skinfold thickness are used. The left side of the body is usually chosen for these measurements. Triceps skinfold thickness is measured halfway down the left upper arm, while the arm is hanging relaxed at the patient's side (Fig. 5.21a).

The subscapular skinfold is measured laterally just below the angle of the left scapula (Fig. 5.21b).

Position A skinfold is held between the investigator's thumb and index finger (subcutaneous fold without muscle). The caliper is placed about 1 mm below the left hand, perpendicular to the skinfold. The caliper is held in the right hand and the measurement is read within 3 seconds (so that pressure does not compress the subcutaneous tissue).

Instruments Special calipers are used for precise measurements. These are constructed to exert a constant pressure of 10 g/mm^2 at the opening and allow an accuracy up to 0.1 mm. Skinfold thickness is measured in millimeters (Figs. 5.18, 5.22 and 5.23).

Remarks The suprailiac skinfold can also be measured (just above the iliac crest in the mid-axillary line) and the sum of the three skinfold measurements (triceps skinfold + suprailiac skinfold + subscapular skinfold) is calculated to give an overall assessment (see Schlueter et al. (1976)).

Pitfalls Too lengthy or too frequently repeated measurements at the same spot will result in compression of the tissue, leading to falsely low measurement.

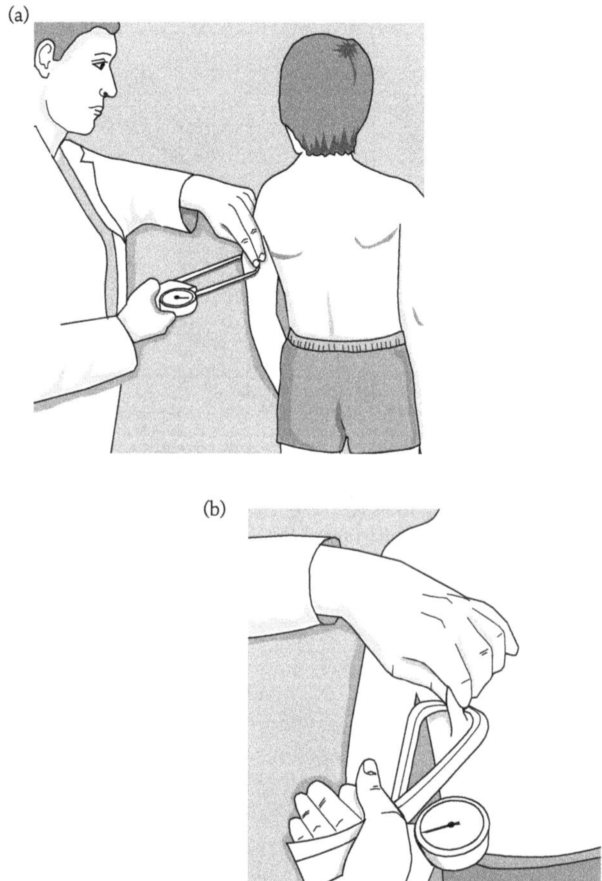

Figure 5.21. Measuring triceps (a) and subscapular skinfolds (b).

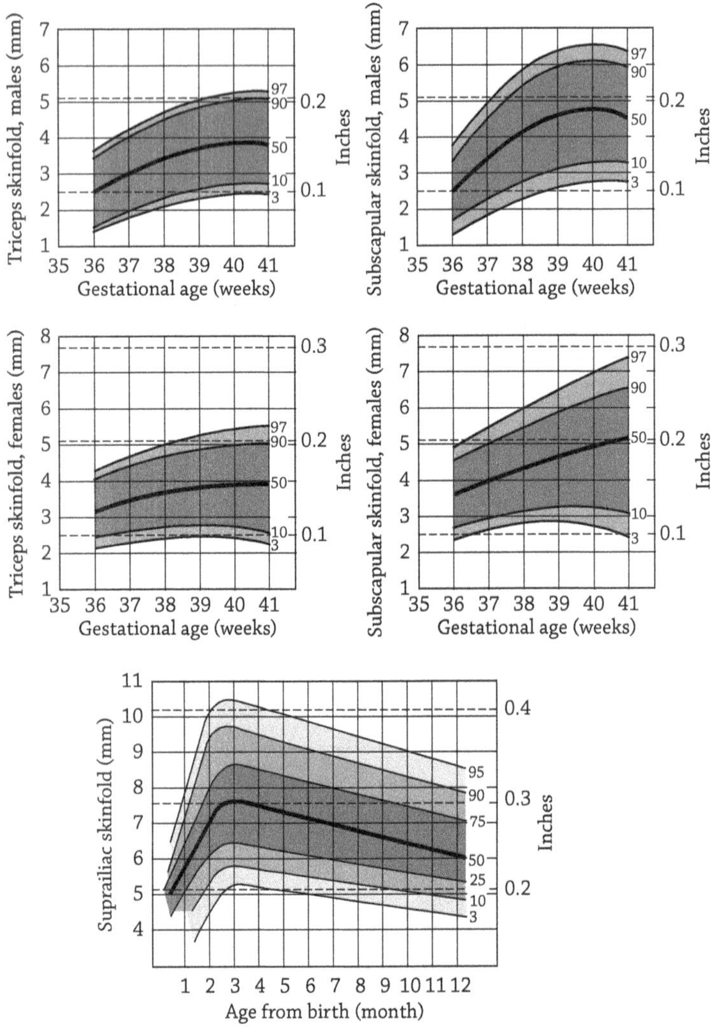

Figure 5.22. Triceps and subscapular (newborn) and suprailiac (birth to 12 months) skinfolds. From Maaser et al. (1972) and Schlueter et al. (1976), by permission.

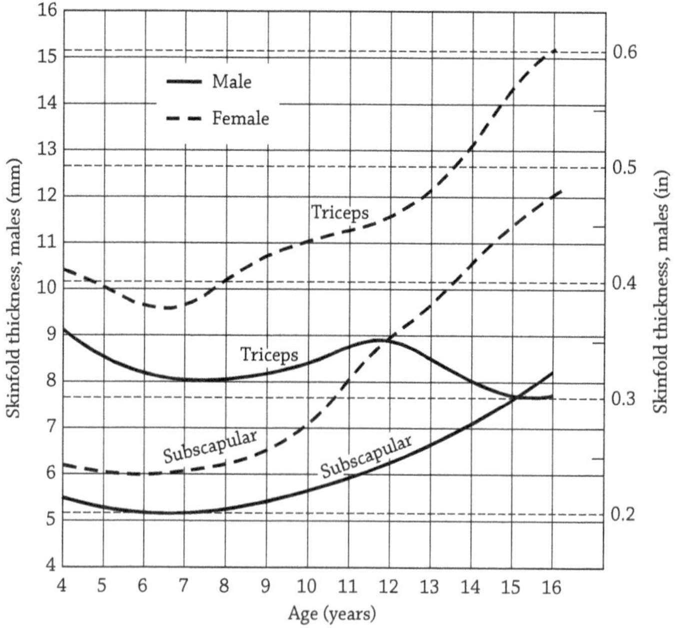

Figure 5.23. Triceps and subscapular skinfolds, males and females, 4 to 16 years. From Maaser et al. (1972) and Schlueter et al. (1976), by permission.

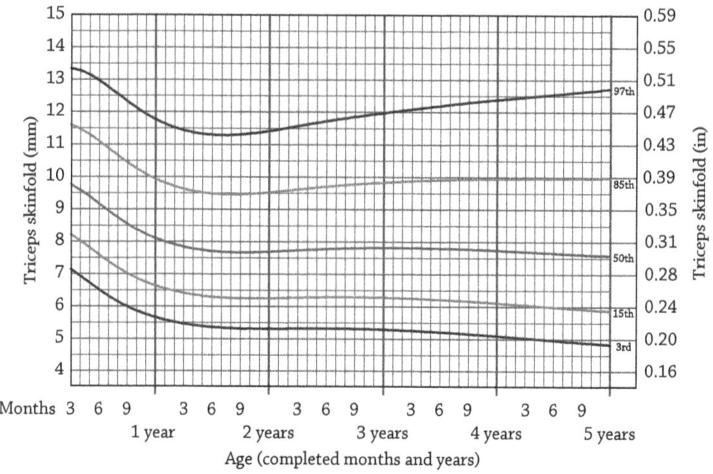

Figure 5.24. Triceps skinfold thickness for age in males. Adapted from http://www.who.int/childgrowth/standards/en/

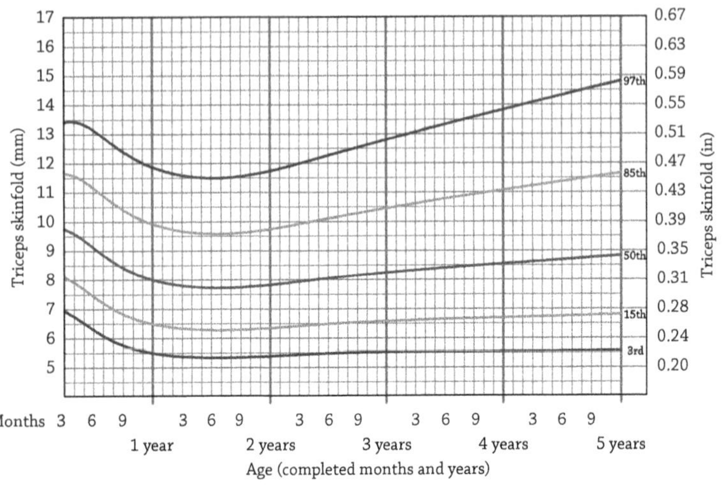

Figure 5.25. Triceps skinfold thickness for age in females. Adapted from http://www.who.int/childgrowth/standards/en/

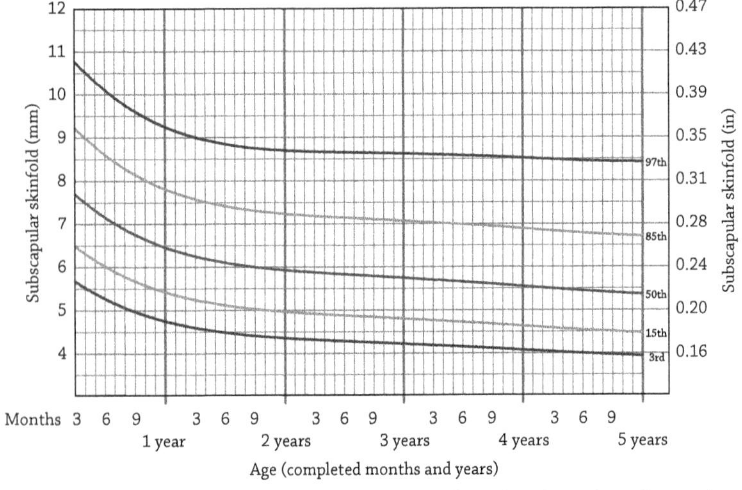

Figure 5.26. Subscapular skinfold thickness for age in males. Adapted from http://www.who.int/childgrowth/standards/en/

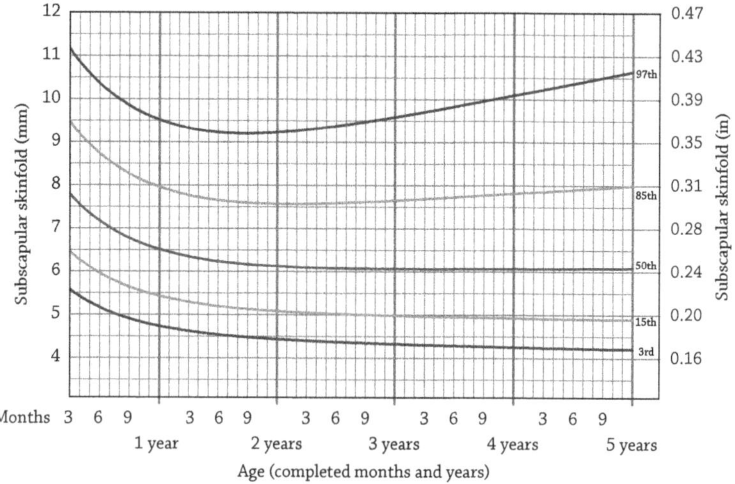

Figure 5.27. Subscapular skinfold thickness for age in females. Adapted from http://www.who.int/childgrowth/standards/en/

BIBLIOGRAPHY

Brandt, I. (1986). Growth dynamics of low-birth-weight infants with emphasis on the prenatal period. In *Human growth: A comprehensive treatise, Vol. 1.* (eds. F. Falkner and J. M. Tanner), pp. 415–475. New York: Plenum.

Brooke, O. G., Butters, F., Wood, C., Bailay, P., and Tudkmachi, F. (1981). Size at birth from 31–41 weeks gestation: Ethnic standards for British infants of both sexes. *Journal of Human Nutrition*, 35, 415–430.

Georgi, M., Schaefer, F., Wuehi, E. and Schaerer, K. (1996). Heidelberger Wachstumskurven. *Monatsschrift Kinderheilkunde*, 144, 813–824.

Hamill, P. V., Drizd, T. A., Johnson, C. L., Reed, R. B., Roche, A. F., and Moore, W. M. (1979). Physical growth: National Center for Health Statistics percentile. *American Journal of Clinical Nutrition*, 32, 607–629.

Hohenauer, L. (1980). Intrauterine Wachtumskurven fuer den Deutschen Sprachraum. *Zeitschrift fuer Geburtshilfe und Perinatologie*, 184, 167–179.

Largo, R. H., Waelli, R., Duc, G., Fanconi, A., and Prader, A. (1980). Evaluation of perinatal growth. *Helvetia Paediatrica Acta*, 35, 419–436.

Maaser, R., Stolley, H., and Droese, W. (1972). Die Hautfettfaltenmessung mit dem Caliper-II. Standardwerte der subcutanen Fettgewebsdicke

2–14 jaehriger gesunder Kinder. *Monaitsschrift fuer Kinderheilkunde*, 120, 350–353.

Olsen, I. E., Groveman, S. A., Lawson, M. L., Clark, R. H., and Zemel, B. S. (2010). New intrauterine growth curves based on United States Data. *Pediatrics*, 125, e214.

Schlueter, K., Funfack, W., Pachalay, J., and Weber, B. (1976). Development of subcutaneous fat in infancy. *European Journal of Pediatrics*, 123, 255–267.

Tanner, J. M. (1978). Physical growth and development. In *Textbook of pediatrics* (eds. J. O. Forfar and G. C. Arneil), pp. 253–303. Edinburgh: Churchill Livingstone.

Tanner, J. M., and Whitehouse, R. H. (1973). Height and weight charts from birth to 5 years allowing for length of gestation. *Archives of Disease in Childhood*, 48, 786–789.

Tanner, J. M., and Whitehouse, R. H. (1976). Clinical longitudinal standards for height, weight, height velocity, weight velocity, and stages of puberty. *Archives of Diseases in Childhood*, 51, 170–179.

Voigt, M., Schneider, K. T. M., and Jaehrig, K. (1996) Analyse des Geburtsgutes des Jahrgangs 1992 der Bundesrepublik Deutschland. Teil 1: Neue Perzentilwerte fuer die Koerpermasse von Neugeborenen. *Geburtshilfe und Frauenheilkunde*, 56, 550–558.

Waelli, R., Stettler, T., Largo, R. H., Fanconi, A., and Prader, A. (1980). Gewicht, Laenge und Kopfumfang neugeborener Kinder und ihre Abhaengigkeit von muetterlichen und kindlichen Faktoren. *Helvetia Paediatrica Acta*, 35, 397–418.

WHO standard growth curves available at http://www.who.int/childgrowth/standards/en/

Chapter 6

Head Circumference (Occipitofrontal Circumference, OFC)

INTRODUCTION

The head circumference (distance around the head) is traditionally measured at the place where the largest measurement is obtained. This practice has given rise to the term *occipitofrontal circumference* (OFC), because those are usually the landmarks of the largest circumference. OFC has become synonymous with head circumference. Care should be taken to obtain the maximum circumference, which is occasionally not at the occiput.

HEAD CIRCUMFERENCE (OFC)

Definition Maximum circumference of the head.

Landmarks The maximum head circumference is measured from just above the glabella area to the area near the top of the occipital bone (opisthocranion) (Fig. 6.1).

Instruments Tape measure.

Position The patient should look straight ahead (Fig. 6.1).

Alternative It is often easier, in young infants, to have them stay seated on an adult's lap while measuring the head circumference and to do the measurement from behind.

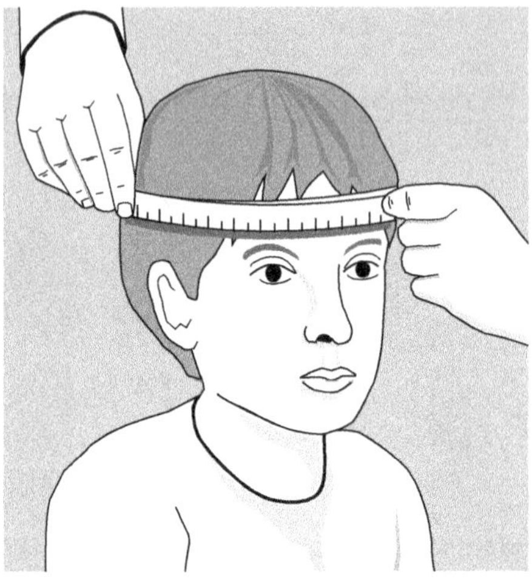

Figure 6.1. Measuring head (OFC) circumference.

Remarks The head circumference measurement should be repeated after completely removing the tape from the head in order to ensure accuracy.

Although height and weight charts after birth are quite different for North American and North European populations, head circumference growth data after birth are not. Therefore, we have included only one figure for neonatal head circumference for males and females, with charts including early gestational ages (Fig 6.2 and 6.3).

As more premature infants with very low birth weights survive, it is appropriate to use special curves for these infants. Most of the catch-up growth for OFC occurs during the first 6 months of life (Fig. 6.4).

Values for North American populations to age 16 years are given in Figs. 6.5–6.8.

Microcephaly is the term used for abnormal smallness of the head, usually as related to age; however, when the head is small it must be evaluated in the context of body size. Hence, a head can be described as microcephalic for age but be normocephalic for body size.

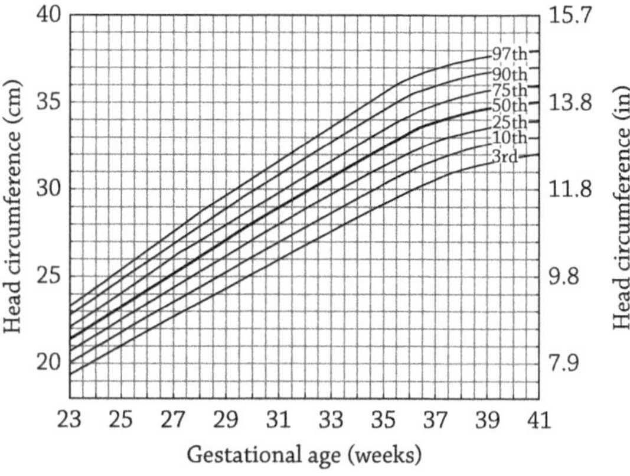

Figure 6.2. Head circumference for males, by gestational age. Adapted from Olsen et al. (2010).

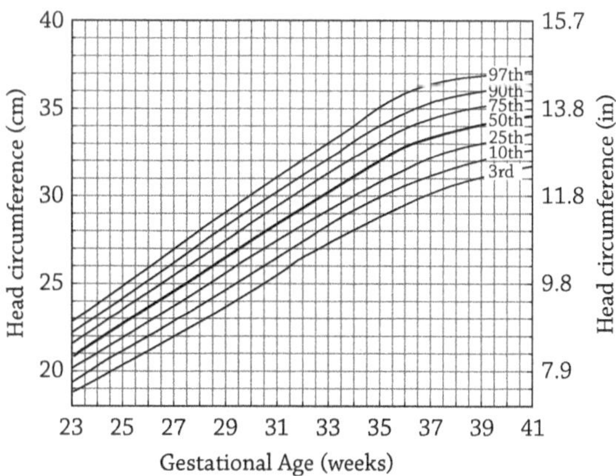

Figure 6.3. Head circumference for females, by gestational age. Adapted from Olsen et al (2010).

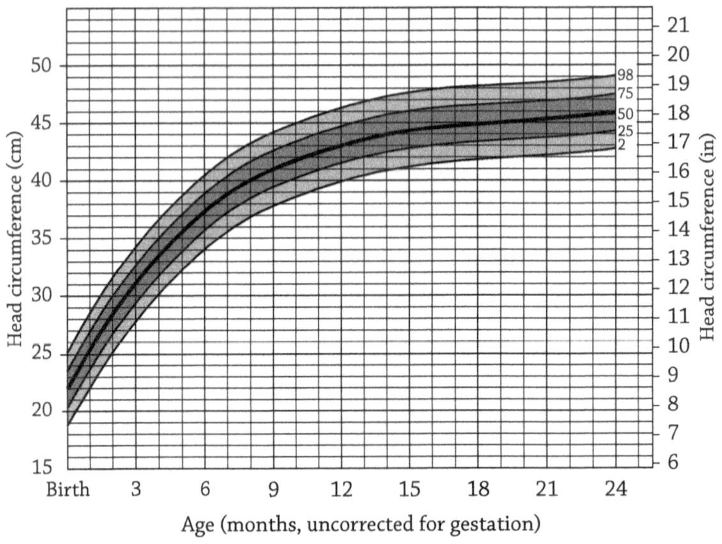

Figure 6.4. Head circumference growth for infants with a birth weight of 501–1000 g, age birth to 24 months. Adapted from Sheth et al. (1995).

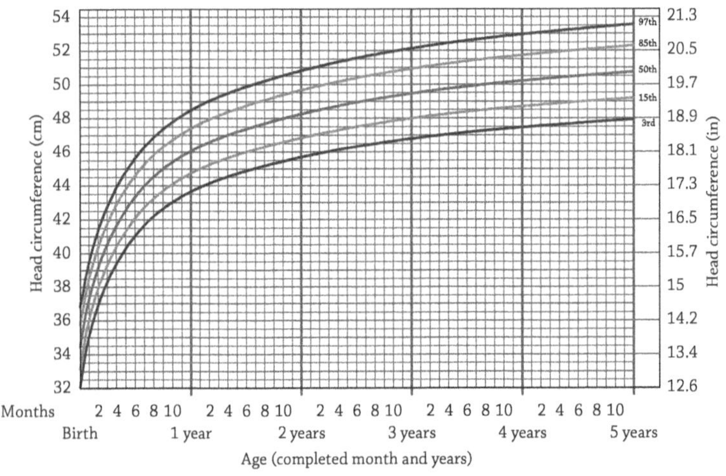

Figure 6.5. Head circumference, males, birth to 5 years. Adapted from http://www.who.int/childgrowth/standards/en/

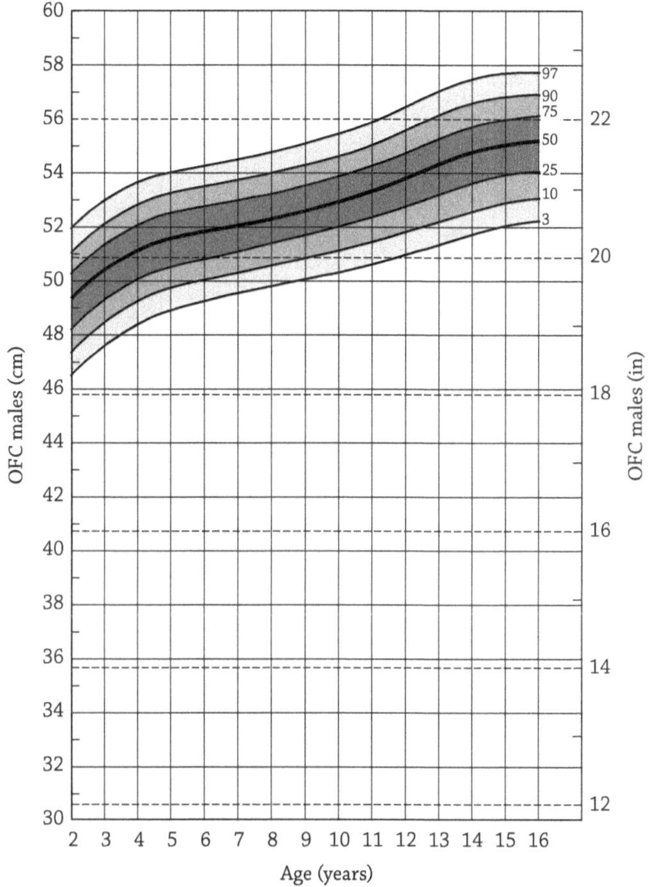

Figure 6.6. Head circumference, males, 2 to 16 years. From Nellhaus (1968) and Tanner (1978), by permission.

Microcranium is the term used for an abnormally small skull. *Macrocephaly* (megalencephaly) is the term for an abnormally large head. Again, macrocephaly must be described in relationship to age and body size. *Macrocranium* is the term for an abnormally large skull.

Pitfalls Thick hair, braids, or big ears can get in the way when measuring head circumference and can lead to falsely elevated OFC values. If the head has an atypical shape, it may be difficult to palpate the landmarks.

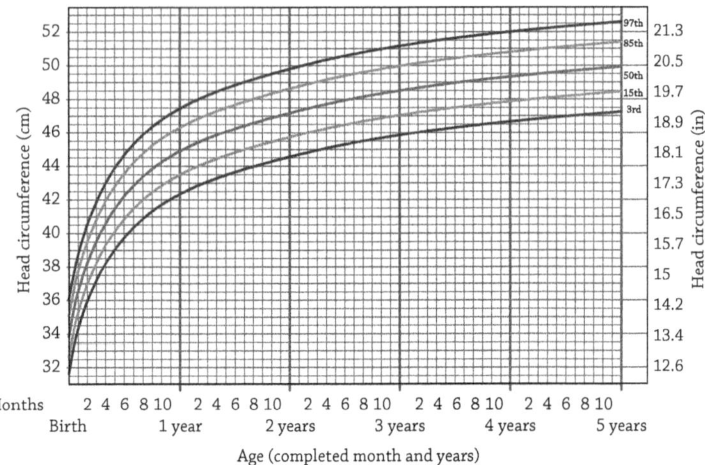

Figure 6.7. Head circumference, females, birth to 5 years. Adapted from http://www.who.int/childgrowth/standards/en/

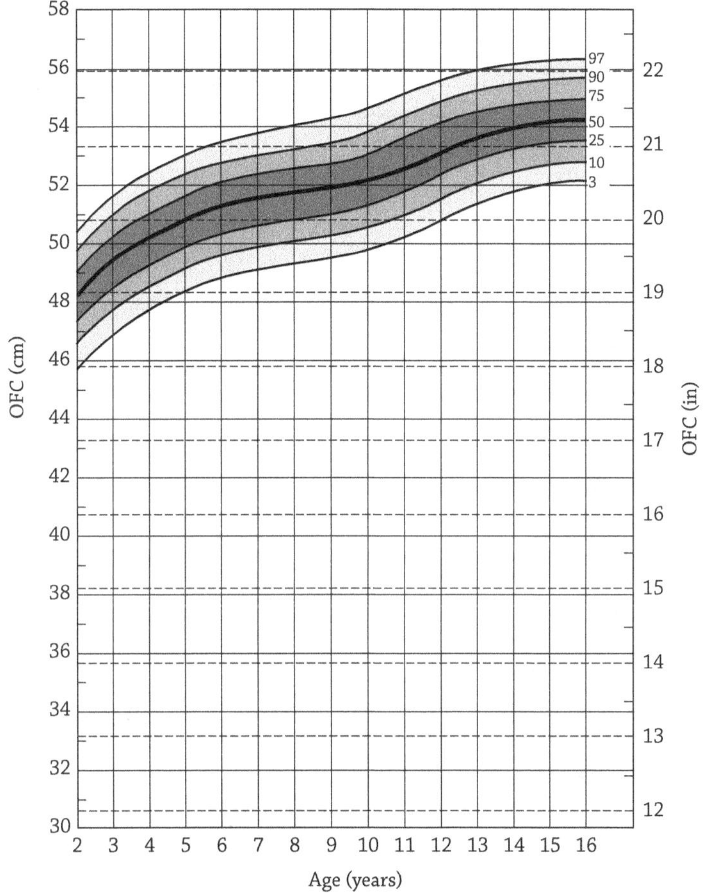

Figure 6.8. Head circumference, females, 2 to 16 years. From Nellhaus (1968) and Tanner (1978), by permission.

In the case of craniosynostosis or an atypical head shape, OFC measurements can give false impressions of micro- or macrocephaly. In those cases, the head width, length, and forehead height are useful parameters. Radiographs should be taken for a more objective estimate of cranial cavity size.

HEAD CIRCUMFERENCE (OFC) VELOCITY

The rate of head size growth decreases after birth. The deceleration is most dramatic in the first year, with the majority of head growth complete by 4 years of age (Fig. 6.9).

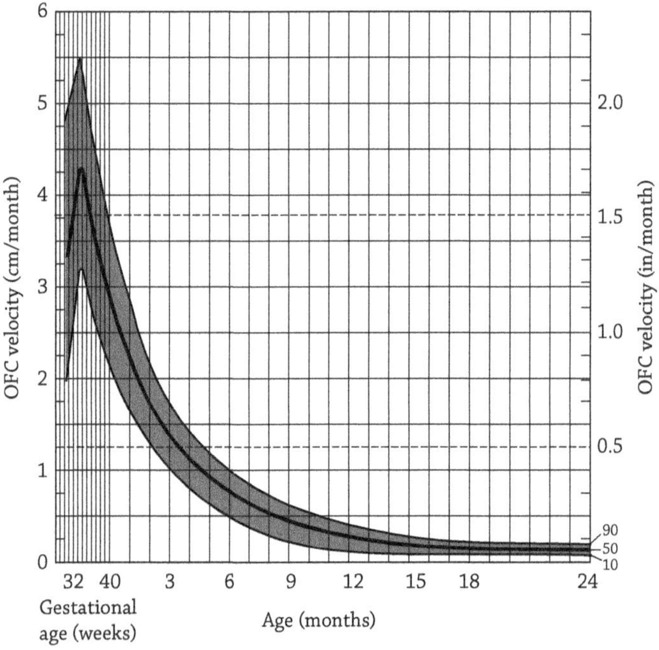

Figure 6.9. Head circumference velocity, both sexes, from 28 weeks to 1 year. From Brandt (1986) and Tanner (1978), by permission.

BIBLIOGRAPHY

Brandt, I. (1986). Growth dynamics of low-birth-weight infants with emphasis on the prenatal period. In *Human growth. A comprehensive treatise, Vol. 1* (eds. F. Falkner and J. M. Tanner), pp. 415–475. New York: Plenum.

Brooke, O. G., Butters, F., Wood, C., Bailay, P., and Tudkmachi, F. (1981). Size at birth from 31–41 weeks gestation: ethnic standards for British infants of both sexes. *Journal of Human Nutrition*, 35, 415–430.

Hohenauer, L. (1980). Intrauterine Wachtumskurven fuer den deutschen Sprachraum. *Zeitschrift fuer Geburtshilfe und Perinatologie*, 184, 167–179.

Nellhaus, G. (1968). Head circumference from birth to eighteen years. Practical composite international and interracial graphs. *Pediatrics*, 41, 106–114.

Olsen, I.E., Groveman, S. A., Lawson, M. L., Clark, R. H., and Zemel, B. S. (2010). New intrauterine growth curves based on United States data. *Pediatrics*, *125*, e214–224.

Sheth, R. D., Mullett, M. D., Bodensteiner, J. B., and Hobbs, G. R. (1995). Longitudinal head growth in developmentally normal preterm infants. *Archives of Pediatric and Adolescent Medicine*, 149, 1358–1361.

Tanner, J. M. (1978). Physical growth and development. In *Textbook of pediatrics* (eds. J. O. Forfar and G. C. Arneil), pp. 253–303. Edinburgh: Churchill Livingstone.

Waelli, R., Stettler, T., Largo, R. H., Fanconi, A., and Prader, A. (1980). Gewicht, Laenge und Kopfumfang neugeborener Kinder und ihre Abhaengigkeit von muetterlichen und kindlichen Faktoren. *Helvetica Paediatrica Acta*, 35, 397–418.

WHO standard growth curves. Available at http://www.who.int/childgrowth/standards/en/

Chapter 7

Craniofacies

INTRODUCTION

The face is unique, both because of variability in size and shape and because of ability to demonstrate personal expression and emotion. Movements around the eyes and mouth contribute to the overall gestalt. Evaluation of the craniofacies is complex.

The development of the shape of the human head and face depends on a variety of interactive genetic and environmental factors. Intrinsic or extrinsic pressure and neuromuscular function contribute to the overall shape. To accurately define what is different in the individual with dysmorphic craniofacial features is a challenge. The nomenclature used to describe facial findings has been standardized (Carey et al., 2009; Hall et al., 2009; Hennekam et al., 2009; Hunter et al., 2009). Comprehensive anthropometric descriptions have become available for many conditions for which data were previously lacking, and standards have been developed for several disorders so that affected children can be compared with their similarly affected peers and normal individuals.

For practical purposes, in this text, we have limited the craniofacial measurements to those we find useful. The reader will find further details in references at the end of this chapter.

Development of the face from five facial primordia appearing around the stomodeum or primitive mouth occurs mainly between the fifth and eighth weeks of gestation. The five facial primordia consist of the frontonasal prominence, the paired maxillary prominences of the first branchial arch, and the paired mandibular prominences of the first branchial arch. The frontonasal prominence forms the forehead and the dorsum and apex of the nose. The alae nasi are derived from the lateral nasal prominences. The fleshy nasal septum and the philtrum are formed by the medial nasal prominences. The maxillary prominences form the upper cheek regions and most of the upper lip. The mandibular prominences give rise to the lower lip, the chin, and the lower cheek regions.

The primitive lips and cheeks are invaded by mesenchyme from the second branchial arch which give rise to the facial muscles. These muscles of facial expression are supplied by the facial nerve. The mesenchyme of the first pair of branchial arches develops into the muscles of mastication, which are innervated by the trigeminal nerve. Abnormal development of the components of the first branchial arch results in various congenital malformations of the eyes, ears, mandible, and palate. Development of the face, lips, tongue, jaws, palate, pharynx, and neck largely involves transformation of the branchial apparatus into adult structures. Most congenital malformations of the head and neck originate during that transformation (e.g., branchial cysts, sinuses, fistulae). The development of the face and palate is complicated and congenital malformations resulting from an arrest of development and/or a failure of fusion of the prominences and processes are not uncommon.

Growth of the face and jaws can coincide with the eruption of the deciduous teeth. These changes are even more marked after the permanent teeth erupt. There is concurrent enlargement of the frontal and facial regions associated with an increase in size of the perinasal air sinuses, which are generally rudimentary or absent at birth. Growth of the sinuses is important in altering the shape of the face.

Measurement of the craniofacies requires only a few standard instruments: sliding and spreading calipers and a tape measure. In addition, a modified protractor and an instrument to determine ear location and angulation are useful but not essential. A general rule when measuring between two soft tissue landmarks is that the hard tips of the calipers touch but do not press on the skin surface. In contrast, when measuring between bony landmarks, the blunt pointers of the calipers are presented against the bony surface. When measuring the circumference, the length, or the width of the head, the examiner must be certain that the metric tape or the tips of the calipers are sufficiently pressed against the skull to eliminate the effect of thick hair cover. Accurate measurement requires correct use of the instrument and knowledge of the landmark. For this reason, we have provided detailed explanations of measurement techniques and pitfalls for each particular parameter.

For measurement of the craniofacies, it is often easiest to have the head resting on a head support from a chair. However, this is not always possible in the clinic. If necessary, an assistant may gently hold the subject's head. Full exposure of the soft nose (alar shape, columella, nasal floor, nostrils) in the frontal plane is facilitated if the head is in the reclining position. Orbital measurements are most easily obtained when the patient's body is supine with the eyes gazing straight up to the ceiling and the plane of the facial profile in the vertical.

The standard orientation of the head for craniofacial measurement is the Frankfort horizontal (FH). In this position, the line connecting the lowest point on the lower margin of each bony orbit (orbitale) and the highest point on the upper margin of the cutaneous external auditory meatus (porion) is horizontal. When the subject is recumbent, the FH becomes vertical.

An alternative head position (the rest position) is determined by the subject's own feeling of the natural head balance. In healthy persons, in the rest position, the inclination of the line connecting the orbitale and the porion (ear opening) is about 5 degrees higher than it is in the FH. Since the subject's head tends to return to the rest position during examination, head position must be rechecked before each measurement. Correct positioning techniques and use of standard landmarks are important not only for the evaluation of the normal face but particularly in the assessment of subjects with a cranial or facial anomaly. The most common palpable landmarks of the craniofacies are shown in Figure 7.1, and a full definition of each of these landmarks is presented in the Glossary.

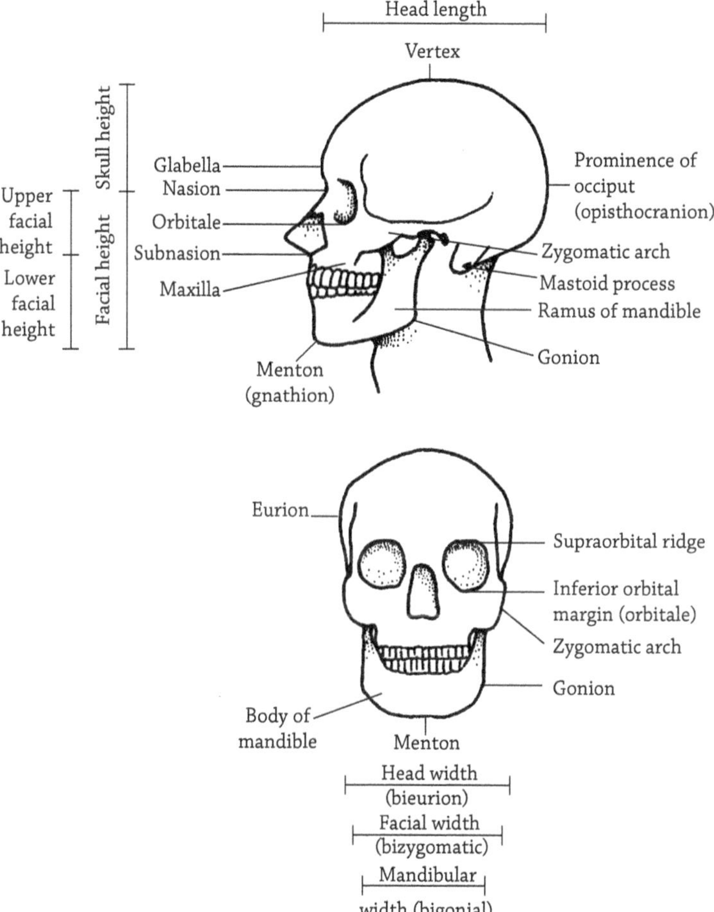

Figure 7.1. Palpable landmarks of craniofacies.

An alternative approach to craniofacial measurement involves a photoanthropometric method using frontal and profile photographs. Photographs are standardized (one-fifth, one-fourth, one-third, one-half, or life-size) for quantification of surface features and to allow scientific, accurate documentations. Some centers prefer to have the patient standing, while other researchers have developed complex machinery to keep the patient in a fixed position at a defined distance from the camera. Details and sources of error are available in articles listed in the Bibliography.

Another approach to craniofacial measurement involves craniofacial pattern profile analysis, which provides a simple and readily understandable method of classifying, illustrating, and comparing pattern deviations from the normal state. Measurements taken from radiographs of the head and face are converted into normalized *z* scores (standard deviation units), and the pattern profile can be presented in a simple graphic form. The reader is directed to the Bibliography at the end of this chapter for further details.

The fourth approach to craniofacial measurement, cephalometry, employs radiography. Further details may be found in the Bibliography at the end of this chapter.

With the advance of three-dimensional reconstruction of computed tomography (CT) images, this technology is increasingly taking the place of two-dimensional cephalometric images (Varghese et al., 2010). Because three-dimensional CT images can be rotated and manipulated on the computer screen, they allow for a more detailed evaluation of craniofacial morphology.

A newer approach to document the three-dimensional surface of the face consists of multiple camera photography. Computerized programs merge the images into a single three-dimensional surface mesh. In addition to image documentation, this approach allows for identification of soft tissue landmarks, distance measurements between landmarks, and calculation of ratios. Software allowing computer image–driven syndrome identification is being developed.

Results of single measurements will indicate the patient's place within or outside the normal range. Repeated measurements allow calculation of changes and growth. Such changes affect the proportions of the face. In both sexes, the vertical profile measurements increase more than horizontal measurements (maximum relative increments occurring earlier in girls than in boys). The upper face seems to grow more rapidly than the lower face up to about the

10th year. After that age, the reverse is apparent. The lower portion of the face, consisting of the mandible, manifests accelerated growth with the result that, at 21 years, the face has the same relative proportions as at 3 years. Growth is generally completed first in the skull, then in the width of the face, and last in the length and depth of the face. Peak growth occurs between 3 and 5 years, followed by continuous deceleration until the 13th year, and then a distinct adolescent acceleration. There is virtually complete cessation of growth of the craniofacies at age 21 years. However, many nasal dimensions, particularly nasal length, continue to increase. With increasing age, most craniofacial dimensions, with the exception of facial width and nasal length, are reduced. This can be ascribed mostly to soft tissue changes.

An approach to measurement of the craniofacies must include comparison with head circumference and height in addition to age. For example, inner and outer canthal distances on the 50th percentile, in the presence of microcephaly, would in fact be abnormal and indicate relative hypertelorism. Various indices comparing two craniofacial measurements are available in the dental and anthropological literature. Few have been included in this text, but references are found at the end of this chapter.

In addition to detailed individual measurements, an evaluation of the craniofacies requires an impression of the overall gestalt of the face both at rest and during movements such as crying, smiling, and frowning. It is important to remember that the shape of the face and its relative proportions change significantly with age, in both normal and dysmorphic individuals. For this reason, the overall gestalt may be quite different at different times during life. This change should be taken into account when a subject is evaluated.

The terminology used to describe the craniofacies is complex and somewhat confusing. A glossary of terms defining specific landmarks and anomalies is provided at the end of this book. A detailed review of the standardized terminology with illustrations is available at http://elementsofmorphology.nih.gov/

SKULL

Introduction

The skull forms from mesenchyme around the developing brain. It consists of two parts—the neurocranium (the protection for the brain) and the viscerocranium (the main skeleton of the jaws). The neurocranium is further divided into cartilaginous and membranous portions. The cartilaginous neurocranium (or chondrocranium) consists initially of the cartilaginous base of the developing skull that forms by fusion of several cartilages. Later endochondral ossification of the chondrocranium forms the bones of the base of the skull. Intramembranous ossification occurs in the mesenchyme at the sides and top of the brain, forming the cranial vault or calvaria. During fetal life the flat bones of the skull are separated by dense, connective tissue membranes called *sutures*. The seven large fibrous areas where several sutures meet are called *fontanelles*. The cartilaginous viscerocranium consists of the cartilaginous skeleton of the first two pairs of branchial arches that will ultimately form the middle ear ossicles, part of the hyoid bone, and the styloid process of the temporal bone. Intramembranous ossification occurs within the maxillary and mandibular prominences of the first branchial arch and subsequently forms the maxillary, zygomatic, and squamous temporal bones and the mandible.

Postnatal growth of the skull occurs because the fibrous sutures of the newborn calvaria permit the skull to enlarge during infancy and childhood. The increase in size is greatest during the first 2 years, the period of most rapid postnatal brain growth. The skull normally increases in capacity until 15 or 16 years of age. After this, a slight increase in size for 3 to 4 years is due to thickening of the bones.

The overall head shape is closely related to the bony structures of the skull and to the shape of the underlying brain. Alterations in head shape can be the result of atypical brain growth, but they may also reflect a number of other factors such as premature synostosis or fusion of the cranial sutures or atypical intrauterine mechanical forces. Abnormal planes of muscle pull, as in torticollis, can cause asymmetric skull growth. The presentation of the individual during delivery also contributes to the shape of the head. Dolichocephaly or scaphocephaly (long narrow head) is a postural deformation of the head that can be associated with intrauterine breech position or prematurity. It generally resolves during infancy with no apparent residual impairment.

Five major sutures are present in the calvaria (Fig. 7.2). Three (the coronal, lambdoidal, and squamosal) are paired, and two (the sagittal and metopic) are single. Cranial growth normally proceeds in a direction perpendicular to each of the major sutures. Increased length of the skull in comparison to width (dolichocephaly or scaphocephaly) and the converse (brachycephaly) can be normal variants. However, both can also occur because of premature synostosis of cranial sutures, where skull growth at the site of the fused suture is inhibited with compensatory expansion at other patent sutural sites (Fig. 7.3). Head shape depends on the sutures that are prematurely fused, the order in which they fuse, and the time at which they fuse. The earlier the synostosis occurs, the more dramatic the effect on subsequent cranial growth and development.

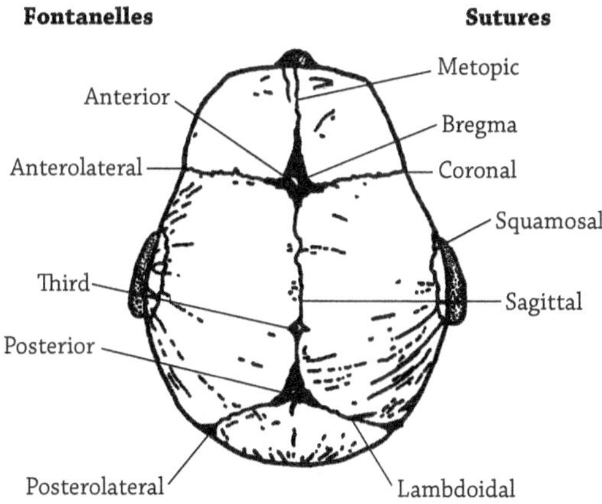

Figure 7.2. Normal fontanelle and suture landmarks. Adapted from Pruzansky (1973).

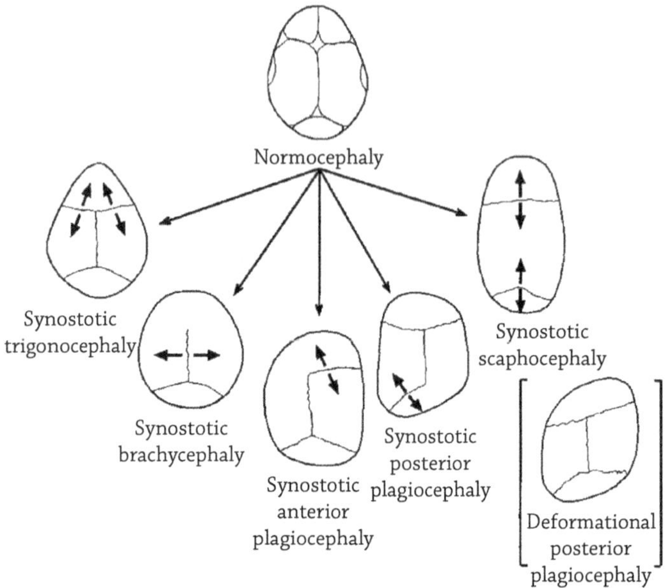

Figure 7.3. Abnormal patterns of suture fusion. Adapted from Cohen and MacLean (2000).

Dolichocephaly can occur with early closure of the sagittal suture, producing a long, narrow cranium. When both sides of the coronal suture are prematurely fused, the head shape is brachycephalic (Fig. 7.3). Unilateral synostosis of the coronal suture results in asymmetry of head shape, termed plagiocephaly (Fig. 7.3). The frontal eminence on the fused side is flattened and the glabella region is underdeveloped. The eyebrows and orbit on the affected side appear elevated. Plagiocephaly resulting from unicoronal synostosis needs to be differentiated from the more common positional plagiocephaly due to deformational forces (Fig. 7.3). Premature closure of one lambdoid suture can also result in plagiocephaly. In trigonocephaly, premature synostosis of the metopic suture results in a triangular prominence of the frontal bone, usually in association with ocular hypotelorism (Fig. 7.3). Metopic ridging may also occur.

When the major determinants of anteroposterior and lateral growth are impeded by coronal and sagittal synostosis, respectively, the cranial vault grows vertically rather than in its normal longitudinal and horizontal directions, resulting in acrocephaly. Acrocephaly is a tall or high skull (vertical index above 77), and the top of the head may be pointed, peaked, or conical in shape. It is also referred to as oxycephaly, turricephaly, or tower skull. A shortened length of the skull compared to its width is referred to as brachycephaly (cephalic index above 81.0); this is typically caused by premature fusion of both coronal sutures (bicoronal synostosis). An elongation of the skull with narrowing from side to side (cephalic index less than 76) is called *dolichocephaly* or *scaphocephaly*, and it is typically caused by premature fusion of the sagittal suture (see Fig. 7.3).

Premature closure of the cranial sutures can occur in isolation or as part of a syndrome, in association with other clinical anomalies.

In addition to describing the skull shape in terms of its length and width, we can also comment on the prominence of various parts of the skull. *Bathrocephaly* is the term used to describe a step-like posterior projection of the skull, caused by external bulging of the squamous portion of the occipital bone. Various craniosynostoses can reduce the depth of the bony orbit, producing proptosis, or prominence of the ocular globe.

Few individuals, if any, have true symmetry of the face, and small differences in the length and width of the palpebral fissures are common.

HEAD LENGTH

Definition Maximum dimension of the sagittal axis of the skull.

Landmarks Measure between the glabella (the most prominent point on the frontal bone above the root of the nose, between the eyebrows) and the opisthocranion (the most prominent portion of the occiput, close to the midline on the posterior rim of the foramen magnum) (Figs 7.1 and 7.4). These landmarks are also critical for measurement of head circumference.

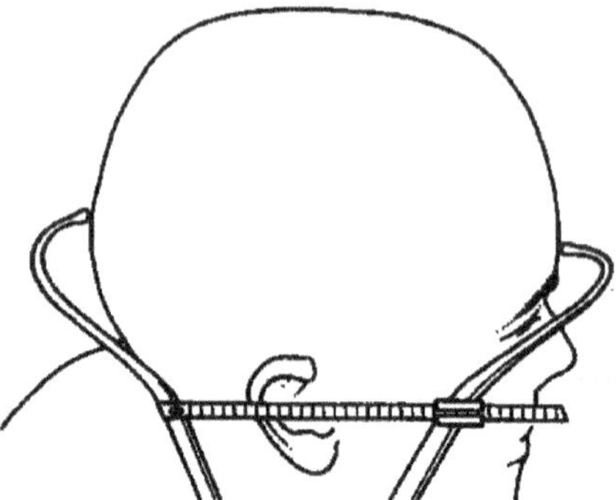

Figure 7.4. Measuring head length with calipers.

Instruments Spreading calipers give the most precise measurement. A tape measure can be used, stretched above or lateral to the head.

Position The patient should be standing or sitting. The examiner views the skull in profile.

Alternative The examiner may stand above the patient and look down on the skull.

Remarks Charts of head length are presented in Figures 7.5 and 7.6. Alterations in skull shape will produce marked variation in this measurement and in head width. Dolichocephaly increases, while brachycephaly reduces, head length. X-ray measurements are more precise but do not take the skin thickness into account.

Pitfalls A bulging forehead or cloverleaf deformity may make it difficult to define the landmarks. One should eliminate the effects of thick hair by applying the caliper tips firmly against the skull.

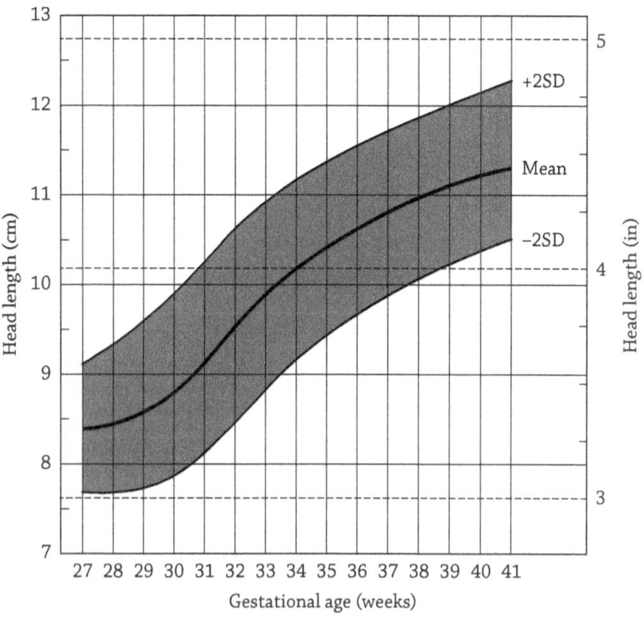

Figure 7.5. Head length, both sexes, at birth. From Merlob et al. (1984), by permission.

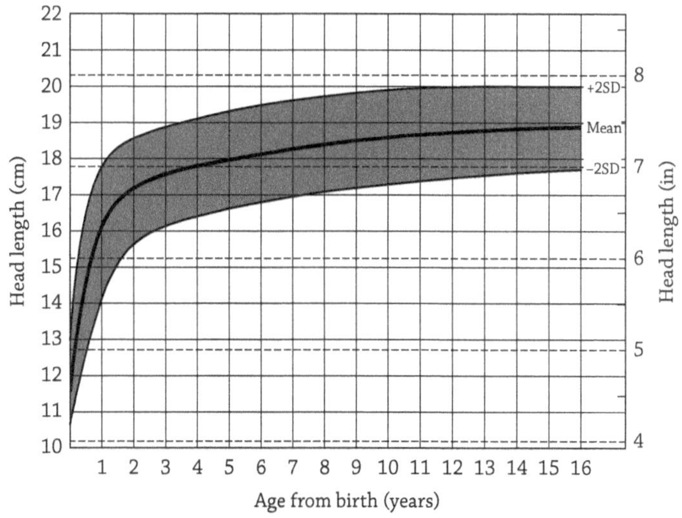

Figure 7.6. Head length, both sexes, birth to 16 years. From Feingold and Bossert (1974) and Farkas (1981), by permission.

Head Width

Definition Maximal biparietal diameter.

Landmarks Measure between the most lateral points of the parietal bones (eurion) on each side of the head (Fig. 7.7).

Instruments Spreading calipers give most accurate measurements. A tape measure held above the head, avoiding the natural curve of the cranial vault, may be substituted.

Position The head should be held erect (in the resting position) with the eyes looking straight ahead.

Alternative Viewing the skull from in front or behind may allow measurement, but the most lateral point of the parietal bone is best judged from above.

Remarks Charts of head width are presented in Figures 7.8 and 7.9. Alteration in skull shape will produce variation in this measurement; for example, dolichocephaly will reduce head width. X-ray measurements are more precise but do not take into account the thickness of soft tissues.

Pitfalls Severe skull deformity and/or asymmetry may distort the measurement of head width. The calipers tips should be firmly applied to the skull to eliminate the effects of thick hair cover.

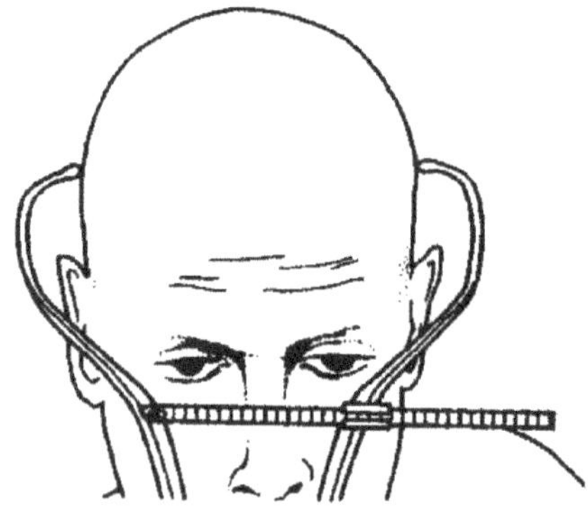

Figure 7.7. Measuring head width with calipers.

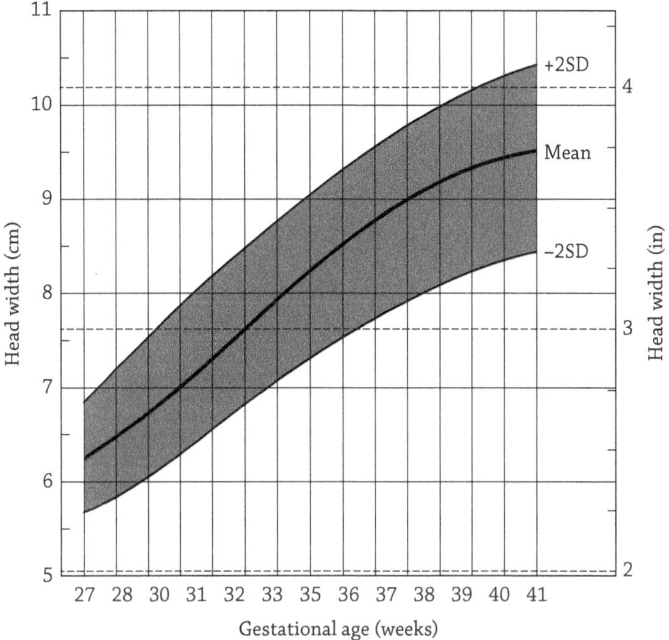

Figure 7.8. Head width, both sexes, at birth. From Merlob et al. (1984), by permission.

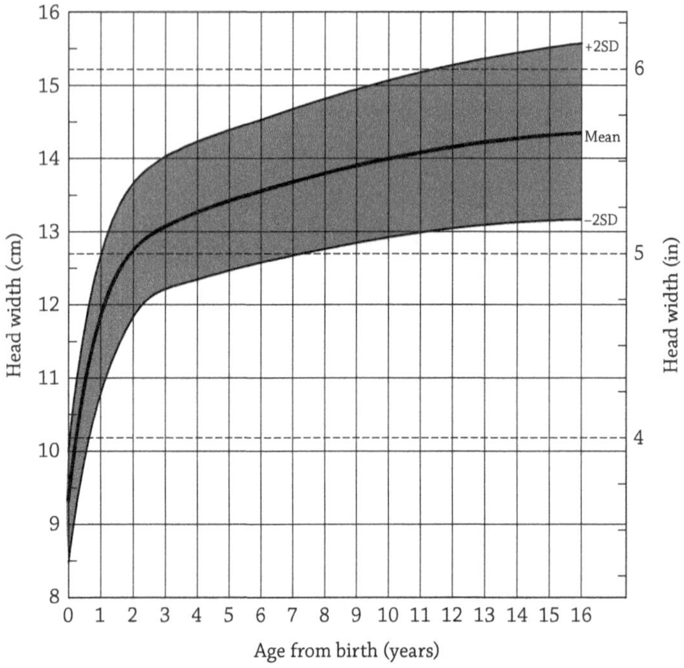

Figure 7.9. Head width, both sexes, birth to 16 years. From Feingold and Bossert (1974), by permission.

Cephalic Index

Definition This index is the ratio of head width, expressed as a percentage of head length.

$$CI = \frac{\text{head width} \times 100}{\text{head length}}$$

Remarks In the "normal" head, the CI is 76%–80.9%. Dolichocephaly: $CI < 76\%$. Brachycephaly: $CI > 81\%$.

Skull Height (Forehead Height)

Definition Distance from the root of the nose (nasion) to the highest point of the head (vertex).

Landmarks Measure from the depth of the nasal root to the superior-most point of the skull in the vertical plane (Figs. 7.1 and 7.10).

Instruments Spreading calipers are most accurate. A tape measure could be used, being held vertically and avoiding the natural curve of the head.

Position The head should be held erect (in the resting position) with the eyes looking straight ahead. The patient should face the examiner.

Alternative The patient may face perpendicular to the examiner.

Remarks Charts of normal skull height are presented in Figure 7.11. Alteration in skull shape will produce marked variation in this measurement. For example, turricephaly will increase the skull height. Radiographic measurements are more precise.

Pitfalls A prominent nasal root may make definition of the nasion difficult and reduce the accuracy of this measurement. If the nasion is poorly defined, measure from a point on the nose at the level of the inner canthi. The vertex is not identical to the bregma, the bony landmark in the middle of the top of the skull where the coronal and sagittal sutures cross.

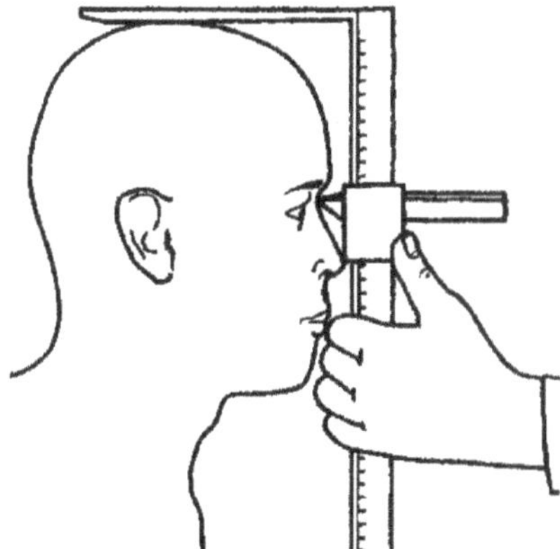

Figure 7.10. Measuring skull height with calipers.

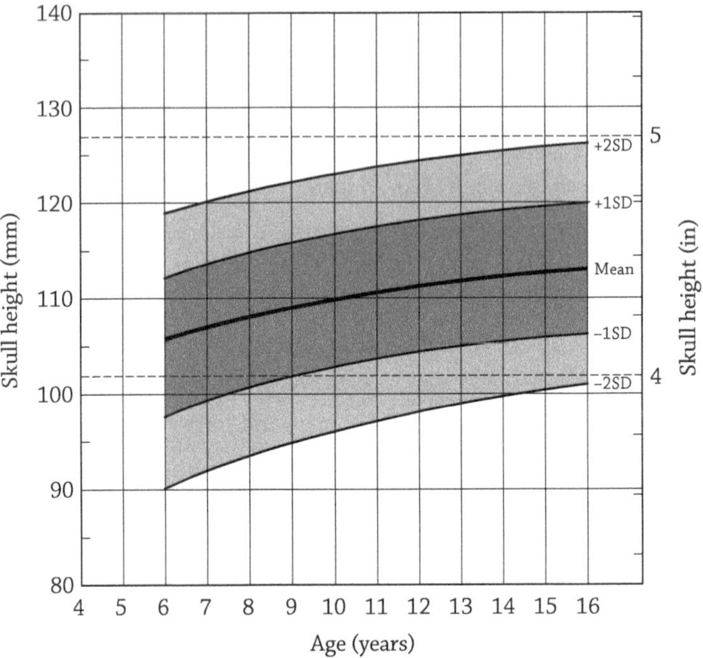

Figure 7.11. Skull height, both sexes, 6 to 16 years. From Farkas (1981), by permission.

Upper Facial Height (Nasal Height)

Definition Distance from the root of the nose (nasion) to the base of the nose (subnasion).

Landmarks Measure from the deepest part of the nasal root (nasion) to the deepest point of concavity at the base of the nose (subnasion), in a vertical plane (Figs. 7.1 and 7.12).

Instruments Sliding calipers are most accurate. A tape measure could be used, avoiding the natural curve of the midface.

Position Frankfort horizontal, with the facial profile in the vertical.

Alternative If the nasal tip is long or pointed down, masking the subnasion, this measurement is best taken from the side.

Remarks Upper facial height corresponds to nasal height (Fig. 7.13).

Pitfalls A prominent nasal bridge may distort the position of the nasion and produce a less accurate measurement.

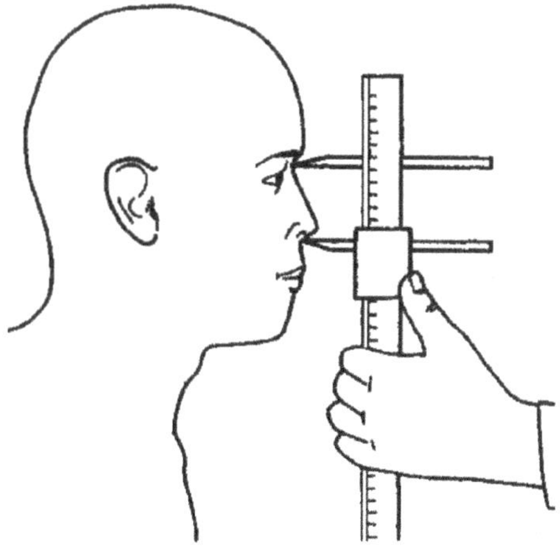

Figure 7.12. Measuring upper facial height with calipers.

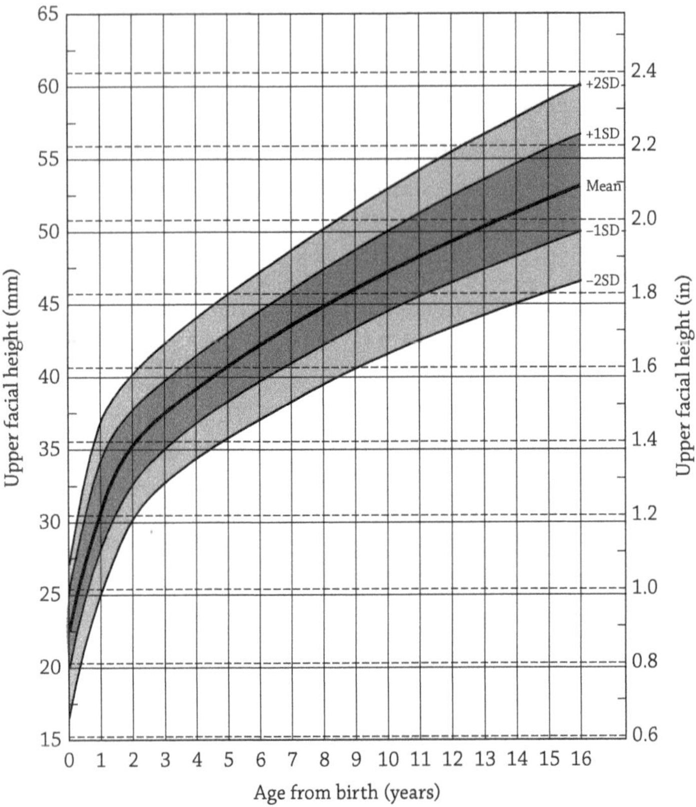

Figure 7.13. Upper facial height, both sexes, birth to 16 years. From Farkas (1981) and Goodman and Grolin ,(1977) by permission.

Lower Facial Height

Definition Length of the lower one-third of the craniofacies (Fig. 7.14).

Landmarks Measure from the base of the nose (subnasion) to the lowest median landmark on the lower border of the mandible (menton or gnathion). The menton is identified by palpation and is identical to the bony gnathion (Figs. 7.1 and 7.14a).

Instruments Tape measure or spreading calipers.

Position Frankfort horizontal, with facial profile in the vertical. The mouth should be closed, with the teeth in occlusion.

Remarks This measurement can also be obtained from a lateral radiograph. The measurement is then taken from the anterior nasal spine (the pointed process extending from the nasal floor, formed by the meeting of both nasal margins at the midline) to the bony gnathion. Spreading calipers are used to measure this distance on a radiograph (Fig. 7.14b).

Pitfalls In comparing cephalometric with anthropometric data, one should remember that cephalometric data do not take into account soft tissue measurements. However, the data from both sources are surprisingly similar, and have been combined in Figure 7.15.

In the presence of a mandibular abnormality such as a cleft, it may be difficult to obtain an accurate measurement of lower facial height. If the mouth is open, the lower facial height will be falsely increased.

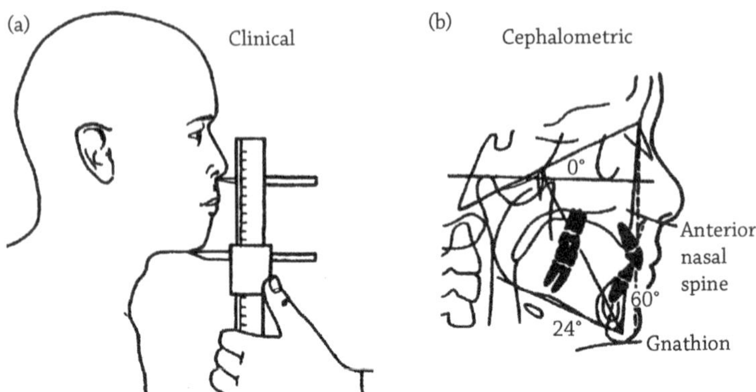

Figure 7.14. Anthrometric (a) and cephalometric (b) measurement of lower facial height.

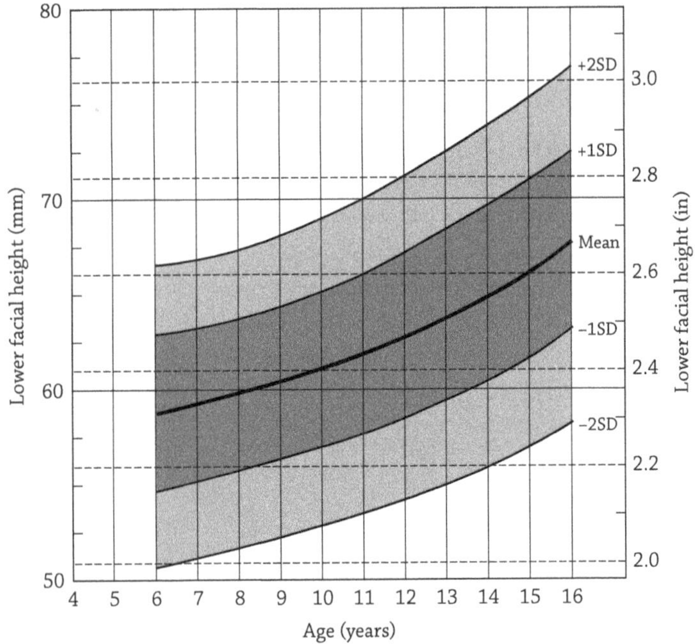

Figure 7.15. Lower facial height, both sexes, 6 to 16 years. From Saksena et al. (1987), McNamara (1984), and Farkas (1981), by permission.

Facial Height

Definition Distance from the root of the nose (nasion) to the lowest median landmark on the lower border of the mandible (menton or gnathion). Lower two-thirds of craniofacies (Fig. 7.16).

Landmarks Measure from the root of the nose (nasion) to the inferior border of the mandible (menton or gnathion) in a vertical plane (Figs. 7.1 and 7.16).

Instruments Spreading calipers give the most reliable measurements. A tape measure can be used but should be held in front of the sagittal axis of the face, in front of the tip of the nose.

Position Frankfort horizontal, with the facial profile in the vertical. The mouth should be closed with the teeth in occlusion.

Alternative Measurements may be obtained from lateral radiographs of the head.

Remarks The facial height chart for children age 4–16 years is provided in Figure 7.17. This measurement is used to calculate the length-to-width ratio of the head (facial index).

Pitfalls Micrognathia or prognathism can make it difficult to find the lower landmark. Prominence of the nasal bridge with a high nasal root may alter the definition of the upper landmark.

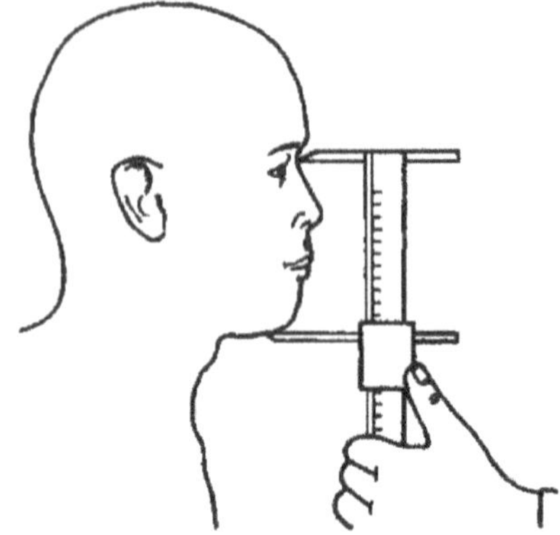

Figure 7.16. Measuring facial height with calipers.

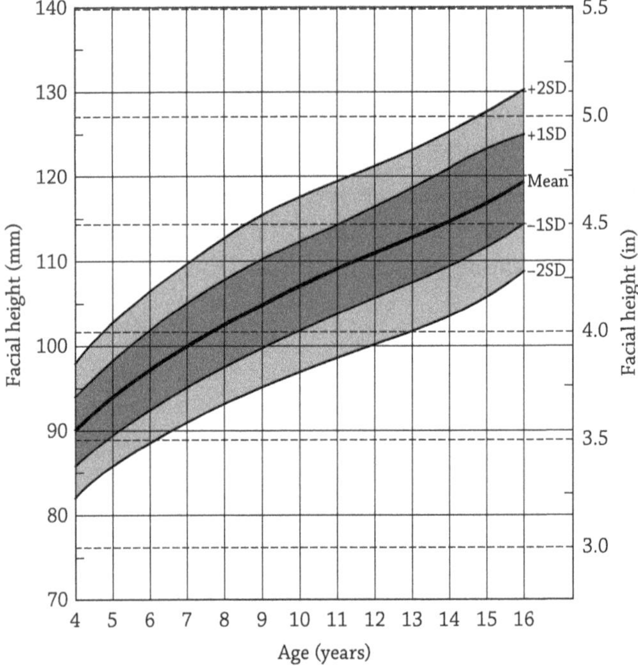

Figure 7.17. Facial height, both sexes, 4 to 16 years. From Farkas (1981) and Saksena et al. (1987), by permission.

Bizygomatic Distance (Facial Width)

Definition The maximal distance between the most lateral points on the zygomatic arches (zygion) (Fig. 7.18).

Landmarks Measure between the most lateral points of the zygomatic arches (zygion), localized by palpation (Figs. 7.1 and 7.18).

Instruments Spreading calipers will give the most precise results. A tape measure can be used, but it should be held in a straight line parallel to the zygomatic arches avoiding the curves of the zygomata.

Position The head should be held erect (in the resting position) with the eyes looking straight in a forward direction.

Remarks The most lateral point of each zygomatic arch is identified by trial measurement, not by anatomical relationship. X-ray measurements will give more exact results but will not take skin thickness into account. Once established, facial width does not change with age (Fig. 7.19).

Pitfalls Conditions in which the first and second branchial arches are abnormal will produce distorted measurements. X-ray films are preferred in this situation.

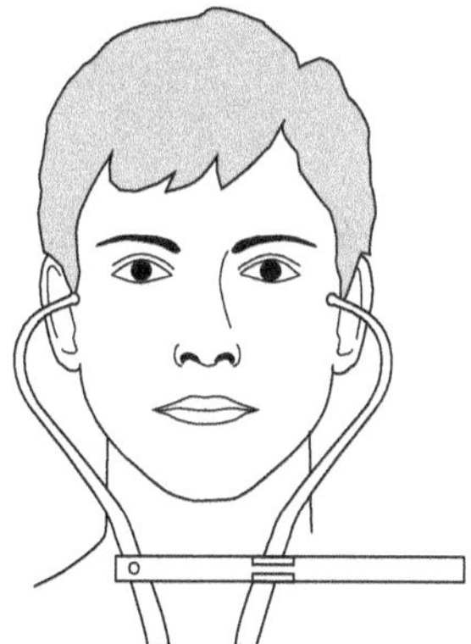

Figure 7.18. Measuring facial width with calipers.

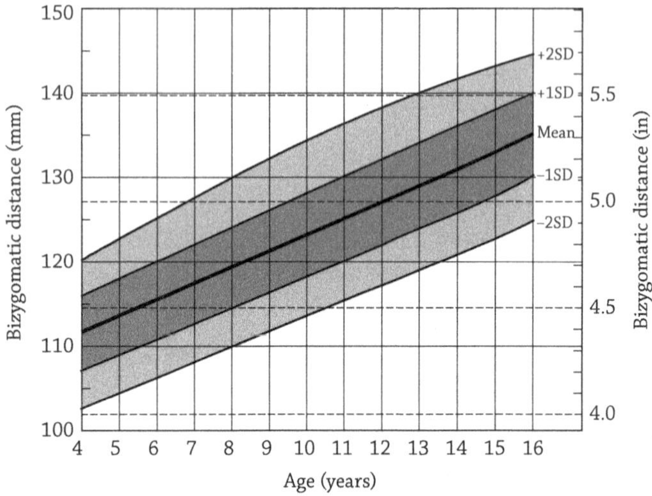

Figure 7.19. Bizygomatic distance, both sexes, 4 to 16 years. From Farkas (1981), by permission.

Facial Index

Definition This ratio utilizes the previous two measurements, facial height (nasion to menton) and bizygomatic distance (facial width), and provides a numerical estimate of facial height compared to width, in order to assess a long, narrow face as compared with a short, wide face (Fig. 7.20).

$$\text{Facial index} = \frac{\text{Facial height (mm)}}{\text{Facial width (mm)}} \times 100$$

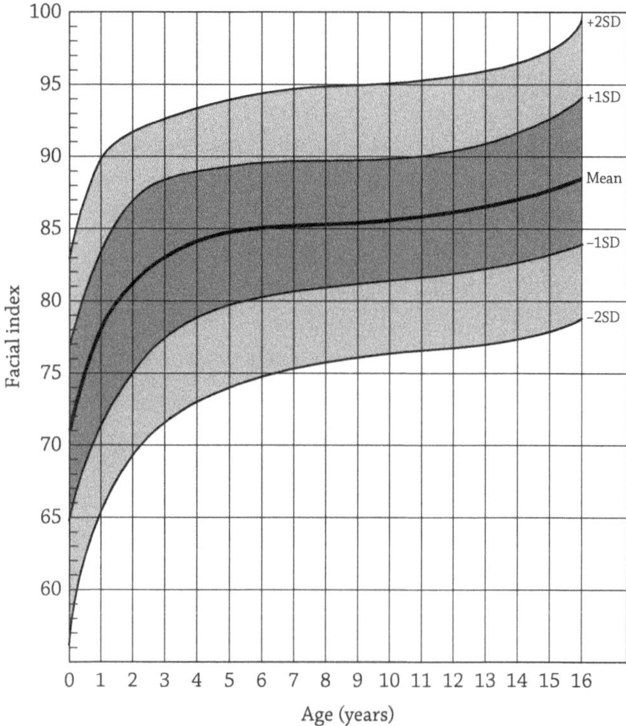

Figure 7.20. Facial index, both sexes, birth to 16 years. From Feingold and Bossert (1974) and Farkas and Munro (1987), by permission.

FONTANELLES

Introduction

Examination of the fontanelles can provide evidence of altered intracranial pressure and is also an index of the rate of development and ossification of the calvaria, which may be altered in a variety of disorders. To utilize fontanelle size and patency as a clue to altered morphogenesis, it is necessary to have normal age-related standards.

Figures 7.21 and 7.22 outline the constant and accessory fontanelles present at birth. The most common accessory fontanelle is the parietal (sagittal) fontanelle, otherwise known as a third fontanelle, which is found in 6.3% of infants and may be more common in infants with Down syndrome. The "metopic" fontanelle represents the extremely long anterior arm of the anterior fontanelle that, in the process of closure, becomes separated from the anterior fontanelle. A metopic fontanelle has been reported in association with craniofacial dysostosis, cleidocranial dysplasia (also known as cleidocranial dysostosis), spina bifida occulta, and meningomyelocoele. It can also

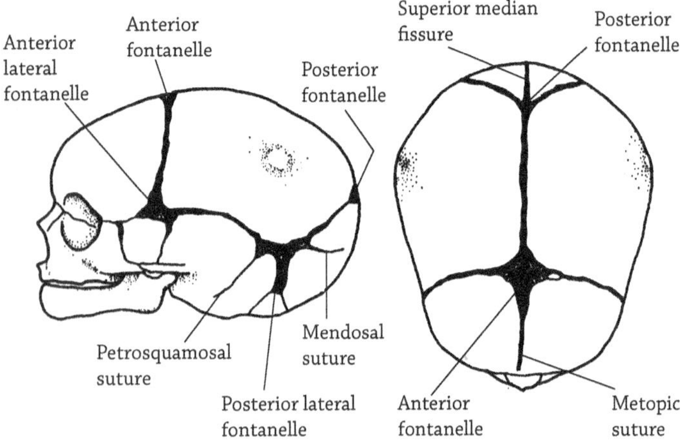

Figure 7.21. Cranium at birth. From Caffey (1978), by permission.

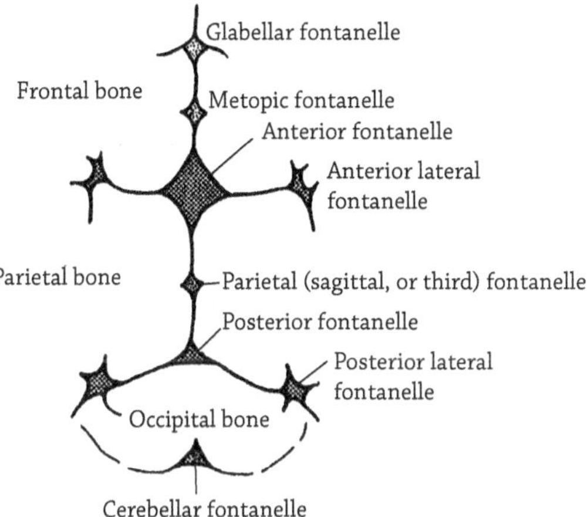

Figure 7.22. Fontanelles at birth (constant and accessory). From Caffey (1978), by permission.

occur as an isolated finding. The incidence of open metopic fontanelles can also be increased in infants with congenital rubella syndrome, Down syndrome, cleft lip with or without cleft palate, and widened sutures. The metopic fontanelle is easy to palpate, and the discovery of its presence during the examination of the newborn infant may be important clinically.

With increasing age, the fontanelles and sutures become smaller and narrower due to the growth of bone into these remnants of the fetal membranous and cartilaginous skull. There is considerable variation in the velocity of this process amongst individuals, and between the two sides of the same skull (Fig. 7.22). The anterior fontanelle is usually reduced to fingertip size by the first half of the second year. The posterior fontanelle may close during the last 2 months of gestation, or the first 2 months following birth. The anterolateral fontanelles disappear during the first 3 months of life, and the posterolateral fontanelles during the second year of life. The frontal (metopic) suture between the two halves of the frontal squamosa begins to close in the second year and is usually completely obliterated during the third year. It persists throughout life in about 10% of individuals. The great sutures of the vault (coronal, lambdoidal, sagittal) persist normally throughout infancy and childhood and do not completely close before the 30th year.

By comparing measurements with age-related fontanelle dimensions in normal persons, the clinician should be able to identify those individuals having either an abnormally large or small fontanelle for age. The presence of an unusually large fontanelle, without increased intracranial pressure, can be a valuable clue in the recognition of a variety of disorders. An unusually small anterior fontanelle may be a secondary feature in disorders that affect brain growth, such as primary microcephaly; it may be due to craniosynostosis, or it may be caused by accelerated osseous maturation secondary to maternal hyperthyroidism or hyperthyroidism in early life. Males have a slightly larger anterior fontanelle than females during the first 6 months of life.

Occasionally, numerous large and small accessory ossification centers may be seen within the sutures. These intrasutural or wormian bones can be mistaken for multiple fracture fragments but are present in the normal healthy individual. However, wormian bones can be associated with inherited disorders such as osteogenesis imperfecta.

Anterior Fontanelle Size

Definition The sum of the longitudinal and transverse diameters of the anterior fontanelle along the sagittal and coronal sutures (Figs. 7.23–7.27).

Landmarks The index finger should be placed as far as possible into each of the four corners of the anterior fontanelle. These four positions may be marked with a dot immediately distal to the fingertip. The longitudinal and transverse diameters may be measured directly, or a piece of white paper can be firmly pressed over the fontanelle to transfer the marks (Fig. 7.24). The points are jointed to form a quadrilateral, and the sum of the longitudinal and transverse diameters along the sagittal and coronal sutures can be measured.

Instruments Spreading calipers, a tape measure, or a ruler may be used.

Position The head should be held erect with eyes looking straight in a forward direction. The examiner should look down on the skull vault from above.

Alternative The infant can be lying prone or supine with the skull again viewed from above.

Closure	Time
Anterior fontanelle	1 year ± 4 months
Posterior fontanelle	Birth ± 2 months
Anterolateral fontanelle	By third month
Posterolateral fontanelle	During second year
Metopic suture	By third year (10%, never)
Clinical closure of sutures	6–12 months
Anatomic closure of sutures	By 30th year

Figure 7.23. Closure of constant and accessory fontanelles and sutures. Adapted from Goodman and Gorlin (1977).

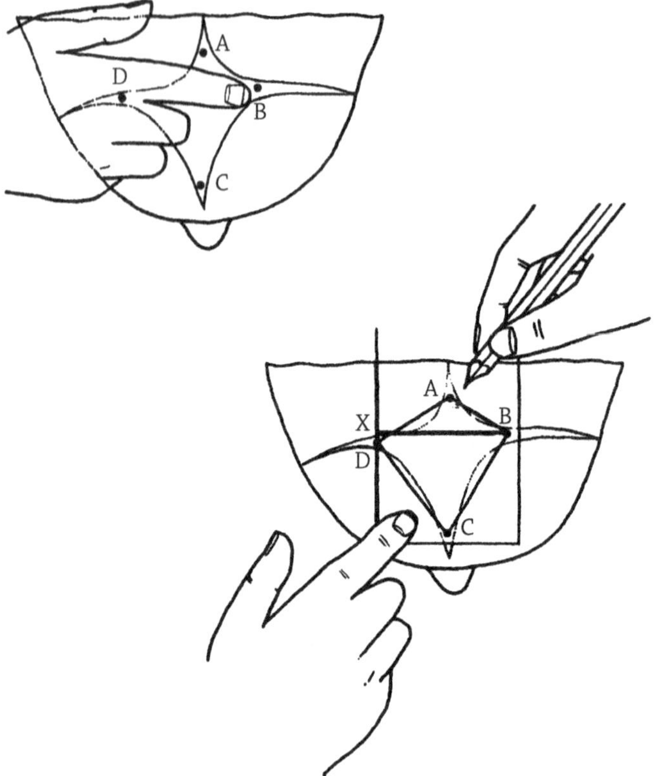

Figure 7.24. Measuring the anterior fontanelle.

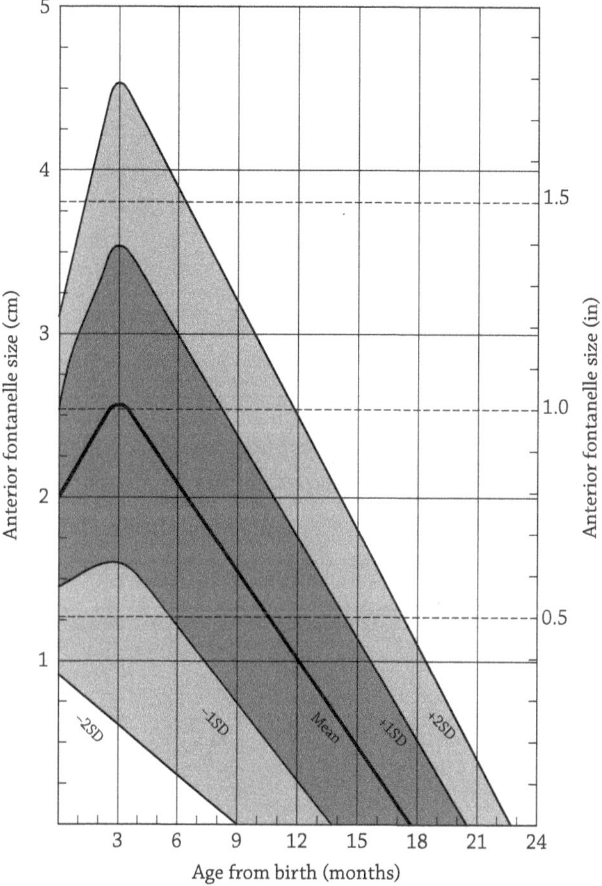

Figure 7.25. Anterior fontanelle size (sum of longitudinal and transverse diameters). From Popich and Smith (1972), by permission.

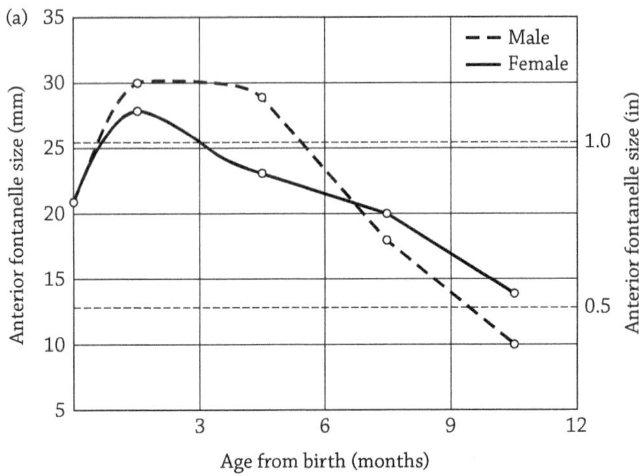

Figure 7.26(a). Anterior fontanelle, comparison of male versus female. From Popich and Smith (1972), by permission.

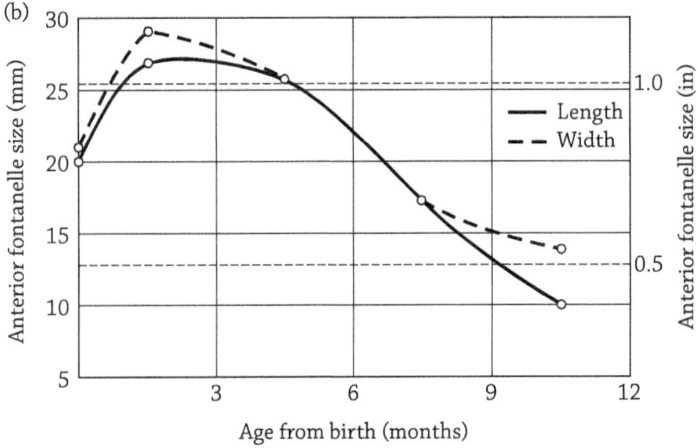

Figure 7.26(b). Anterior fontanelle, comparison of length versus width. From Popich and Smith (1972), by permission.

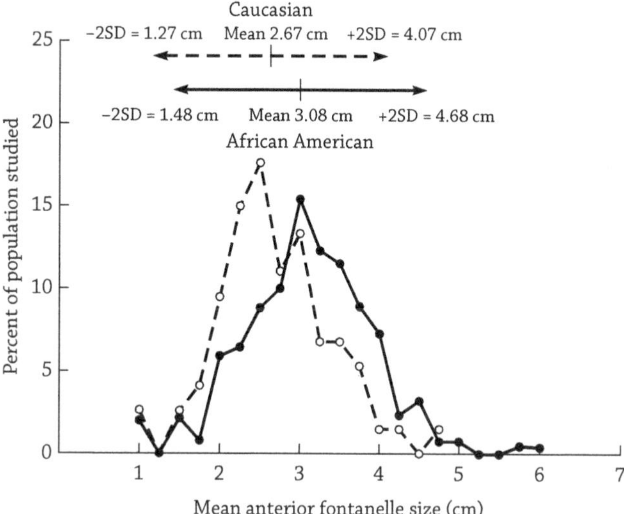

Figure 7.27. Comparison of mean anterior fontanelle size in African American and Caucasian American populations, both sexes, at birth. From Faix (1982), by permission.

Remarks An alternative method for determining fontanelle size is to calculate the area of the fontanelle $(AC \times BX)/2$ in square millimeters (Fig. 7.24). An atypically small anterior fontanelle may be caused by craniosynostosis involving the coronal and/or sagittal sutures. Males have a slightly larger anterior fontanelle than females for the first 6 months of life.

Pitfalls Occasionally, in a young child, the sagittal suture is widely patent and communicates with the posterior fontanelle, making definition of the landmarks more difficult. The anterior fontanelle may extend anteriorly into an open metopic suture.

Posterior Fontanelle Size

Definition Length of the posterior fontanelle (Fig. 7.28).

Landmarks The posterior fontanelle is a triangular structure. Measure from the anterior corner (A) to the midpoint (B) on a line connecting the two posterolateral margins created by the occipital bone (Fig. 7.28).

Instruments Spreading calipers or a tape measure can be used.

Position The head should be held erect with the eyes facing forward.

Alternative The neonate may lie prone.

Remarks The posterior fontanelle is usually closed in neonates and only 3% of normal newborn infants have a posterior fontanelle that measures more than 2 cm. A third (or parietal) fontanelle may be found in about 5% of normal infants about 2 cm anterior to the posterior fontanelle. It occurs with greater frequency in Down syndrome and in congenital rubella syndrome. Figure 7.29 shows normal values for posterior fontanelle size in African American and Caucasian American children at birth.

Pitfalls If the sagittal suture is widely patent, the anterior border of the posterior fontanelle may be difficult to distinguish.

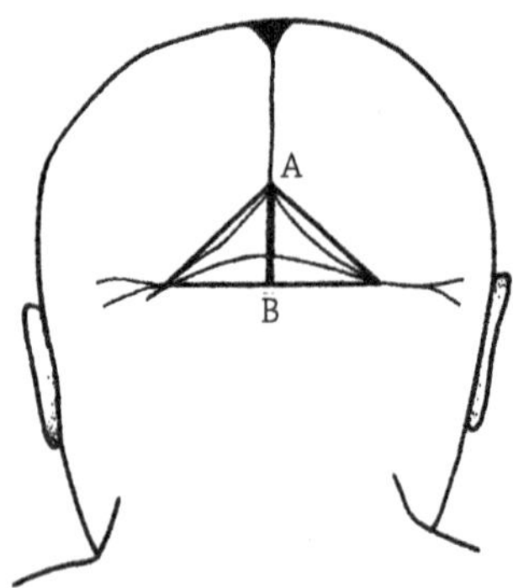

Figure 7.28. Measuring posterior fontanelle size.

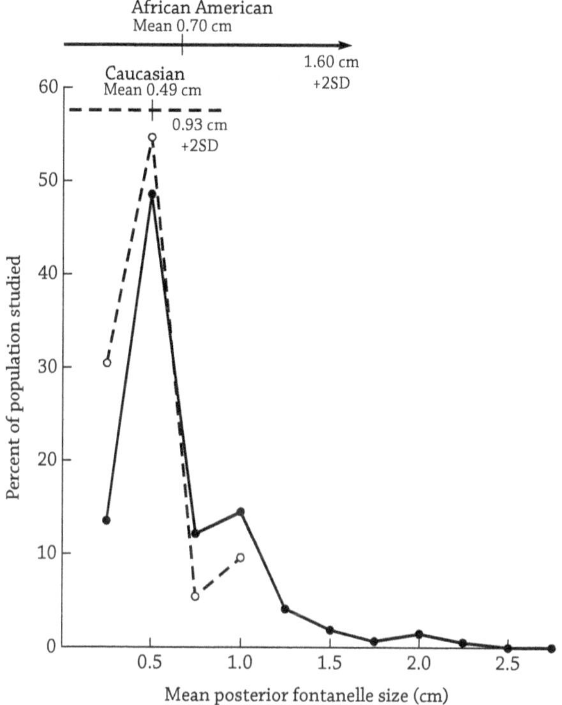

Figure 7.29. Comparison of posterior fontanelle size in African American and Caucasian American populations, both sexes, at birth. From Faix (1982), by permission.

SCALP AND FACIAL HAIR PATTERNING

Hair directional slope is secondary to the plane of stretch exerted on the skin by the growth of underlying tissues during the period of down-growth of the hair follicles at around 10–12 weeks gestation. The posterior parietal hair whorl is interpreted as the focal point from which the growth stretch is exerted by the dome-like outgrowth of the brain during the time of hair follicle development. Malformations that precede hair follicle development, such as encephalocele, produce anomalies in scalp patterning. Eighty-five percent of patients with primary microcephaly have altered scalp hair patterning, indicating an early onset of abnormal brain development. Aberrant scalp patterning is also found frequently in association with established syndromes such as Down syndrome. Thus, aberrant scalp hair patterning may be utilized as one indicator of altered size and/or shape of the brain prior to 12 weeks gestation. Early anomalies in development of the eye and of the face can secondarily affect hair patterning over the eyebrow and frontal area, as can gross anomalies in development of the ear, which will secondarily affect hair patterning, especially in the preauricular area. Full details of hair patterning anomalies plus quantitative differences in hair are found in Chapters 11 and 12.

EYES

Introduction

The critical period of human eye formation is during developmental stages 10–20 (22–50 days). Because of the complexity of eye development, many congenital abnormalities can occur.

Examination of the eye should include a review of periorbital structures (Hall et al., 2009). Are the supraorbital brows prominent, pugilistic, heavy, or hypoplastic? Is there periorbital edema? Is there excessive pigmentation? Are the eyes deeply set or prominent? Are there deep creases under the eyes?

The spacing of the eyes is discussed in greater detail in the measurement section. Although one might assume that the clinical impression concerning whether the eyes are too near or too far apart might be consistent with the actual measurement, experience does not bear this out. The clinician may be misled by the width of the face, glabella shape, the presence of epicanthal folds and the width and shape of the nasal bridge. In addition, the spacing of the eyes must be compared to the head circumference for valid interpretation. True ocular hypertelorism, or wide spacing of the eyes, occurs with an increased interpupillary distance (IPD) or increased bony interorbital distance. With lateral displacement of the inner canthi and lacrimal punctae (primary telecanthus), there may be a false impression of widely spaced eyes. An approximate clinical impression of whether there is lateral displacement of the lacrimal puncta can be obtained by seating the individual directly in front of the observer and drawing an imaginary vertical line through the inferior lacrimal point. If this line cuts the iris, there is lateral displacement of the inner canthus. The differences between telecanthus and pure hypertelorism are documented in Figure 7.30. Soft tissue measurements of eye spacing are less precise than bony measurements obtained from a standard radiograph. The bony interorbital distance is discussed, in detail, in the measurement section.

The eyelids develop from two ectodermal folds containing cores of mesenchyme. The eyelids meet and adhere by about the 10th week and remain adherent until about the 26th week of pregnancy. A defect of the eyelid, termed palpebral or eyelid coloboma, is characterized by a notch in the upper or lower eyelid.

Evaluation of the eyelid includes an assessment of the length of the palpebral fissure. There may be a discrepancy in the length of the palpebral fissure between the two eyes, although this is generally

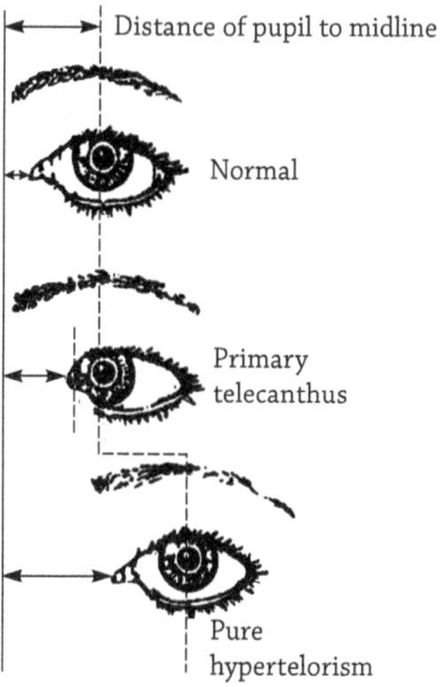

Figure 7.30. Comparison of telecanthus and ocular hypertelorism. From Pashayen (1973), by permission.

minor. Palpebral fissure length may be reduced in Dubowitz syndrome and fetal alcohol spectrum disorder. The width of the palpebral fissure, that is, the degree of opening of the eye, may also vary and may be asymmetric. Frank ptosis, or drooping of the eyelid, is generally caused by weakness of levator palpebrae superioris. Ptosis is frequently found in association with multiple congenital anomaly syndromes such as Smith–Lemli–Opitz syndrome, Noonan syndrome, and Freeman–Sheldon syndrome. Obliquity of the palpebral fissures is discussed in detail in the measurement section. One refers to upward-slanting or upslanting palpebral fissures if the lateral margin is superior to the medial margin, and downward-slanting or downslanting palpebral fissures if the lateral margin is inferior to the medial margin.

An epicanthal or epicanthic fold is a lateral extension of the skin of the nasal bridge down over the inner canthus, covering the inner angle of the palpebral fissure. The upper end of the fold can begin at the eyebrow, at the skin of the upper lid, or at the tarsal fold (Fig. 7.31). Approximately 30% of individuals of Caucasian ethnicity under six months of age have epicanthal folds in association with normal depression of the nasal root. Only 3% of individuals of Caucasian ethnicity between 12 and 25 years of age have epicanthal folds because the root of the nose is less depressed in adulthood and the nasal bridge becomes more prominent. Epicanthal folds are more frequent in people of Asian ancestry. Epicanthus inversus refers to an epicanthal fold originating from the lower lid.

The thickness and length of the eyelashes should be evaluated. Eyelashes are ingrown in entropion and everted in ectropion. Extremely long eyelashes requiring trimming occur in Costello syndrome due to *HRAS* p.Gly13Cys and may be referred to as dolichocilia. Distichiasis is the term for double rows of eyelashes—one row in the normal position, the other behind it and located at the site of the openings of the meibomian glands. These glands are hypoplastic or absent in such cases. All four lids can be affected.

The configuration of the eyebrows is useful in syndrome diagnosis. Evaluation should include position, shape, texture of hair, and the distribution of the eyebrows. A medial flare is seen in association

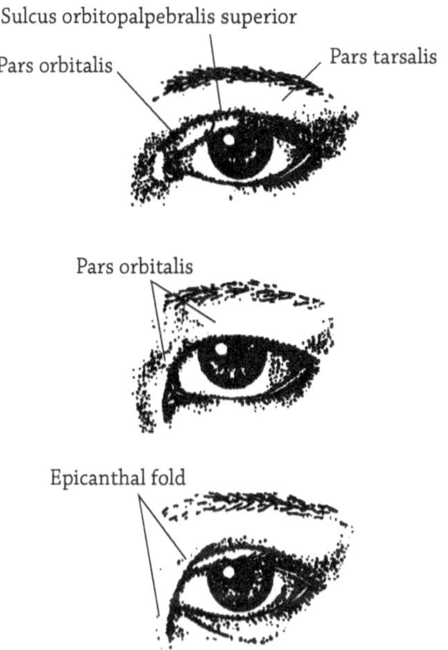

Figure 7.31. Epicanthal variations. From Goodman and Gorlin (1977), by permission.

with Williams syndrome. A diamond shape with an arch laterally is seen in Noonan syndrome. Synophrys is the term used for eyebrows which grow or fuse together over the nasal root, as seen in Cornelia de Lange syndrome. Fullness of the lateral aspect of the brow can be seen in Noonan syndrome, Williams syndrome, and hypothyroidism.

Many anomalies of iris color and structure are found. Unilateral or patchy altered pigmentation or hypopigmentation can occur, producing heterochromia iridis. A prominent pattern of the iris stroma radiating out from the pupil is known as a stellate iris. Brushfield spots are elevated white, or light yellow, iris nodules. They are best seen in blue irides, but are as frequent in brown irides. They are commonly present in the midzone of the iris in a ring, associated with peripheral iris hypoplasia in Down syndrome. They can be seen more peripherally in normal individuals. Lisch nodules are small, gray-tan hamartomata of the iris. Careful slit-lamp examination is usually required to see them. Multiple Lisch nodules are seen in neurofibromatosis type 1. Colobomas, or a defect in the closure of the optic fissure, can also occur in the iris, giving the pupil a keyhole appearance. The gap or notch may be limited to the iris or may extend deeper and involve the ciliary body and retina.

Variation in size and shape of the pupil should be described. Pupil size varies under ordinary conditions in proportion to the amount of light that reaches the inner eye. Pupillary asymmetry, or anisocoria, may be congenital or may result from defects of the eye or in the neural pathways. Aniridia, congenital absence of the iris, may be an isolated finding or part of a syndrome (e.g., Wilms tumor–aniridia–genitourinary malformation, intellectual disability [WAGR] syndrome).

The cornea may vary in size and shape. Microcornea consists of a reduction in size of the cornea to a diameter of 10 mm or less, in association with growth failure of the anterior part of the eye and incomplete development of the iridocorneal angle. Approximately 20% of patients with microcornea will develop glaucoma in later life. Megalocornea is a corneal diameter of 13–18 mm and may occur as an isolated malformation. If the anomaly is limited to the anterior portion of the globe, visual acuity can be normal. Megalocornea is frequently associated with subluxation of the lenses, cataracts, enlargement of the ciliary ring, and noticeable iridodonesis. Iridodonesis is a shimmering of the iris when the eye is moved rapidly from side to side in the presence of a dislocated or absent lens. Keratoconus is an obtuse conical shape to the cornea, with the vertex in or near the corneal center. It produces abnormal refraction and is seen with an increased frequency in Down syndrome. It may also be associated with retinitis pigmentosa and Alport syndrome. The cornea can appear cloudy in various storage disorders, particularly the mucopolysaccharidoses. Corneal clouding is best appreciated from the side of the eye or through a slit-lamp. Kayser–Fleischer rings are areas of greenish-yellow pigmentation in Descemet's membrane at the corneal periphery as seen in Wilson's disease.

Abnormalities of the conjunctiva include telangiectasia, which are dilatations of capillary vessels and minute arteries forming a variety of angiomas, and pterygia, which are patches of thickened conjunctiva, usually fan shaped, with the apex toward the pupil.

The sclera is generally white. It may be blue-gray in the neonate and in disorders such as osteogenesis imperfecta.

Inner Canthal Distance

Definition The distance between the inner canthi of the two eyes.

Landmarks Measure from the innermost corner of one eye to the innermost corner of the other eye, in a straight line avoiding the curvature of the nose (Fig. 7.32).

Instruments A graduated transparent ruler is most accurate; however, a tape measure or blunt calipers can be used.

Position The head should be held erect (in the resting position) with the eyes facing forward.

Remarks Charts of inner canthal distance are provided in Figures 7.33 and 7.34. Without accurate measurement, the distance between the eyes may appear greater or less than the mean, depending upon the width of the face, the form of the glabella area, the presence of epicanthal folds, and the width and shape of the nasal bridge. As with all other measurements, the inner canthal distance should be related to the head circumference for interpretation.

Pitfalls In the presence of epicanthal folds, inner canthal distances are not easily ascertained.

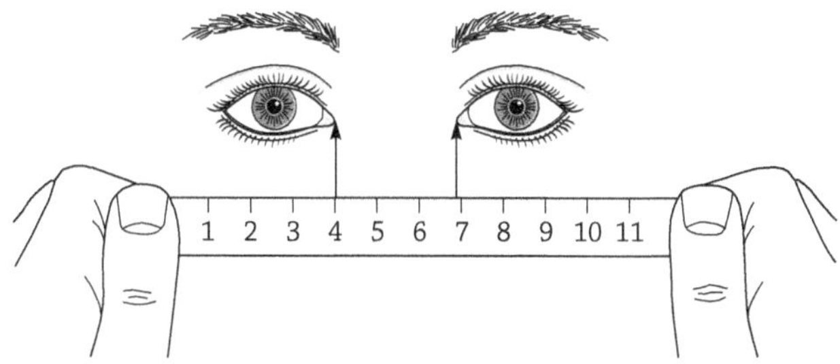

Figure 7.32. Measuring inner canthal distance.

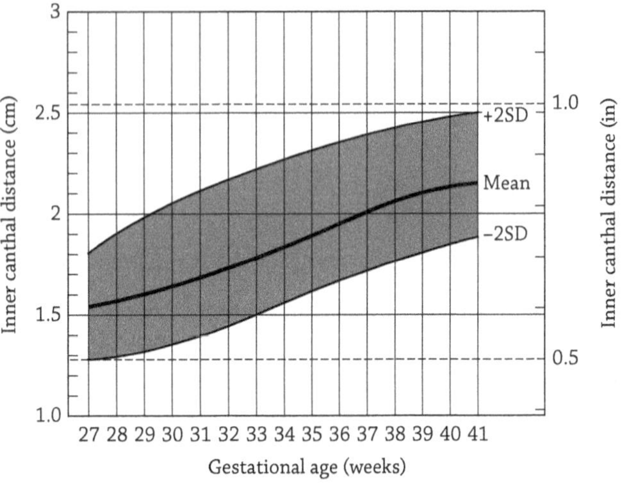

Figure 7.33. Inner canthal distance, both sexes, at birth. From Merlob et al. (1984), by permission.

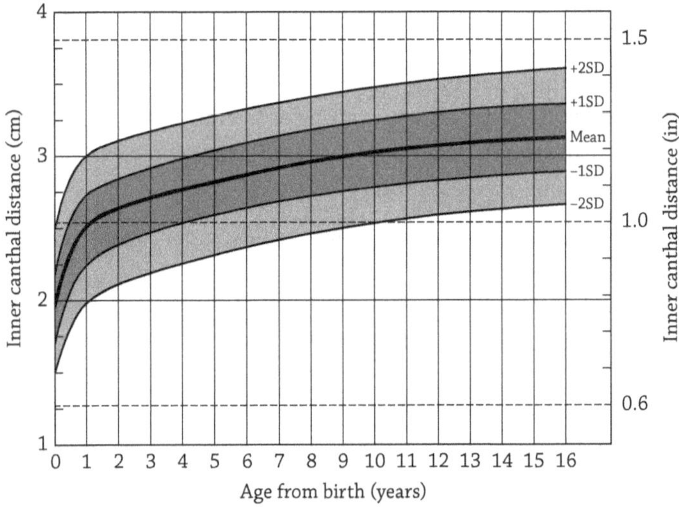

Figure 7.34. Inner canthal distance, both sexes, birth to 16 years. From Laestadius et al. (1969) and Feingold and Bossert (1974), by permission.

Outer Canthal Distance

Definition The distance between the outer canthi of the two eyes.

Landmarks Measure from the most lateral corner of one eye to the most lateral corner of the other eye, in a straight line avoiding the curvature of the face (Fig. 7.35).

Instruments A graduated transparent ruler is most accurate; however, a tape measure or blunt calipers can be used.

Position The head should be held erect (in the resting position) with the eyes open and facing forward.

Remarks As with any other measurement, the outer canthal distance should be compared to the overall head circumference for interpretation.

Pitfalls If the eyes are not fully open, or in the presence of ptosis, definition of the outer canthus may be difficult.

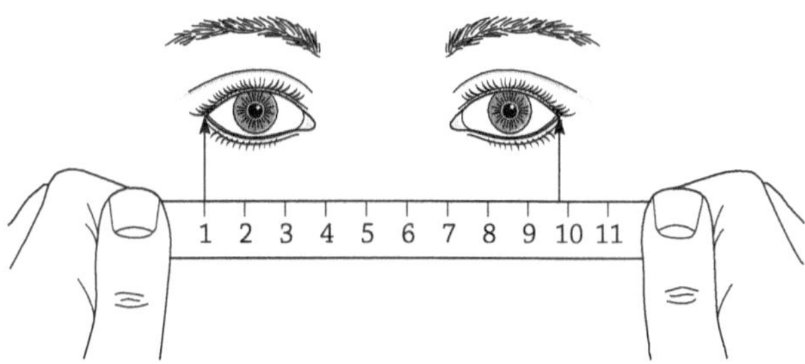

Figure 7.35. Measuring outer canthal distance.

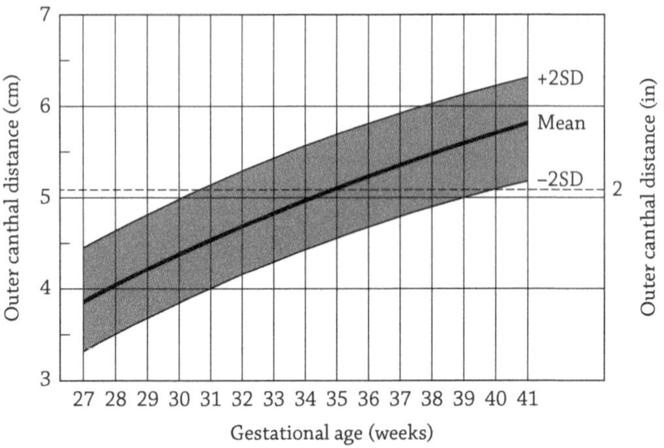

Figure 7.36. Outer canthal distance, both sexes, at birth. From Merlob et al. (1984), by permission.

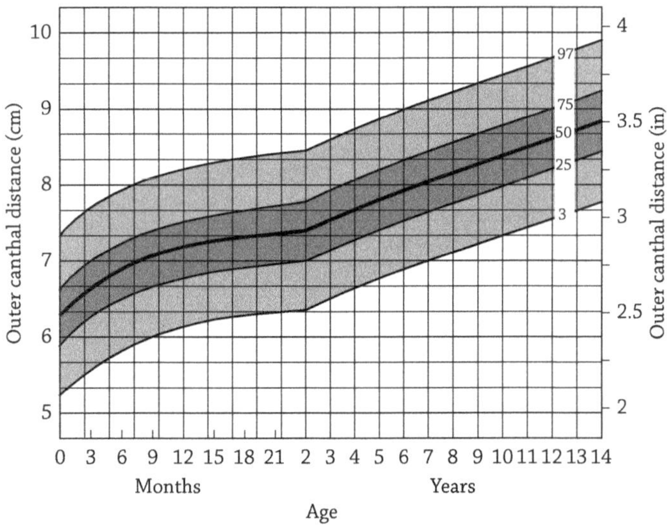

Figure 7.37. Outer canthal distance, both sexes, birth to 16 years. From Feingold and Bossert (1974), by permission.

Interpupillary Distance

Definition The distance between the centers of the pupils of the two eyes.

Landmarks Measure between the centers of both pupils (Fig. 7.38).

Instruments A graduated transparent ruler is most accurate. A tape measure can be used stretched in a straight line to avoid curvature of the face.

Position The head should be held erect (in the resting position) with the eyes facing straight forward. This is easiest when the patient is reclining, the eye fissures are horizontal, and the eyes are gazing straight upward. A young child may need to be restrained for accurate measurement.

Alternative The child or infant may lie supine.

Remarks Charts of interpupillary distance are provided in Figures 7.39 and 7.40. Since the measurement of interpupillary distance requires the eyes to be fixed, this is not an easy task in the infant or young child. Feingold and Bossert, by means of multiple linear regression techniques, have suggested the use of the following formula: $IP = 0.17 + 0.59IC + 0.41OC$, where IP is the interpupillary distance, IC is the inner canthal distance, and OC is the outer canthal distance (Fig. 7.41). The reason for distinguishing increased interpupillary distance from increased inner canthal distance is to distinguish between true hypertelorism and telecanthus or lateral displacement of the lacrimal punctae. A rough clinical impression of whether there is lateral displacement of the lacrimal puncta can be obtained by seating the individual directly in front of the examiner and drawing an imaginary vertical line through the inferior lacrimal point. If this line cuts the iris, then there is lateral displacement of the inner canthus. If the inner canthal distance divided by the interpupillary distance is greater than 0.6, then lateral displacement of the inner canthus, also known as dystopia canthorum, is present.

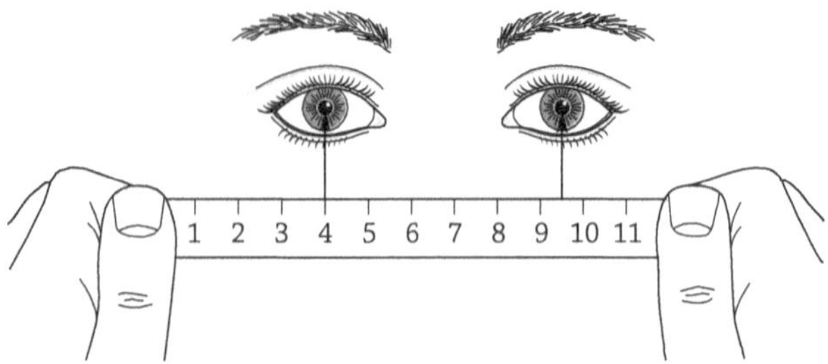

Figure 7.38. Measuring interpupillary distance.

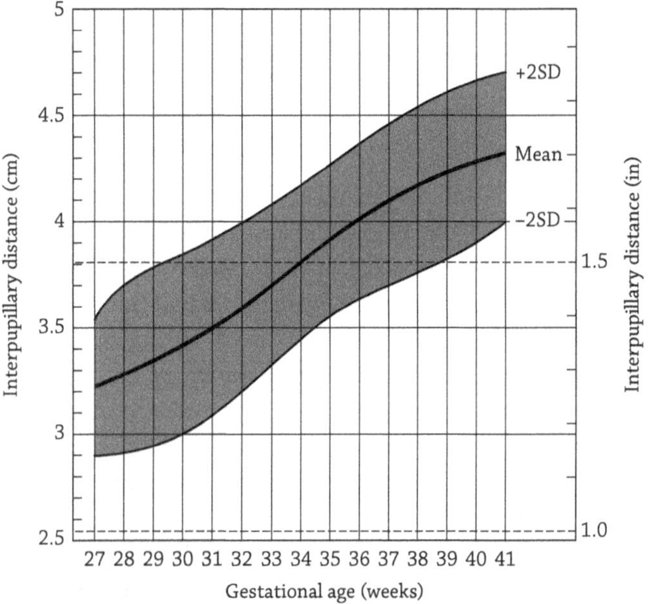

Figure 7.39. Interpupillary distance, both sexes, at birth. From Merlob et al. (1984), by permission.

Pitfalls Unless the individual can keep the eyes perfectly still, it is impossible to measure interpupillary distance. The formula outlined earlier can be used instead.

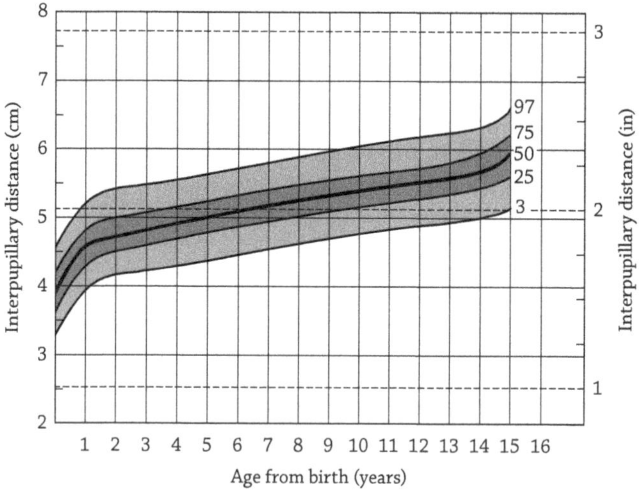

Figure 7.40. Interpupillary distance, birth to 16 years. From Feingold and Bossert (1974), by permission.

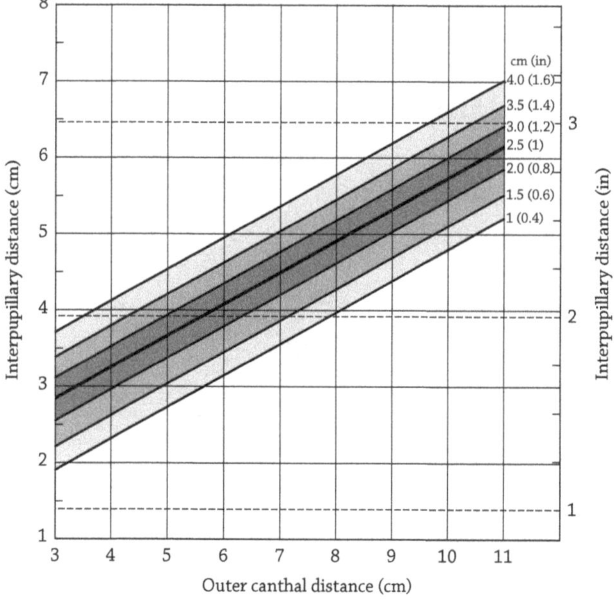

Figure 7.41. Interpupillary distance calculated from inner and outer canthi. From Feingold and Bossert (1974), by permission.

Palpebral Fissure Length

Definition Distance between the inner and outer canthus of one eye.

Landmarks Measure from the inner to the outer canthus of the right eye. Repeat on the left eye (Fig. 7.42).

Instruments A graduated transparent ruler or blunt calipers is most accurate; however, a tape measure can be used.

Position The head should be held erect (in the resting position) with the eyes open and facing forward.

Alternative The infant or young child can lie supine.

Remarks Charts of palpebral fissure length from birth to age 16 years are presented in Figures 7.43 and 7.44. A difference in the length of the two palpebral fissures occurs in about 30% of individuals, but it is rarely in excess of 1 mm. As a rough guide, the palpebral fissure length is approximately equivalent to the inner canthal distance. Blepharophimosis describes a decrease in the width of the palpebral fissures without fusion of the eyelids. Ethnic variation occurs in palpebral fissure length (Fig. 7.45).

Pitfalls In the presence of epicanthal folds, the palpebral fissure length is not easily ascertained.

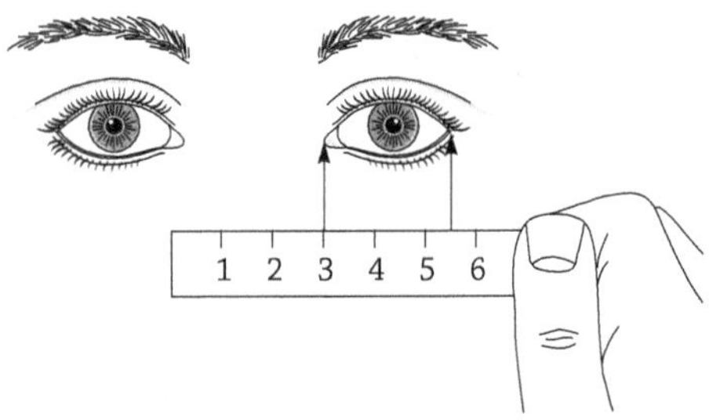

Figure 7.42. Measuring palpebral fissure length.

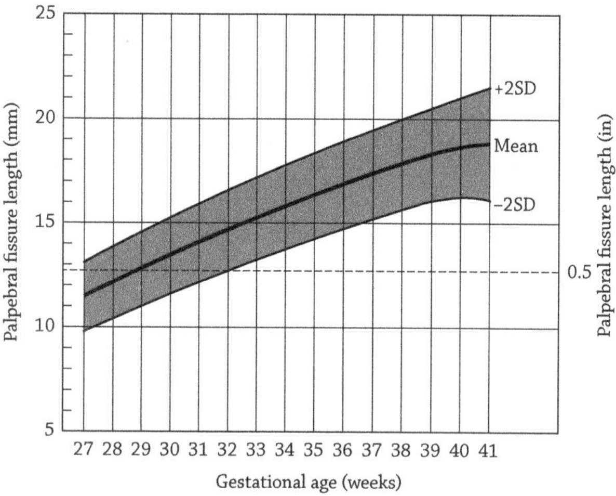

Figure 7.43. Palpebral fissure length, both sexes, at birth. From Mehes (1974) and Merlob et al. (1984), by permission.

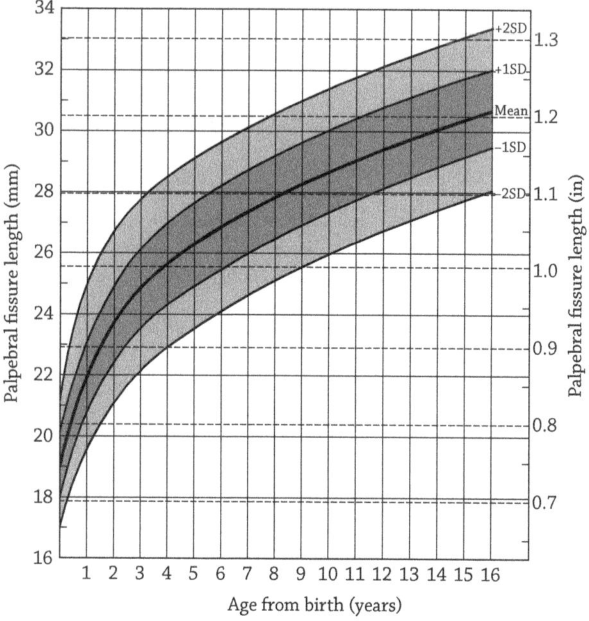

Figure 7.44. Palpebral fissure length, both sexes, birth to 16 years. From Farkas (1981), Chouke (1929), Laestadius et al. (1969), and Thomas et al. (1987), by permission.

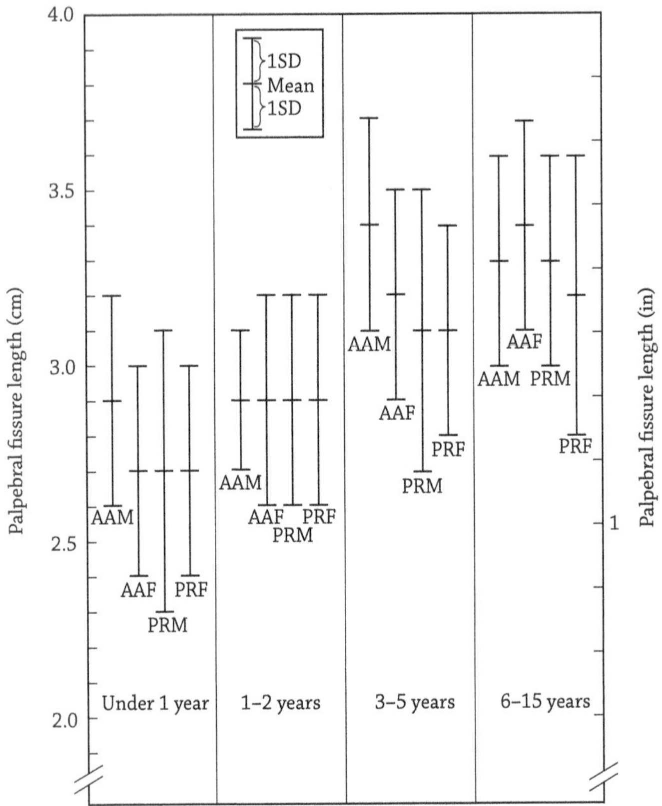

Figure 7.45. Palpebral fissure length, ethnic differences in African American and Puerto Rican children (AAF, African American female; AAM, African American male; PRM, Puerto Rican male; PRF, Puerto Rican female). From Iosub et al. (1985), by permission.

Obliquity (Inclination or Slant) of the Palpebral Fissure

Definition Angle of slant of the palpebral fissure from the horizontal (Fig. 7.46).

Landmarks A comparison between two lines is necessary. One line connects the inner canthus and outer canthus of the eye. The second line connects the two inner canthi and is projected laterally. The slant of the palpebral fissure is the angle between the two lines (Fig. 7.46).

Instruments A commercial angle meter, protractor, or goniometer is a useful instrument for this measurement. One edge is placed along the line joining the inner canthi; the other straight side follows the line between the commissures of each eye.

Position The standard orientation of the head is the Frankfort horizontal (FH), which in practice is achieved if the head is held with the facial midline vertical, the neck neither flexed nor extended, and the patient looking straight ahead at the observer.

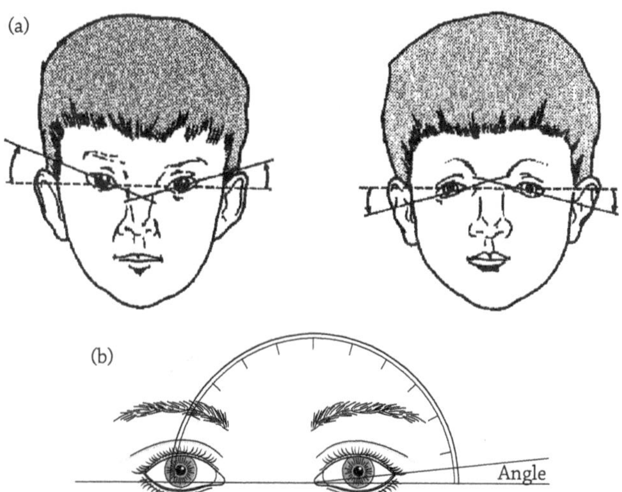

Figure 7.46. The obliquity of the (a) palpebral fissure can be measured with (b) a transparent protractor.

Alternative A rough angle meter or protractor can easily be made on firm transparent material such as X-ray film. A horizontal line on this device is aligned with the FH in the patient and the angle of obliquity of the palpebral fissure is read according to the position of the outer canthus. A rough estimate of this horizontal can be made by joining a line between the two inner canthi and extending this laterally; however, the FH is more accurate.

Remarks This is a particularly difficult measurement unless the patient can be kept perfectly still. Palpebral fissure inclinations for ages 6–18 years are shown in Figure 7.47.

Pitfalls The eyes should be open and relaxed, since the outer canthus is lower than the inner canthus when the eye is closed. The presence of epicanthal folds makes it difficult to locate the inner canthi. The presence of ectropion or lateral supraorbital fullness may create a false illusion of down-slanting palpebral fissures.

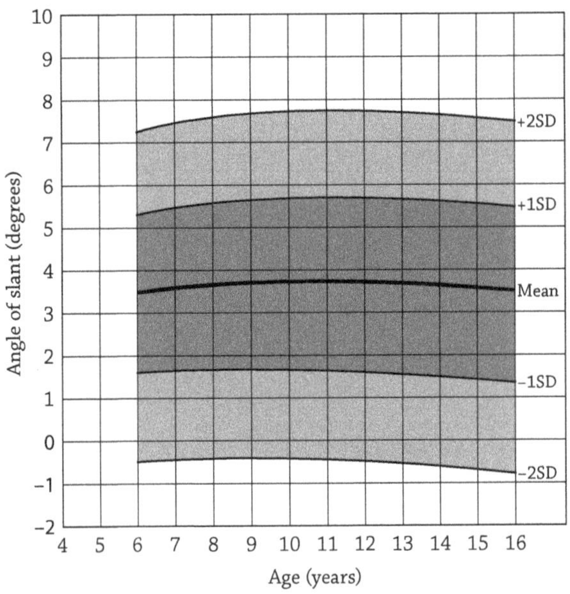

Figure 7.47. Palpebral fissure inclination, both sexes, 6 to 18 years. From Farkas (1981), by permission.

Orbital Protrusion

Definition Degree of protrusion of the eye (exophthalmos).

Landmarks The calibrated end of a Luedde exophthalmometer is held firmly against the lateral margin of the orbit. The long axis of the instrument is held parallel to the long axis of the eyeball. The examiner sights the anterior margin of the cornea through the calibrated scale and reads the distance in millimeters (Fig. 7.48).

Instruments A Luedde exophthalmometer; for details, see Gerber et al. (1972). A transparent calibrated ruler can be substituted.

Position Frankfort horizontal, with the facial profile in the vertical. The patient should be viewed from the side.

Remarks A Luedde ruler is easy to use and not frightening to children. Orbital protrusion will vary during puberty. Normal protrusion is between 13 and 22 mm for children and adults.

Pitfalls In the presence of ptosis, it may be difficult to estimate the anterior margin of the cornea.

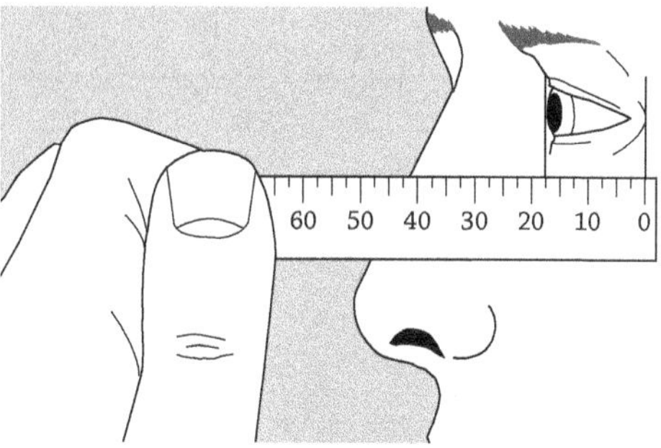

Figure 7.48. Measuring orbital protrusion.

Corneal Dimensions: Transverse Diameter

Definition Transverse diameter of the cornea.

Landmarks Measure between the medial and lateral borders of the right iris, which, for practical purposes, represent the edges of the cornea. Repeat measurements on the left eye (Fig. 7.49a).

Instruments Spreading calipers, a transparent ruler, or tape measure may be used.

Position The standard orientation of the head is the Frankfort horizontal.

Remarks The cornea is relatively large at birth and almost attains its adult size during the first and second years. Practically all of its postnatal growth occurs in the second 6 months of life, although some increase in size may be evident up to the end of the second year. Although the eyeball as a whole increases its volume almost three times from birth to maturity, the corneal segment plays a relatively small part in this growth. The transverse diameter of the cornea increases roughly from 10 mm in the infant to a value slightly less than 12 mm in the adult. In the infant, values of less than 10 or more than 11 mm require further evaluation. Average values for the transverse diameter (external diameter of horizontal base) are found in Figure 7.49b.

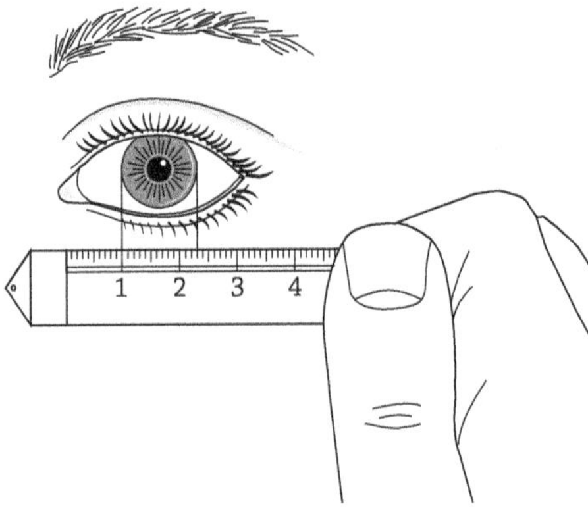

Figure 7.49(a). Measuring transverse diameter of the cornea.

Transverse diameter	Newborn (mm)	Adult (mm)
External diameter of horizontal base	10.0	11.8
External diameter of corneal arc	14.0	18.2
Internal diameter of corneal arc	11.0	16.4
Mean thickness	0.8	0.9
Oblique thickness	1.1	1.6
External height	3.0	3.4
Internal height	1.1	2.7

Figure 7.49(b). Corneal dimensions, both sexes, at birth and adult. From Duke-Elder (1963), by permission.

A more recent measurement methodology to examine corneal diameter used photographs taken from children with a paper ruler taped to their foreheads (Lagrèze and Zobor, 2007). With this technique, corneal diameter was measured to be 9.98 mm directly after birth for males and females, increasing to a plateau of 11.51 mm within the first 24 months of life (Lagrèze and Zobor, 2007).

EARS

Introduction

The ear consists of three anatomical parts—external, middle, and internal or inner ear. The external and middle parts are concerned mainly with transferring sound waves from the environment to the internal ear. The internal ear contains the vestibulocochlear organ, which is concerned with equilibrium and hearing.

The external auricle develops from six swellings called *auricular hillocks* (Fig. 7.50), which arise around the margins of the first branchial groove. The swellings are produced by proliferation of mesenchyme from the first and second branchial arches. As the auricle grows, the contribution of the first branchial arch becomes relatively reduced. The lobule is the last part of the auricle to develop. The external ears begin to develop in the upper part of the future neck

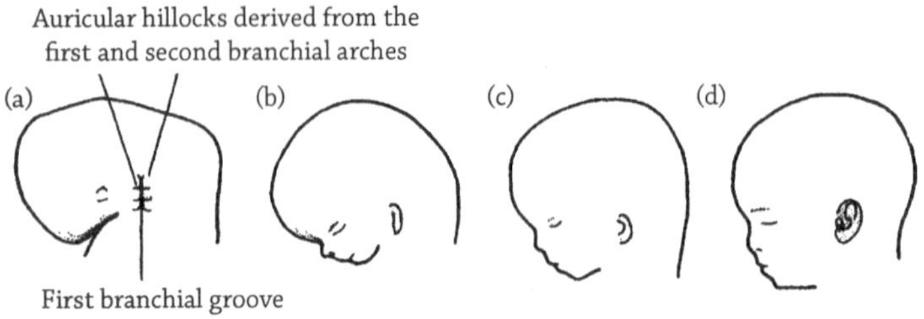

Auricular hillocks derived from the first and second branchial arches

(a) (b) (c) (d)

First branchial groove

Figure 7.50. Embryonic development of the ear.

region, but, as the mandible develops, the auricles move to the side of the head and ascend to the level of the eyes.

The human usually has three external auricular muscles and six intrinsic muscles. A protruding or cupped auricle is usually the consequence of a defect in the posterior auricular muscle. A "lop ear" refers to a defect of the superior auricular muscle. Abnormalities of the intrinsic ear muscles may lead to abnormal ear creases and anatomy—for example, a prominent antihelix, or the crumpled ear of Beal syndrome. Absence of the superior crus is correlated with an increased risk for hearing impairment.

Ears are almost as distinctive as fingerprints, and much has been written about their variation in form, size, and position (Hunter et al., 2009). The main anatomical landmarks are noted in Figure 7.51.

Evaluation of the ears should include an assessment of

1. both preauricular regions looking for skin appendages, fistulae, and pits;
2. the tragus, looking at the size in proportion to the size of the ear;
3. the external auditory meatus, whether normal, narrow, or atretic;
4. the shape of each ear and its symmetry; whether it has a free or attached ear lobe;
5. the anterior and posterior surface of each ear or helix;
6. the position and angulation of the ear;
7. the relative positions of the tragi, to see whether they are on the same level.

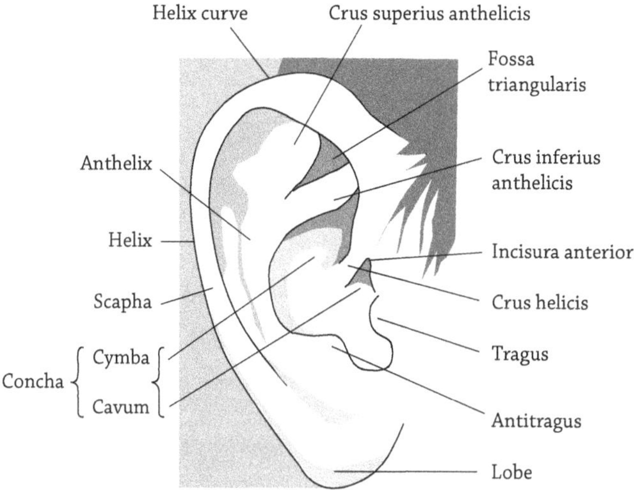

Figure 7.51. Landmarks of the external ear.

The right auricle is usually slightly larger than the left in both height and width. Discrepant growth can also occur secondary to pressure phenomena. In severe torticollis, compression of one ear against the ipsilateral shoulder will cause increased growth of the ear. The same situation can occur in utero. The frequency of missing or attached ear lobes varies with ethnicity, but in individuals with Caucasian ethnicity, it averages about 20%–25%. Complete absence of the auricle, or anotia, is extremely rare. In microtia, vestiges of the external ear are present, and a graded classification is applied. Type I or first-degree microtia (Fig. 7.52a) consists of a small external ear retaining the typical overall structure. Type II or second-degree microtia (Fig. 7.52b) describes a more severe anomaly with a longitudinal cartilaginous mass. In type III or third-degree microtia (Fig. 7.52c) the rudimentary cartilaginous or soft tissue mass does not resemble a pinna. In type IV, or anotia (Fig. 7.52d), no soft tissue mass is present. In cryptotia, there is abnormal adherence of the upper part of the auricle to the head, as the skin of the postauricular region directly joins the skin of the upper portion of the auricle. Cryptotia, defined as an invagination of the superior part of the auricle under a skin

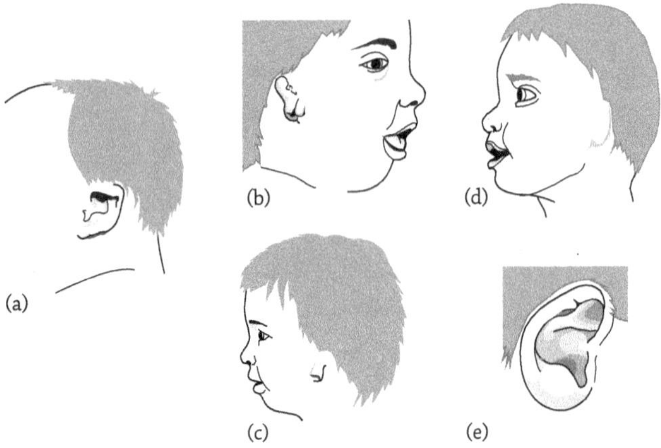

Figure 7.52. Microtia classification type I (a), II (b), III (c), and IV (d), and cryptotia (e).

fold, (Fig. 7.52e) is attributed to the persistence of fetal attachment of the auricle to the underlying skin.

Many variations in shape can be observed in the helix and antihelix. The Darwinian tubercle is a small projection arising from the descending part of the helix and is considered a normal variant. Anterior ear lobe creases are seen in Beckwith–Wiedemann syndrome. In this condition, there may also be scored grooves or notches on the posterior aspect of the superior helix or lobe.

Variations in ear position and angulation are discussed in detail in the measurement section. Subjective assessment of ear position and angulation is extremely imprecise and is influenced by the position of the patient's head, the size of the cranial vault, and the size of the neck and mandible. There are several different methods for objective assessment of ear position and angulation, which are detailed in the next section.

Auricular appendages or tags are relatively common and result from the development of accessory auricular hillocks. They are usually anterior to the auricle and more often unilateral than bilateral. The appendages consist of skin but may also contain cartilage. They vary greatly in size and may be sessile or pedunculated. The most frequent location is the line of junction of the mandibular and hyoid arches. Less frequently, they occur in the line of junction of the mandibular and maxillary processes, on the cheek, between the auricle and the angle of the mouth. Appendages in this area are more often associated with microtia or oblique facial fissures.

Ear Length

Definition The maximum distance from the superior aspect to the inferior aspect of the external ear (pinna).

Landmarks Measure from the superior aspect of the outer rim of the helix to the most inferior border of the earlobe or pinna (Fig. 7.53).

Instruments Tape measure or transparent, calibrated ruler.

Position The head should be held erect (in the resting position) with the eyes facing forward. The head should not be tilted forward or backward. The facial profile should be vertical and the patient viewed from the side.

Alternative A young infant or child can be held prone with the head turned to one side.

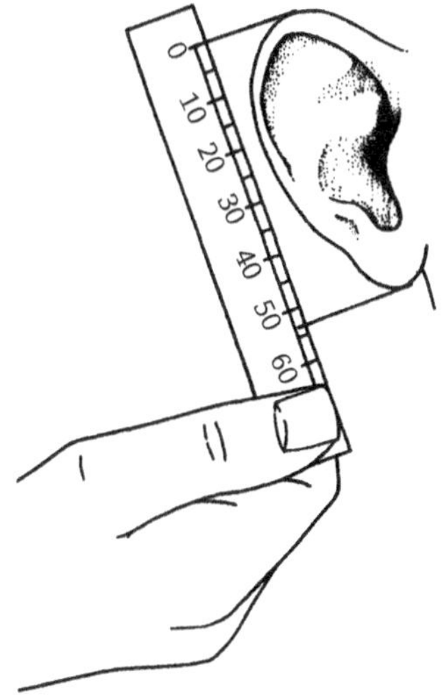

Figure 7.53. Measuring ear length.

Remarks Ear defects are important in syndrome diagnosis, particularly in the newborn infant. Small ears have been found to be a consistent clinical characteristic of Down syndrome and are the most clinically apparent malformation in Treacher Collins syndrome and hemifacial microsomia. External ear abnormalities are common in the 22q11.2 microdeletion syndrome and in CHARGE syndrome. The ear is one of the few organs that continue to grow in length during adulthood, although ear width changes little after 10 years of age. The ear is generally longer in males than in females and the sex difference increases with age. Charts of ear length from birth to 16 years of age are presented in Figures 7.54 and 7.55.

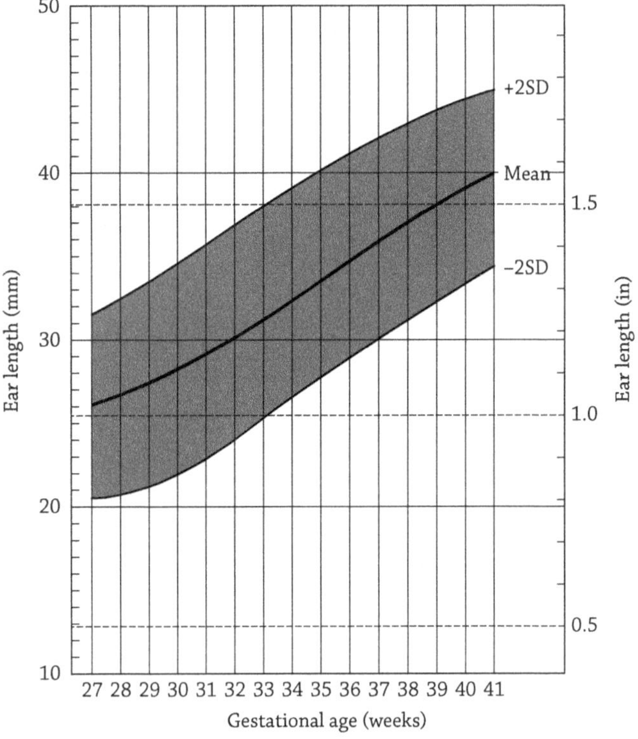

Figure 7.54. Ear length, both sexes, at birth. From Merlob et al. (1984), by permission.

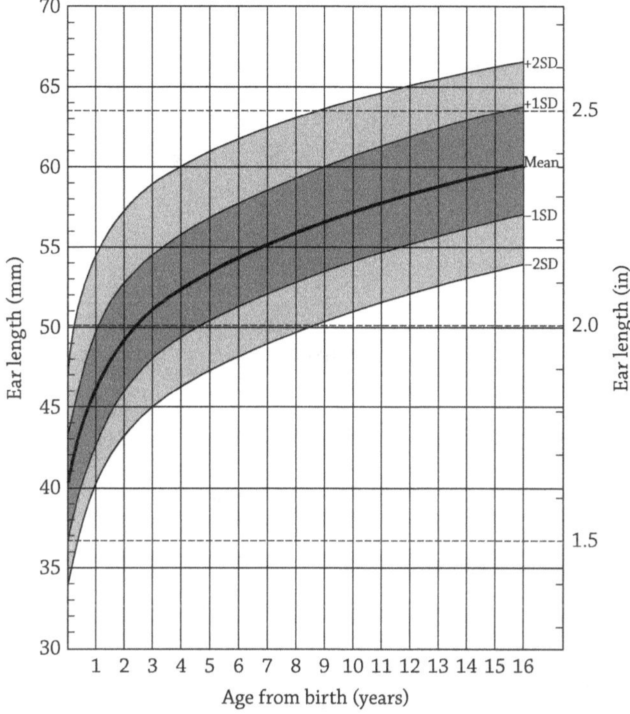

Figure 7.55. Ear length, both sexes, birth to 16 years. From Farkas (1981) and Feingold and Bossert (1974), by permission.

Pitfalls In the presence of a posteriorly angulated ear, the measurement should still be taken from the most superior portion of the helix to the inferior portion of the pinna, even though the axis of this measurement is not in the vertical plane. If the superior aspect of the helix is overfolded, do not unfold it to measure the length.

Ear Width

Definition Width of the external ear (pinna).

Landmarks Measure transversely from the anterior base of the tragus, which can be palpated, through the region of the external auditory canal to the margin of the helical rim, at the widest point (Fig. 7.56).

Instruments Tape measure, calibrated transparent ruler, or calipers may be used.

Position The head should be held erect (in the resting position) with the eyes facing forward.

Alternative The infant or young child may be lying prone with the head tilted to one side.

Remarks Normal ear width is shown in Figure 7.57. Ear width changes little after 10 years of age.

Pitfalls The observer should be careful to take this measurement in the transverse dimension; otherwise, a falsely elevated value will be obtained. With cupped or protuberant ears, the most accurate measurement is obtained with the ear pressed firmly against the head.

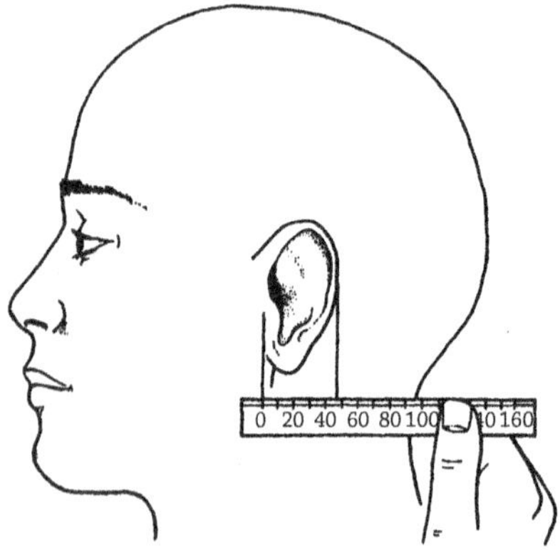

Figure 7.56. Measuring ear width.

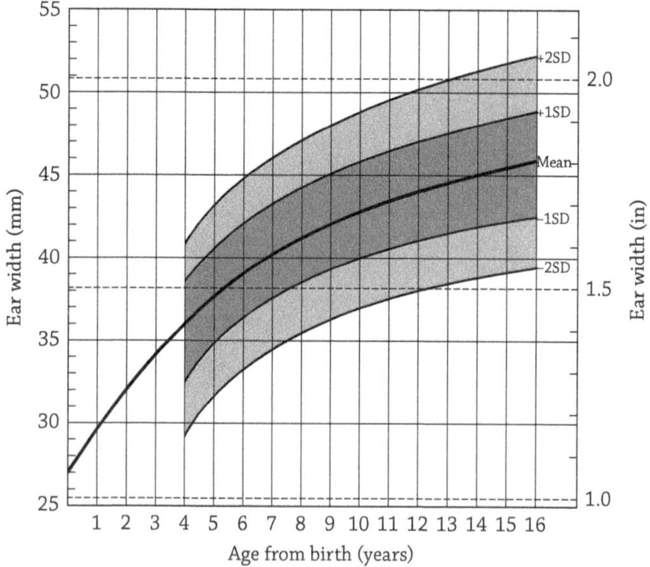

Figure 7.57. Ear width, both sexes, birth to 16 years. From Goodman and Gorlin (1977) and Farkas (1981), by permission.

Ear Protrusion

Definition Protrusion of each ear is measured as the angle subtended from the posterior aspect of the pinna to the mastoid plane of the skull. The typical range for this angle is shown in Figure 7.59.

Landmarks Measure between the posterior aspect of the pinna and the mastoid plane of the skull. The zero mark of the protractor is placed above the point of attachment of the helix in the temporal region, and its straight side is pressed against the subject's head. The extent of the protrusion is indicated on the curved side of the protractor (Fig. 7.58).

Instruments Transparent protractor.

Position The head should be held erect with eyes facing forward.

Alternative A linear measurement can be made with a tape measure, calipers, or transparent ruler if a protractor is not available. If

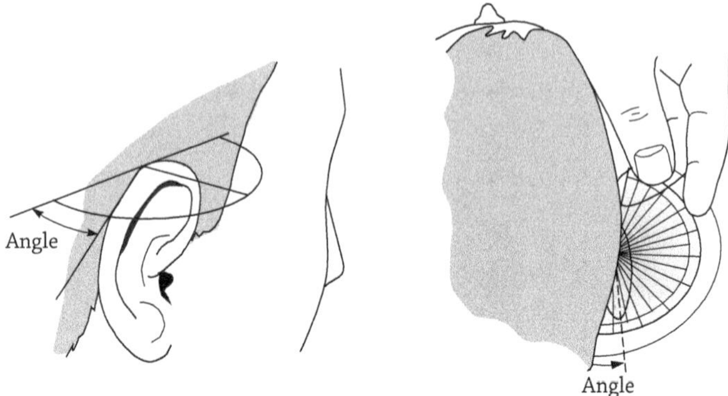

Figure 7.58. Measuring ear protrusion.

the greatest linear distance between the external ear and the temporal region of the skull is more than 2 cm, then excessive protrusion of the ear is considered to be present.

Remarks Ear protrusion values are shown in Figure 7.59. Ear protrusion can indicate a weakness of the posterior auricular muscles, as can be found in myopathies. By contrast, a "lop ear" denotes weakness of the superior auricular muscles, and a "cup ear" generally reflects weakness of all three external auricular muscles.

Pitfalls Several measurements should be taken in order to ascertain the maximum angle or maximum distance between the ear and the mastoid area.

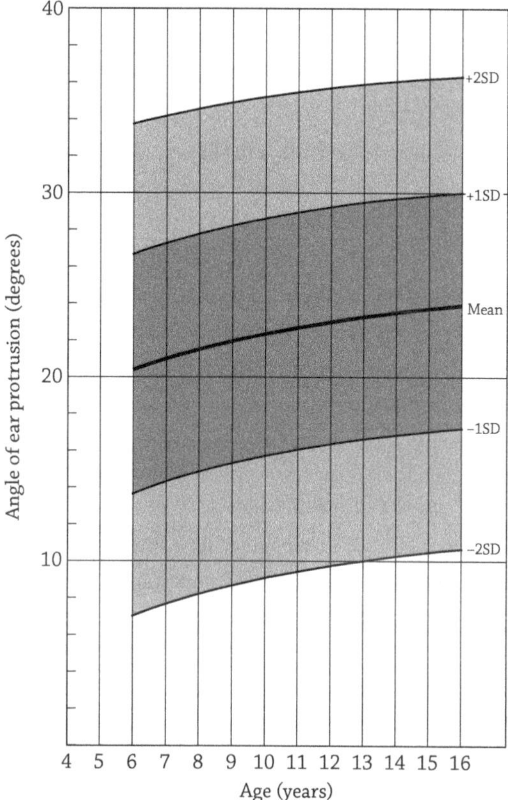

Figure 7.59. Ear protrusion angle, both sexes, 6 to 16 years. From Farkas (1981), by permission.

Ear Position

Definition Location of the superior attachment of the pinna. Note: the size and angulation of the external ear are not relevant.

Landmarks Four methods to determine the position of attachment of the ear are outlined.

1. Draw an imaginary line between the outer canthus of the eye and the most prominent part of the occiput. The superior attachment of the pinna should be on or above this line (Fig. 7.60a).
2. Draw an imaginary line through the inner and outer canthi and extend that line posteriorly. The superior attachment of the pinna should lie on or above that line (Fig. 7.60b).
3. Draw an imaginary line between both inner canthi and extend that line posteriorly. The superior attachment of the pinna should lie on or above that line (Fig. 7.60c).
4. Anthropologists determine the position of the ear according to a proposal by Leiber. The highest point on the upper margin of the cutaneous (external) auditory meatus (porion) is the landmark used to determine position, rather than the superior attachment of the pinna. A profile line that touches the glabella and the most protruding point of the upper lip is imagined. A straight line is drawn from the porion to meet this profile line at 90 degrees (Fig. 7.60d). The area of the face between the free margin of the lower eyelid and the upper edge of the nasal ala must be crossed by the line drawn from the ear canal if it is to be considered at normal level. In a high-set ear, this line meets the profile line above the free margin of the lower eyelid, and in a low-set ear, this line meets the profile line below the upper edge of the nasal ala.

Instruments A tape measure, flexible transparent ruler, or graduated piece of X-ray film can be used to define the horizontal plane for the first three methods outlined earlier. For Leiber's method, a special instrument that can be held along the facial profile line with

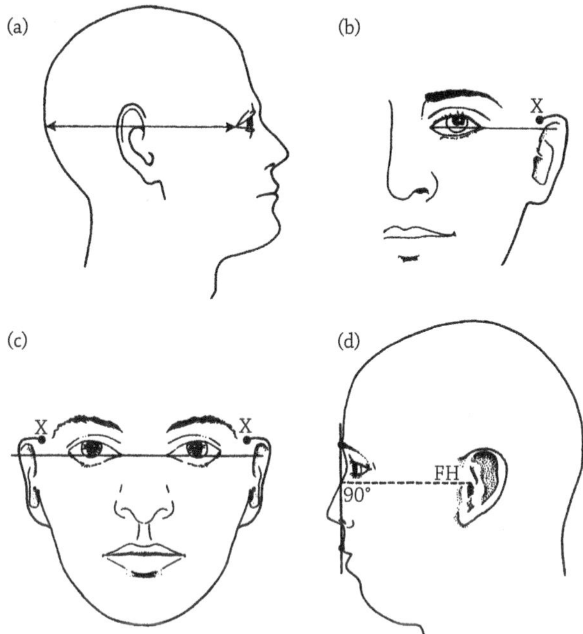

Figure 7.60(a–d). Methods of measuring ear position.

a perpendicular arm that can be moved up and down until it touches the porion can be used.

Position The head should be held erect with eyes facing forward.

Remarks The landmarks used to determine ear position are among the most controversial in clinical dysmorphology. None of them is perfect, and the reader is advised to become acquainted with one method that is comfortable and to use this method constantly. Although we prefer to use the superior attachment of the pinna as a landmark, other clinical dysmorphologists and anthropologists may assess ear position based on the level of the porion. Photographs are useful to assess ear position only if all landmarks are shown.

Pitfalls Subjective impression of ear placement seems to be influenced by the position of the person's head relative to that of the observer. In the frontal view, the ears are subject to parallax. If the neck is extended, they appear low. If it is flexed, they seem high. In the lateral view, ear position seems to be judged in relation to the vertex above, and the chin and level of the tip of the shoulder below. A high ratio between these distances gives the impression of low-set ears. This may explain why the ears of a small infant appear to be set lower than those of an older child. The infant's neck and mandible are relatively small compared to the cranium. The inclination of the auricle also affects the observer's impression of ear level. The ears look lower set when the auricles are tilted posteriorly. For this reason, ear length and position should be validated by quantitative criteria such as those outlined previously.

Ear Angulation

Definition Angulation of the median longitudinal axis of the external auricle (pinna).

Landmarks Inclination of the medial longitudinal axis of the ear from the vertical is measured by placing the long side of an angle meter along the line connecting the two most remote points of the medial axis of the ear (see section on measurement of ear length). The vertical axis is then established in one of two ways.

1. The most accurate measurement of the vertical is a line perpendicular to the Frankfort horizontal plane (FH), which connects the highest point on the upper margin of the cutaneous auditory meatus (porion) and the lowest point on the bony lower margin of each orbit (orbitale). The angle between the median longitudinal axis of the ear and the Frankfort horizontal can be measured directly; however, this value can be estimated from the angle between the vertical axis and the median longitudinal axis of the ear (Fig. 7.61a).
2. The vertical axis can be estimated by imagining a line perpendicular to a line connecting the outer canthus of the eye and

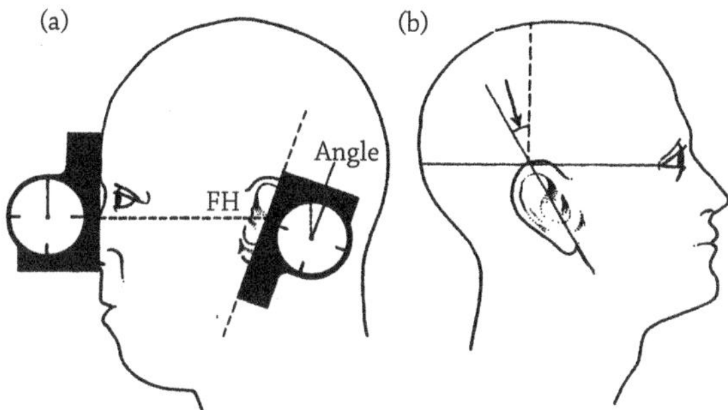

Figure 7.61. Methods of measuring ear angulation.

the most prominent point of the occiput. Once again angulation of the ear is that angle subtended between the median longitudinal axis of the ear and the vertical axis (Fig. 7.61b).

Instruments A special protractor with pointer is the ideal instrument. However, a tape measure or transparent flexible ruler can be used to define landmarks, utilizing a protractor to measure the angle of angulation. Alternatively, graduated X-ray film can be used.

Position Frankfort horizontal, with the facial profile in the vertical.

Remarks As in the assessment of ear position, there is considerable controversy about the method of choice for defining ear angulation. Both of the aforementioned methods are practical. We recommend that the reader choose one method and become familiar with it.

Normal angulation is between 17 and 22 degrees (range: 10–30 degrees) (Fig. 7.62).

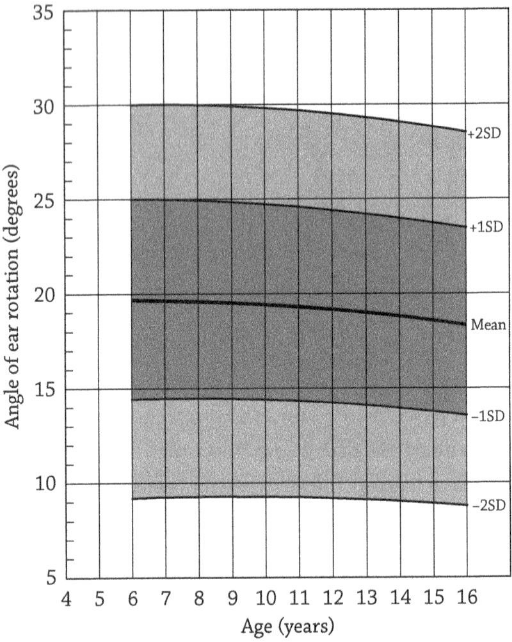

Figure 7.62. Ear angulation, both sexes, 6 to 16 years. From Farkas (1981), by permission.

NOSE

Introduction

The nose is remarkable in its variability, in profile, frontal plane, and from the undersurface. Details and definitions of the soft tissue and bony landmarks are available in the references at the end of this chapter or in Hennekam et al. (2009), and they are illustrated in Figure 7.63a. A qualitative assessment of the nose should include the following:

1. the nasofrontal angle: is it normal, flat, or deep;
2. the nasal root protrusion: is it average, high, or low;
3. the nasal bridge: is it high, low, broad, beaky, or bulbous;
4. the nasal tip: is it normal, flat, or bifid;

5. the shape of each nasal ala: is it normal, slightly flat, markedly flat, slightly or markedly angled;
6. the nasal ala configuration: is it cleft, hypoplastic or hypertrophic; is there a coloboma;
7. the type and size of the nostrils: are they symmetric, asymmetric, and what type are they according to the Topinard classification (Fig. 7.63b).

The Topinard classification describes seven types of nostrils, three of which are intermediate (Fig. 7.63b). Type 7 is characteristic of nostrils in patients with a repaired cleft lip. More than half of the general

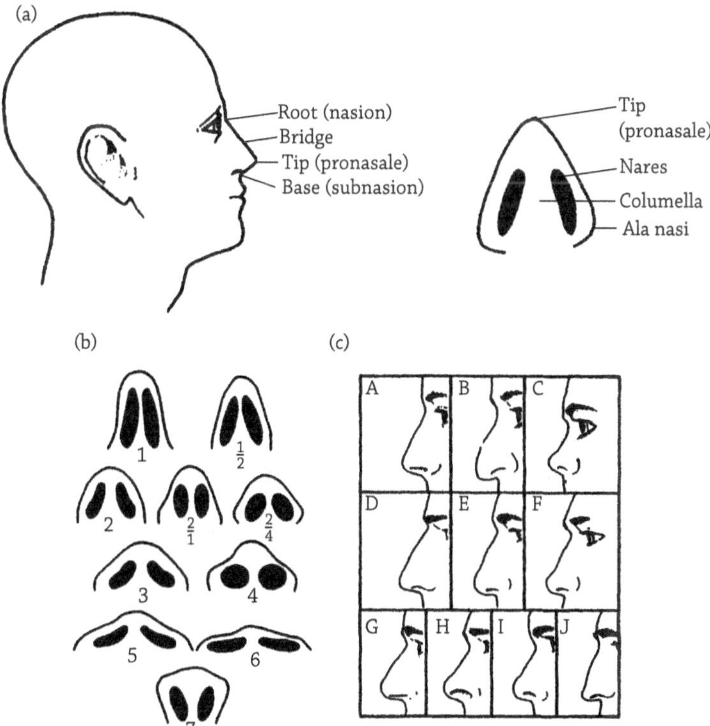

Figure 7.63 (a). Landmarks for measurements of the nose. (b) Topinard classification of nostrils. (c) Common variables in nose shape.

population have Type 2 nostrils; a quarter have Type 1 nostrils, with the other types being less frequent. The Topinard classification outlines some of the variability in size and shape of the alae nasi, nares, and columella.

Common variations in nose shape are shown in Figure 7.63c. Attempts to quantify changes in nose shape with age have rarely been documented. However, it is well known that the nasal root is depressed in the infant and young child, associated with a scooped-out nasal bridge. With increasing age, the nasal bridge rises, producing a more prominent root. Nostril type also varies with age. The prevalence of Topinard Type 4 decreases significantly after age 18.

Most nasal measurements are soft tissue measurements. However, many alternatives are available from radiographs. These will not be described in detail here, and the interested reader is referred to the literature cited at the end of this chapter.

The horizontal measurements of the nose, particularly the width of the nasal root and the interalar distance, provide information about midline development in the same way that the measurements of eye spacing reflect midline development. The nasal tip may be broad, grooved, cleft, or actually bifid with increasing width of the nose. A bifid nose results when the medial nasal prominences do not merge completely. In this situation, the nostrils are widely separated and the nasal bridge is bifid. This type of malformation may be part of a spectrum known as frontonasal dysplasia.

Unlike most vertical facial dimensions, nasal length continues to increase throughout life.

NASAL HEIGHT

Definition The distance from the nasal root (nasion) to the nasal base (subnasion).

Landmarks Measure from the deepest depression at the root of the nose to the deepest concavity at the base of the nose, in a vertical axis (Fig. 7.64).

Instruments Spreading calipers are most accurate. A tape measure could be used if held straight in a vertical plane, avoiding the contours of the face.

Position Frankfort horizontal, with the facial profile in the vertical. The patient can be observed from the front or from the side.

Remarks Nasal height is the same as upper facial height, which has been documented in a previous section (Fig. 7.65).

Pitfalls If the nasal root is high with a prominent nasal bridge, the actual position of the nasion may be difficult to place. If the nasal tip is pointed, long, and overhangs the upper lip, then the position of the subnasion may be difficult to place, particularly from an anterior view.

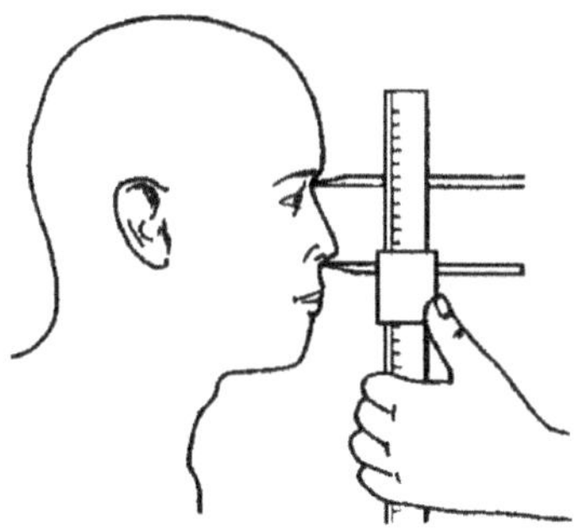

Figure 7.64. Measuring nasal length.

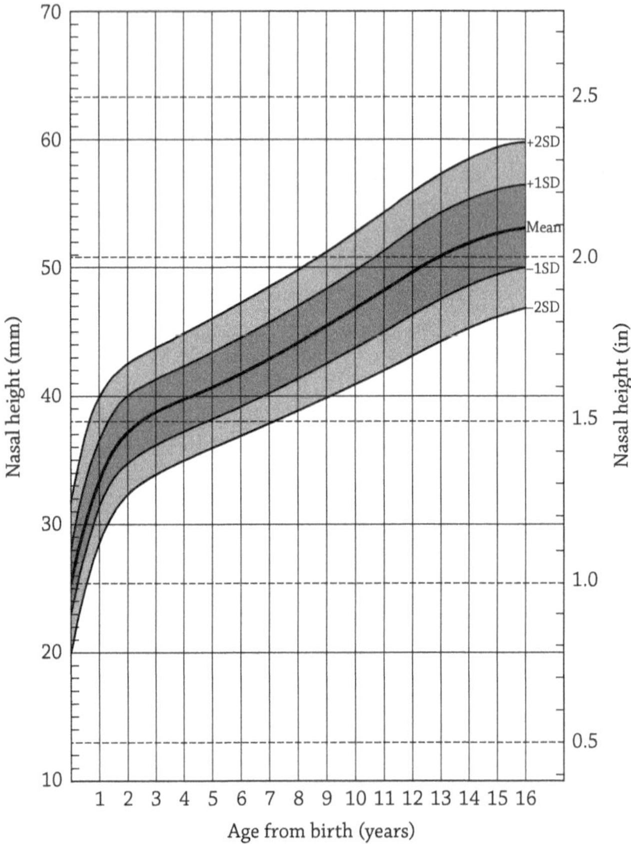

Figure 7.65. Nasal height (upper facial length), both sexes, birth to 16 years. From Goodman and Gorlin (1977), Farkas (1981), and Saksena et al. (1987), by permission.

LENGTH OF COLUMELLA

Definition Length of the most inferior aspect of the nasal septum.

Landmarks Measure along the crest of the columella from the base of the nose (subnasion) to the most anterior point of the columella at the level of the tip of each nostril (Fig. 7.66).

Instruments Tape measure or sliding calipers.

Position The patient should recline with the midfacial plane in the vertical.

Remarks Normal columella length for children age 6–16 years is shown in Figure 7.67. It is important to note that this measurement does not extend to the tip of the nose but only to the anterior-most part of the nostril. The measurement from the subnasion to the tip of the nose is that of nasal protrusion.

Pitfalls The columella may be curved rather than linear. It is important that a tape measure is used and worked along the skin surface of the columella in the presence of a curve, since a linear measurement with sliding calipers would falsely reduce this measurement.

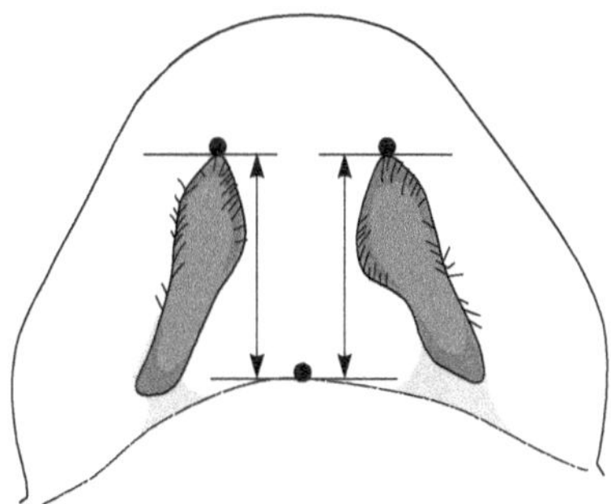

Figure 7.66. Measuring columella length.

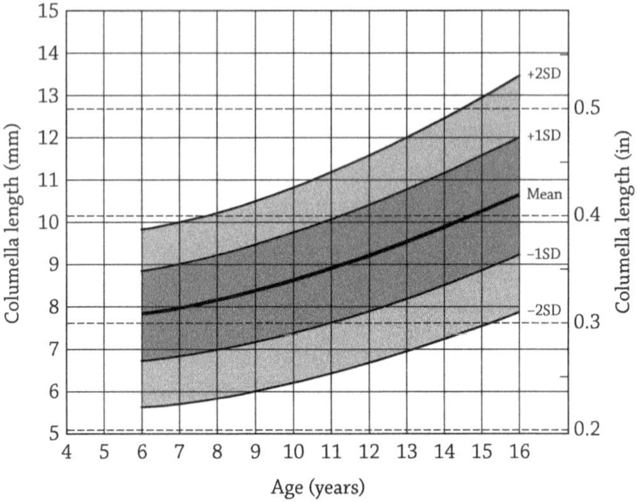

Figure 7.67. Columella length, both sexes, 6 to 16 years. From Farkas (1981), by permission.

NASAL PROTRUSION

Definition Nasal protrusion or depth.

Landmarks Measure from the tip of the nose (pronasale) to the deepest concavity at the base of the nose (subnasion) in a straight line (Fig. 7.68).

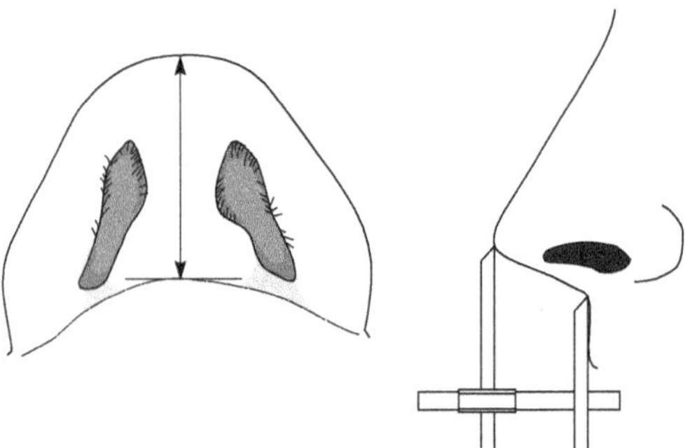

Figure 7.68. Measuring nasal protrusion.

Instruments Spreading calipers are most accurate. A transparent graduated ruler can be substituted.

Position The patient should be reclining in order that the nose is observed from its inferior aspect.

Alternative Nasal protrusion can be assessed from the side with the patient perpendicular to the observer.

Remarks The shape of the nose, seen from its inferior aspect, is tremendously variable both within and between ethnic groups. (Details are found in the introduction to this section.) Variability in the length of the columella accounts for part of the variability in protrusion of the nose (Fig. 7.69).

Pitfalls Occasionally the columella and nasal septum protrude below the plane of the alae nasi. Measurement of nasal protrusion should not be made along the surface of the nasal septum following its curve to the nasal tip but should be linear.

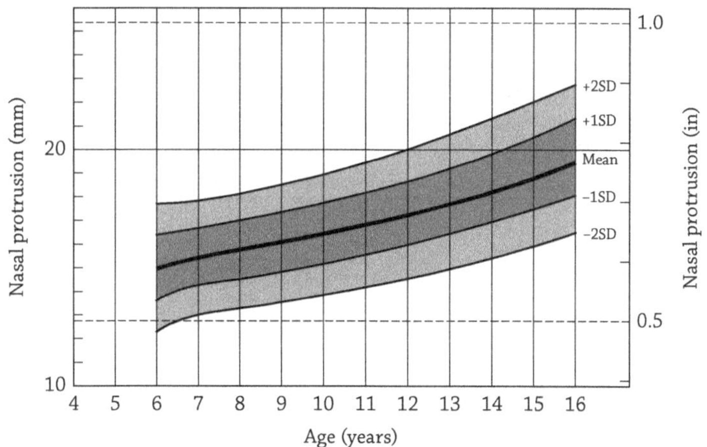

Figure 7.69. Nasal protrusion, both sexes, 6 to 16 years. From Farkas (1981), by permission.

INTERALAR DISTANCE (NASAL WIDTH)

Definition Distance between the most lateral aspects of the alae nasi.

Landmarks Measure from the lateral-most aspect of one ala nasi to the lateral-most aspect of the ala nasi (Fig. 7.70).

Instruments Spreading calipers are the most accurate instruments, although a transparent calibrated ruler or tape measure can be substituted.

Position The patient should be reclining, with the vertical.

Remarks Values for nasal width from birth to age 16 years are shown in Figure 7.71. There is tremendous variation both within and between ethnic groups in the interalar distance. Nasal width continues to increase with age, mainly due to soft tissue changes.

Pitfalls The nostrils should be held in the position of rest when this measurement is taken.

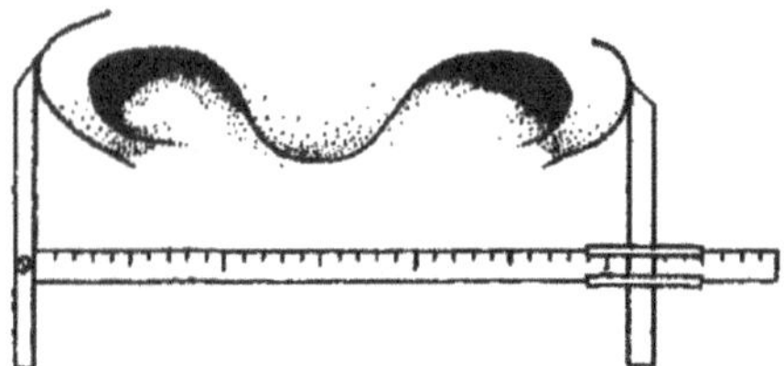

Figure 7.70. Measuring nasal width.

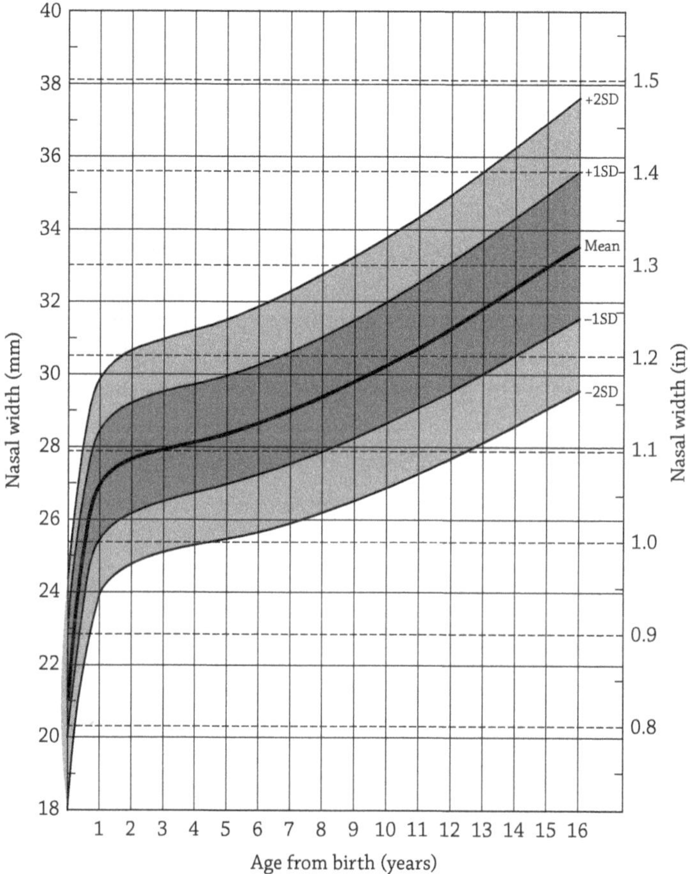

Figure 7.71. Interalar distance (nasal width), both sexes, birth to 16 years. From Goodman and Gorlin (1977) and Farkas (1981), by permission.

PHILTRUM

Introduction

The philtrum, or vertical groove in the central part of the upper lip, extends from the base of the nose to the superior aspect of the vermilion border of the lip. In some individuals, the philtrum is poorly demarcated, while in others, the cutaneous elevations that mark its lateral borders or pillars are easily discernible. The enclosed area is usually depressed. The philtral margins or pillars may be parallel or divergent. Although adequate graphs are available for philtral length, normal philtral width has been of little concern to the clinician; however, increased width and flattening are subjectively established in fetal alcohol spectrum disorder and Cornelia de Lange syndrome.

Length of the Philtrum

Definition Distance between the base of the nose and the border of the upper lip, in the midline.

Landmarks Measure from the base of the nose (subnasion) to the superior aspect of the vermilion border of the lip, in the midline (Fig. 7.72).

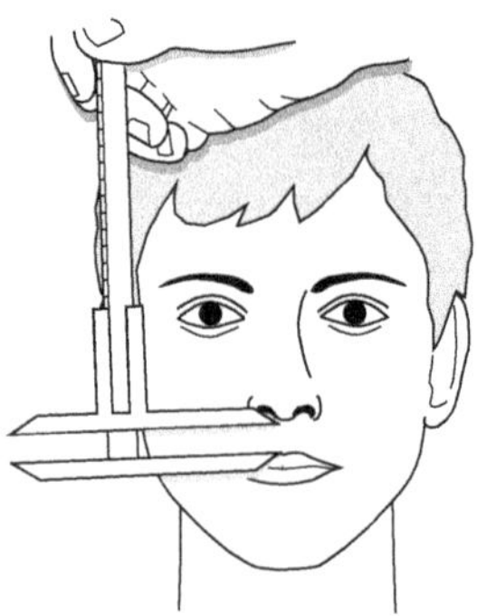

Figure 7.72. Measuring philtrum length.

Instruments Ideally, the philtral length is measured with spreading calipers; however, a calibrated transparent ruler could be used.

Position The head should be held (in the resting position) erect with the eyes facing forward. The observer should be positioned on the side of the patient, so that the face is in profile.

Alternative A young infant or child could lie supine with the head held.

Remarks Variation in philtrum length is shown in Figures 7.73 and 7.74.

Pitfalls In the newborn with a cleft lip, either unilateral or bilateral, this measurement may not be reliable. Facial expression, particularly smiling, will alter this measurement. Thus, the patient's facial expression should be neutral.

Philtrum smoothness and upper lip thinness are measured in five-point Likert pictorial scales by holding the lip-philtrum guide next to the patient's face and assigning each feature the Likert rank of the photograph that best matches each feature (Fig. 7.75).

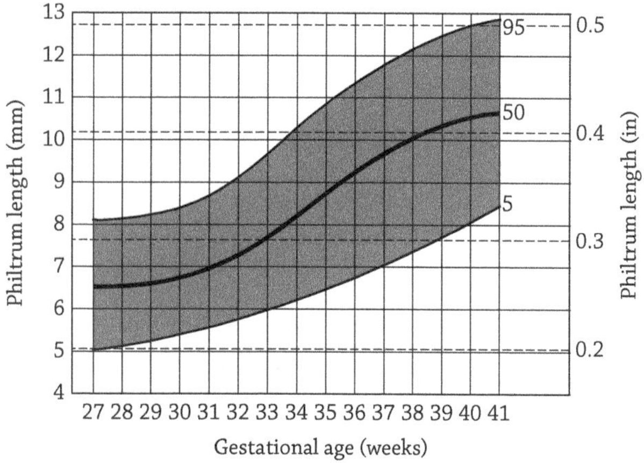

Figure 7.73. Philtrum length, both sexes, at birth. From Merlob et al. (1984), by permission.

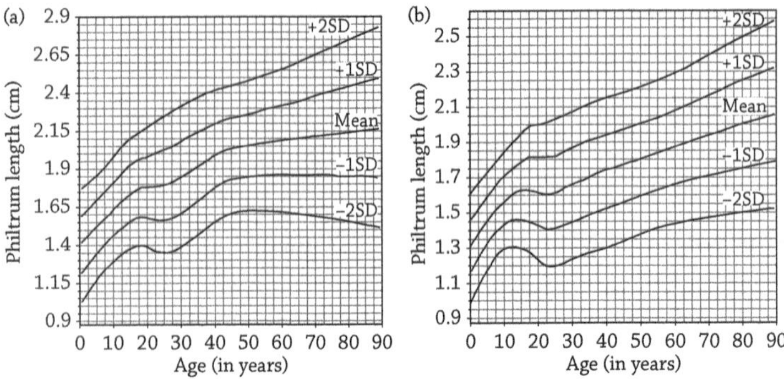

Figure 7.74. Philtrum length in males (a) and females (b) by age. Adapted from Zankl et al. (2002).

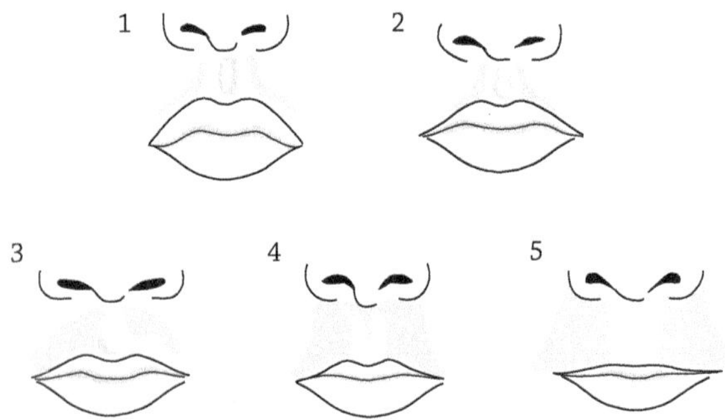

Figure 7.75. Pictorial example of the five-point Likert scale. From Astley and Clarren (1995), by permission.

MOUTH

Introduction

Variation in the size of the mouth is well documented, and detailed graphs are provided in the measurement section. It is far more difficult to evaluate the lips objectively. However, with the aid of calipers and a cooperative, relaxed patient, the visible vermilion of the upper lip can be measured. In Caucasians, the middle of the lip to the aperture ranges from 3–3.5 mm in the newborn to 4.7–4.8 mm in the 1-year-old, to approximately 6 mm in the adult. Corresponding lower lip measurements are 3.6–4.7, 5.9–6.3, and 9–10 mm, respectively. Further variation in lip shape is associated with differences in philtral development. A well-formed, deeply grooved philtrum is usually associated with wide-spaced peaks to the vermilion border of the upper lip. Conversely, a poorly formed, flat philtrum is usually associated with a relatively thin, even surface to the vermilion border. A tented upper lip often results from long-standing, bilateral, facial muscle weakness, such as that seen in congenital myotonic dystrophy.

Congenital pits or recesses of the lips are present in 2%–3% of neonates. They usually occur in the lower lips, where they may be bilateral or unilateral, showing a well-defined circular depression on the vermilion border. In the upper lip, where they are rare, they are found lateral to the philtrum. They represent the orifices of mucous tracts that extend into the substance of the lip. A double lip is a deformity that consists of redundant tissue in the mucosal portion of the lip just inside its vermilion border. The anomaly, which can occur in the upper or in the lower lip, has been observed in both males and females and is individually rare. It is more conspicuous in the upper lip because the mucosal duplication, which shows a median notch, hangs down and partly covers the incisors. Double lip may be associated with relaxation of the supratarsal fold (blepharochalasis) and with thyroid enlargement (Ascher syndrome).

Width of the mouth is a difficult soft tissue measurement to assess. Macrostomia, or large mouth, may be caused by lateral or transverse facial clefts running from the mouth toward the ear. This abnormality results from failure of the lateral mesenchymal masses of the maxillary and mandibular prominences to merge. Congenital microstomia is a small mouth, and in severe cases, microstomia may be associated with mandibular hypoplasia. A small mouth, with pursed lips, may also result from perioral fibrosis.

Frenulae are strands of tissue extending between the buccal and alveolar mucosae. Abnormal numbers of frenulae may be associated with various craniofacial syndromes, most commonly oral-facial-digital (OFD) syndrome. An assessment of alveolar ridge thickness should be included in the evaluation of the mouth. Thickening may be congenital or acquired, for example, following prolonged therapy with antiepileptic medications.

The reader is referred to the references at the end of this chapter for further information.

•

Intercommissural Distance (Mouth Width)

Definition Mouth width at rest.

Landmarks Measure from one cheilion (corner of the mouth) to the other cheilion (Fig. 7.76).

Instruments Spreading calipers are best. A tape measure held straight or a calibrated transparent ruler may be substituted.

Position The head should be held erect (in the resting position) with the eyes facing forward and the mouth held close and in a neutral position.

Alternative The young infant or child may lie supine.

Remarks The intercommissural distance has been estimated by several authors, despite the intrinsic difficulties in measuring soft tissue points (Figs. 7.77 and 7.78).

Pitfalls The mouth should be at rest, as grimacing, crying, smiling, or any other facial expression will distort the measurement.

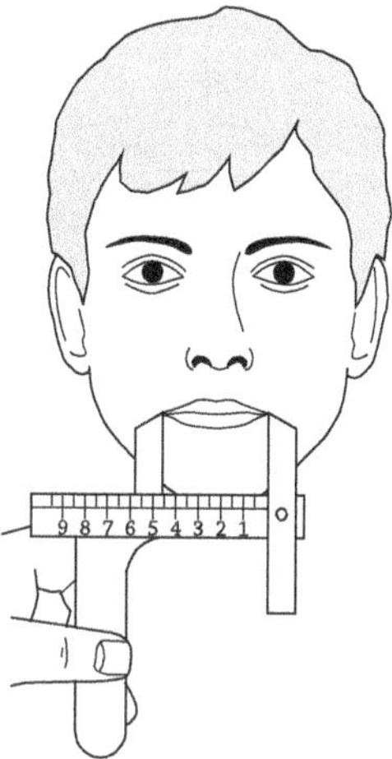

Figure 7.76. Measuring mouth width. Adapted from Garn et al. (1984).

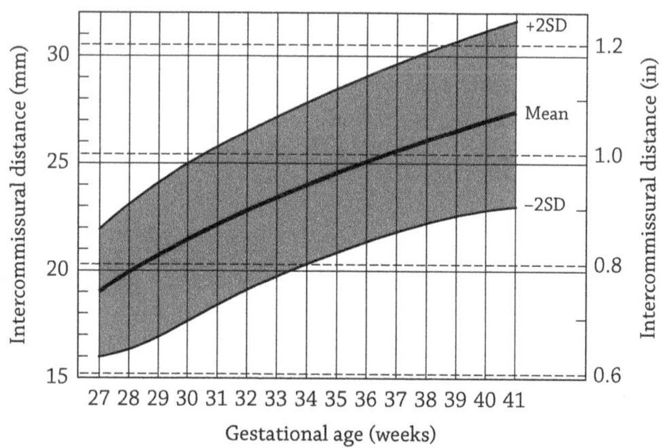

Figure 7.77. Intercommissural distance, both sexes, at birth. From Merlob et al. (1984), by permission.

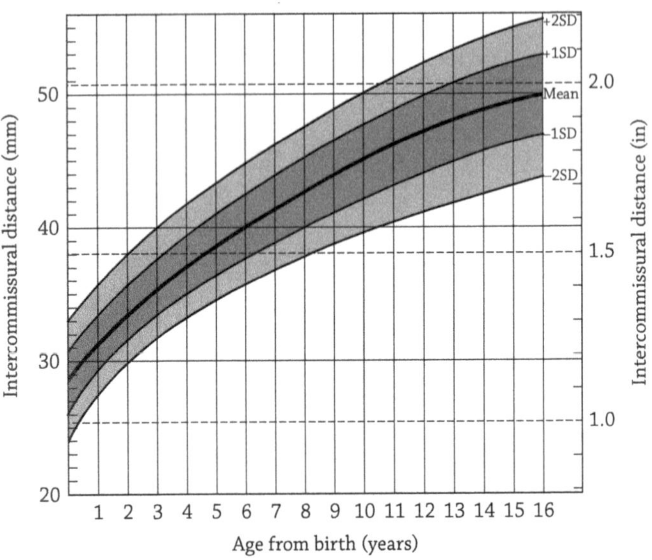

Figure 7.78. Intercommissural distance, both sexes, birth to 16 years. From Feingold and Bossert (1974) and Farkas (1981), by permission.

PALATE

Introduction

Simple devices have been designed to measure directly palatal height, width, and length. For detailed study, these data may be ascertained from plaster casts. Length of the palate can also be assessed from X-rays. Physicians may find it easier to use a rough estimate of palate height in the clinic. If the maximum height of the palate is greater than twice the height of the teeth, it can be considered abnormal.

Unusually prominent lateral palatine ridges are a nonspecific feature of a variety of disorders in which there is either neuromuscular dysfunction or an anatomic defect that prevents or limits tongue thrust into the palatal vault. The lateral palatine ridges are normally more prominent during prenatal life and infancy. With increasing age, they become progressively flattened by the moulding forces of the tongue and usually disappear by 5 years of age. Prominent lateral palatine ridges may be misinterpreted as a true “narrow high arched palate,” which is a much less common anomaly.

Palate Length: Cephalometric

Definition Length of the palate.

Landmarks Measure from the anterior to the posterior nasal spine (Fig. 7.79).

Instruments Spreading calipers are used to measure the distance on a radiograph taken with a “cephalostat.”

Position Standard cephalometry; see general introduction to Chapter 7 for details.

Remarks Values for cephalometric measurement of the palate length are shown in Figure 7.80. Soft tissue measurement of palate length is difficult and requires special instrumentation (Shapiro et al., 1963). With this instrument, palate length is defined as the distance from the labial point of the incisive papilla to the midline of the junction of the hard and soft palates (Fig. 7.81). The majority of clinical dysmorphologists will not have access to such instrumentation.

The palate is generally longer in males than females. This sex difference is accentuated with increasing age.

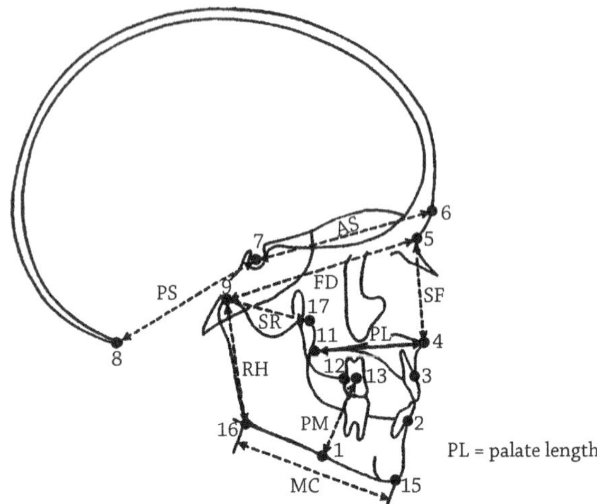

Figure 7.79. Radiographic landmarks for measuring palate length (PL). AS, anterior skull base length; FD, facial depth; RH, ramus height; PM, palate-mandible height; PS, posterior skull base length; SF, superior facial height; SR, superior ramus length. Adapted from Garn et al. (1984).

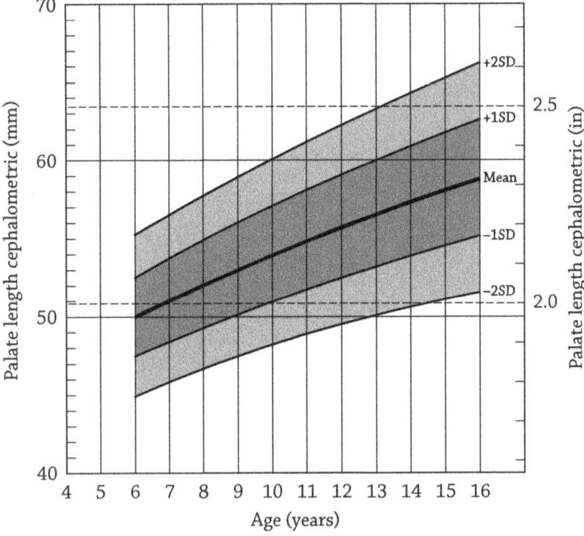

Figure 7.80. Palate length (cephalometric), both sexes, 6 to 16 years. From Garn et al. (1984), by permission.

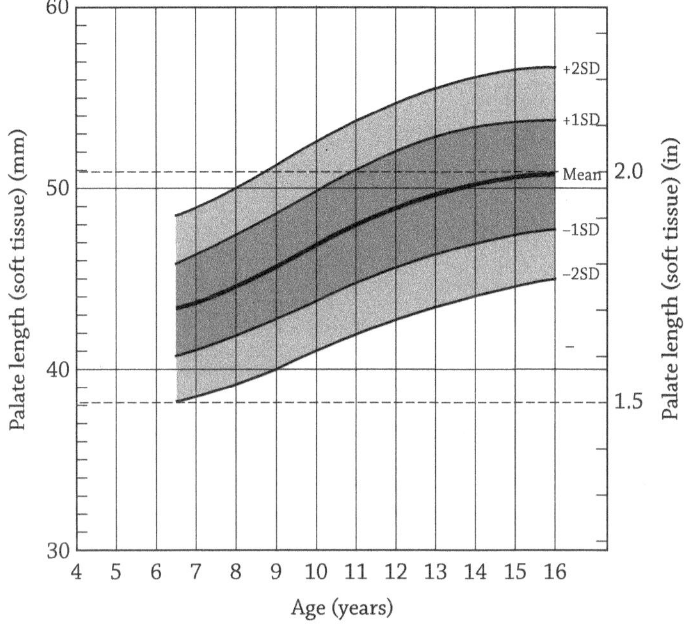

Figure 7.81. Palate length (soft tissue), both sexes, 6 to 16 years. From Redman (1963), by permission.

Palate Height

Definition Height of the palate.

Landmarks Measure the shortest distance between the midline of the junction of the hard and soft palates and the plane established by other reference points as outlined in palate length and palate width (Fig. 7.82).

Instruments A palatal measuring device is necessary (Shapiro et al., 1963).

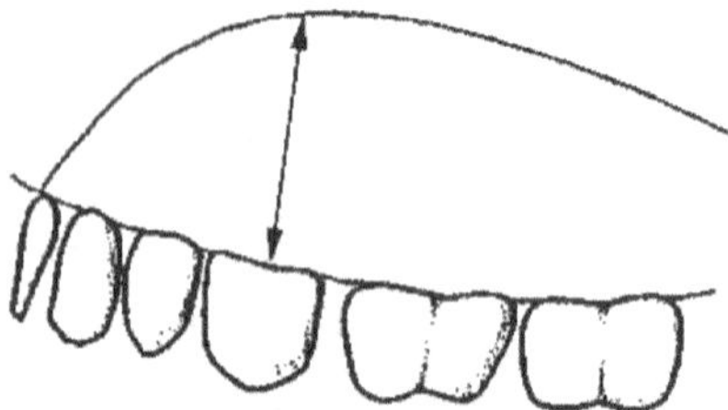

Figure 7.82. Measuring palate height.

Remarks Most clinicians will not have access to a palatal measuring device, but an assessment of the height of the palate is vital if deviation from normal palatal shape is to be defined. We suggest, as a rough guide, that when maximum palate height is greater than twice the height of the teeth, it should be considered abnormally high.

Pitfalls Thickened palatine and alveolar ridges producing narrowness of the palate can give a false impression of increased palate height.

Palate Width

Definition Width of the palate.

Landmarks Measure the distance between the maxillary first permanent molar on the right side and the maxillary first permanent molar on the left side at the lingual cervical line (Fig. 7.83), and compare to the standard measurements in Fig. 7.84.

Remarks Palate width is once again measured with a specific device that is not generally available to clinicians.

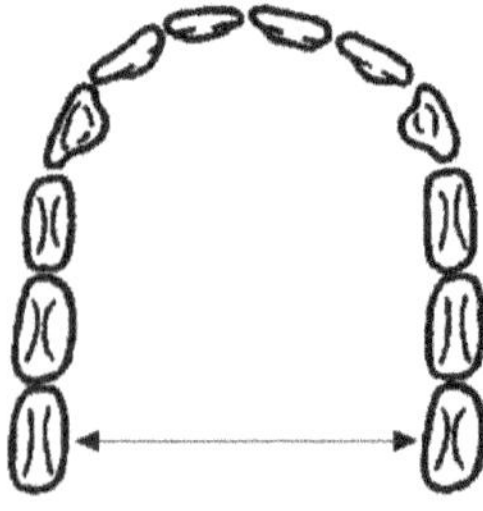

Figure 7.83. Measuring palate width.

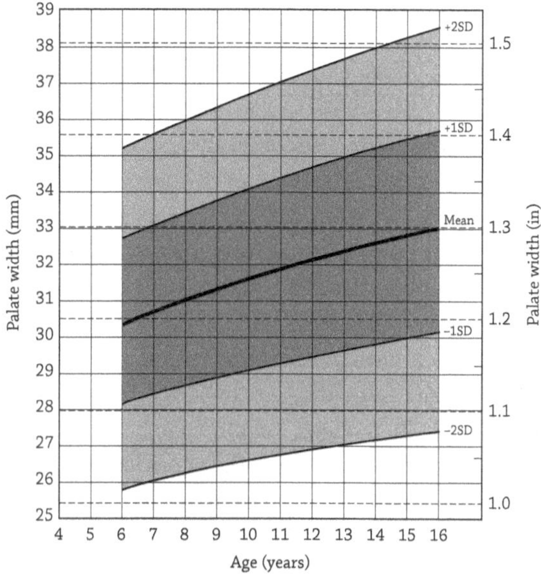

Figure 7.84. Palate width, both sexes, 6 to 16 years. From Redman (1963), by permission.

TONGUE

Introduction and Landmarks

Around the end of the fourth week of gestation, a median, somewhat triangular elevation appears in the floor of the pharynx just rostral to the foramen caecum. This elevation, the median tongue bud, gives the first indication of tongue development. Soon, two oval distal tongue buds (lateral lingual swellings) develop on each side of the median tongue bud. These elevations result from proliferation of mesenchyme in the ventromedial parts of the first pair of branchial arches. The distal tongue buds rapidly increase in size, merge with each other, and overgrow the median tongue bud. The merged distal tongue buds form the anterior two-thirds or oral part of the tongue. The posterior third or pharyngeal part of the tongue is initially indicated by two elevations that develop caudal to the foramen caecum, the copula from the second branchial arches, and the hypobranchial eminence from the third and fourth branchial arches. Branchial arch mesenchyme forms the connective tissue and the lymphatic and blood vessels of the tongue and probably some of its muscle fibers. Most of the tongue musculature, however, is derived from myoblasts that migrate from the myotomes of the cervical somites. The hypoglossal nerve accompanies the myoblasts during their migration and innervates the tongue musculature when it develops.

The papillae of the tongue appear at about 54 days of gestation. All the papillae will develop taste buds.

Tongue landmarks are outlined in Figure 7.85.

Remarks Congenital malformations of the tongue include congenital cysts and fistulae derived from remnants of the thyroglossal duct, ankyloglossia (tongue-tie), in which the frenulum from the inferior surface of the anterior part of the tongue extends to near the tip of the tongue and interferes with free protrusion; cleft tongue, caused by incomplete fusion of the distal tongue buds posteriorly; and bifid tongue, in which there is complete failure of fusion of the distal tongue buds.

There is variation in the size of the tongue among individuals, and no normal measurements have been established. Most

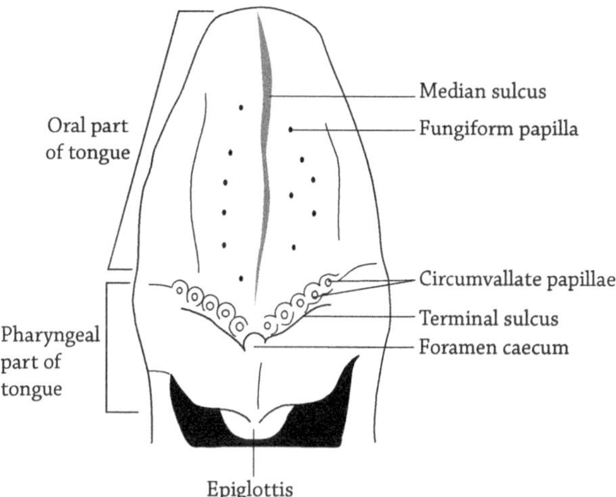

Figure 7.85. Landmarks of the tongue.

pediatricians, however, have established their own norms for children. A large tongue (macroglossia) or a relatively large tongue may be important for the diagnosis of congenital hypothyroidism, Beckwith-Wiedemann syndrome, or Down syndrome in the neonatal period. The tongue may be large if it is the site of a congenital vascular malformation. Acquired forms of macroglossia include trauma and allergic reactions, for example, angioneurotic edema. When considering the tongue in facial diagnosis, one should remember that largeness is not necessarily the same as protrusion.

Diminished bulk of the tongue may be associated with an atrophic process. Tongue atrophy is a very important clinical sign and usually indicates a lower motor neuron lesion or disturbance of the intrinsic tongue musculature. One should distinguish between bilateral atrophy and unilateral atrophy. The term *aglossia* refers to absence of the tongue, although usually some rudiments of the tongue are present. Aglossia may be seen in association with limb anomalies.

One should look for abnormal postures of the tongue or an inability to protrude the tongue. Topographic tongue abnormalities, such as a furrowed tongue or geographic tongue, should be noted.

TEETH

Introduction

The teeth develop from ectoderm and mesoderm. The enamel is produced by cells derived from oral ectoderm. All other dental tissues develop from mesenchyme. The mandibular teeth usually erupt before the maxillary teeth, and girls' teeth usually erupt sooner than boys' teeth. As the root of the tooth grows, the crown gradually erupts through the oral mucosa. The part of the oral mucosa around the erupted crown becomes the gum or gingiva.

Eruption of the deciduous teeth usually occurs between 6 and 24 months after birth (Fig. 7.86). The permanent teeth develop in a manner similar to that just described. As a permanent tooth grows, the root of the corresponding deciduous tooth is gradually resorbed by osteoclasts. Consequently, when the deciduous tooth is shed, it consists only of the crown and the uppermost portion of the root. The permanent teeth usually begin to erupt during the sixth year and continue to appear until early adulthood. They are often serrated initially and become smooth with time. The chronology of onset of prenatal and postnatal enamel formation is illustrated in Figure 7.87. Details of dental age are provided in Chapter 13.

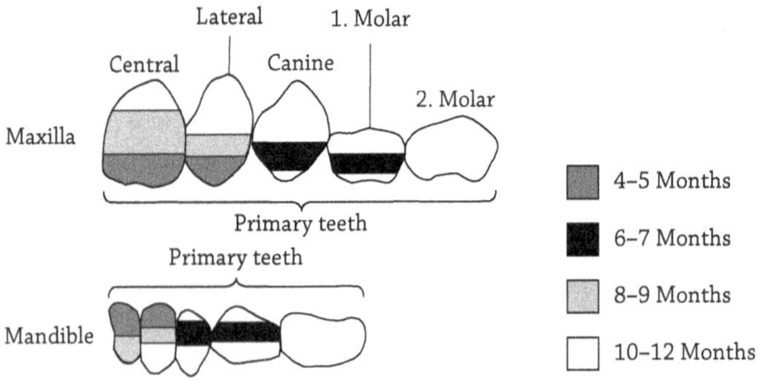

Figure 7.86. Tooth eruption.

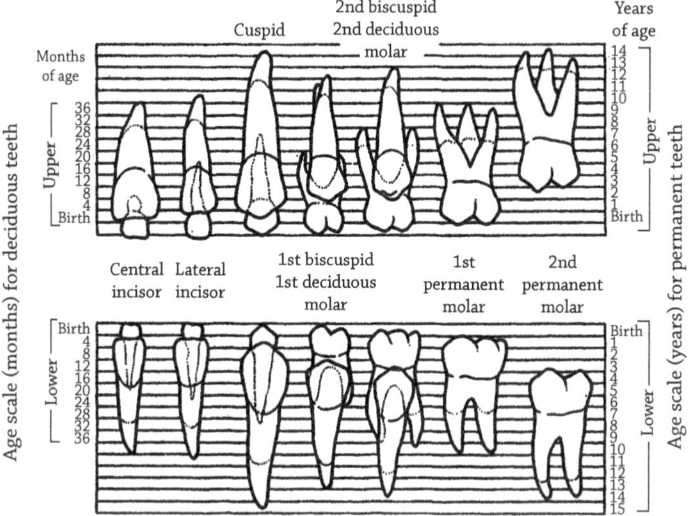

Figure 7.87. Tooth enamel development.

Remarks Defective enamel formation results in grooves, pits, or fissures on the enamel surface. These defects result from temporary disturbances in enamel formation. Various factors may injure the ameloblasts, for example, nutritional deficiency, tetracycline therapy, and infections such as measles. Rickets is probably the most common cause of enamel hypoplasia. In amelogenesis imperfecta, the enamel is soft and friable because of hypocalcification, and the teeth are yellow to brown in color. This genetic trait affects about one in every 20,000 children. In dentinogenesis imperfecta, a condition relatively common in Caucasian children, the teeth are brown to gray-blue with an opalescent sheen. The enamel tends to wear down rapidly, exposing the dentin. Foreign substances incorporated into the developing enamel will cause discoloration of the teeth. Hemolysis and tetracycline therapy are among the causes of tooth discoloration. The primary teeth are affected if tetracyclines are given from 18 weeks of gestation to 10 months postnatally, and the permanent teeth may be affected if exposure occurs between 18 weeks prenatally and 16 years of age.

Abnormally shaped teeth are relatively common. Occasionally, spherical masses of enamel called *enamel pearls or drops* are attached to the tooth. They are formed by aberrant groups of ameloblasts. The maxillary lateral incisor teeth may assume a slender tapering shape (peg-shaped lateral incisors). Congenital syphilis affects the differentiation of the permanent teeth, resulting in screwdriver-shaped incisors with central notches in their incisive edges, called Hutchinson teeth.

The most common dental anomaly present at birth is premature eruption of one or more of the deciduous teeth, usually the mandibular incisors. One or more supernumerary teeth may develop, or the normal number of teeth may fail to form. Supernumerary teeth usually appear in the area of the maxillary incisors, where they disrupt the position and eruption of normal teeth. The extra teeth commonly erupt posterior to the normal ones. In partial anodontia, one or more teeth are absent. In total anodontia, no teeth develop. This very rare condition is usually associated with an ectodermal dysplasia.

Disturbances during the differentiation of teeth may result in gross alterations in dental morphology, for example, macrodontia (large teeth) and microdontia (small teeth). Taurodontia is a variation in tooth form involving all or some of the primary and secondary molars, marked by elongation of the body of the tooth producing large pulp chambers and small roots. Taurodontia is found in association with several chromosomal abnormalities.

MAXILLA

Introduction

The lateral parts of the upper lip, most of the maxilla, and the secondary palate form the maxillary prominences of the first branchial arch. These prominences merge laterally with the mandibular prominences.

Unilateral maxillary absence is a rare condition and is due to failure of development of one maxillary process. Absence of the premaxillary area is found in cyclopia when the frontonasal process does not form. Subtle hypoplasia of the maxilla is best appreciated on a radiograph and is an important feature to be looked for in first-degree relatives of patients with Treacher Collins syndrome.

In the measurement section that follows, the maxilla is chiefly evaluated by cephalometric means. Clinical evaluation of the maxilla is extremely subjective and is best performed in profile, looking at the prominence of the maxilla in comparison to the prominence of the supraorbital ridges, malar area, and mandible. No objective clinical measurements appear to be available.

Effective Midfacial Length: Cephalometric

Definition Size and prominence of the maxilla (Fig. 7.88).

Landmarks Measure from the condylion of the mandible (the most posterosuperior point of the condylar outline) to point A (the deepest midline point on the maxilla between the anterior nasal spine and the prosthion, which is the inferior labial termination of the cortical plate just above the maxillary incisors) (Fig 7.89).

Instruments Spreading calipers are used to measure this distance on a radiograph taken with "cephalostat."

Position Standard cephalometry—see introduction to Chapter 7.

	6 years		9 years		12 years		14 years		Adults	
	Mean	SD	Mean	SD	Mean	SD	Mean	SD	Mean	SD
Male	81.7	3.4	87.7	4.1	92.1	4.1	95.2	3.2	98.8	4.3
	81.7	3.4	87.7	4.1	92.1	4.1	95.2	3.2	99.8	6.0
	80.5	2.4	84.9	2.5	90.3	3.6	93.9	4.6		
Female	79.7	2.2	85.0	2.3	89.6	2.4	92.1	2.7	90.7	5.2
	79.8	2.2	85.0	2.3	89.6	2.4	92.1	2.7	91.0	4.3
	78.6	3.1	88.3	4.0	87.3	4.6	89.2	5.2		

Figure 7.88. Effective midfacial length (mm), both sexes, 6 to 18 years. From McNamara (1984) by permission.

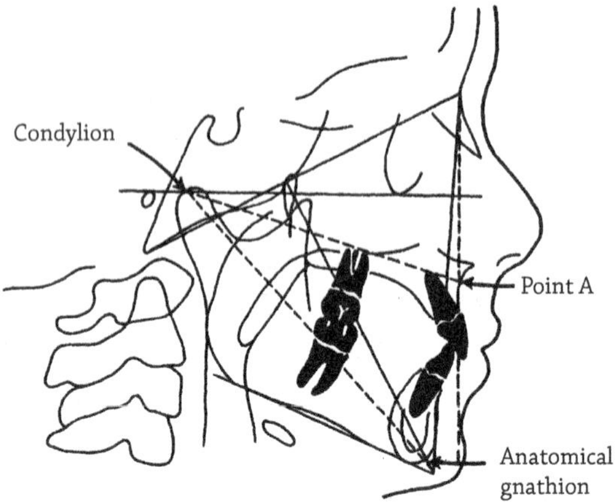

Figure 7.89. Cephalometric measurement of effective midfacial length.

Remarks Unfortunately, clinical evaluation of the maxilla and malar area is difficult and subjective. Relative prominence or flattening of the malar area is best appreciated in profile, relative to the prominence of supraorbital region. Similarly, prominence of the maxilla, in profile, should be relative to the mandible.

Outer Canthal, Nasal, Outer Canthal (ONC) Angle

Definition The angle subtended by the base of the nose in the midline to the outer canthi of the eyes.

Landmarks Draw an imaginary line from the outer canthus of the right eye to the base of the nose (base of the columella) in the midline. Draw a second imaginary line from the outer canthus of the left eye to the same point at the base of the nose. Measure the angle between those two lines (Fig. 7.90).

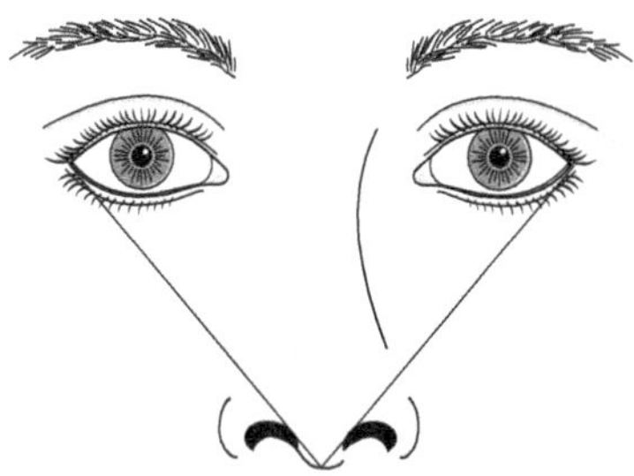

Figure 7.90. Measuring ONO angle.

Instruments Two fixed measures such as a tape measure or flexible ruler and protractor are necessary.

Position The head should be held erect (in the resting position) with the patient facing forward.

Alternative A young infant or child should be lying supine.

Remarks This angle is best measured from a full frontal photograph taken at a fixed distance from the patient (Fig. 7.91). It provides an estimate of both the spacing of the eyes and the upper facial height, and thus it will vary in the presence of hypo- or hypertelorism or an increase or reduction in upper facial height. Although best appreciated from a photograph, it can still provide useful information during clinical evaluation.

Pitfalls Depending on the prominence of the nose, it may be very difficult to draw a straight line between the outer canthus and the base of the nose in the midline. In this situation, photographic estimation is advised.

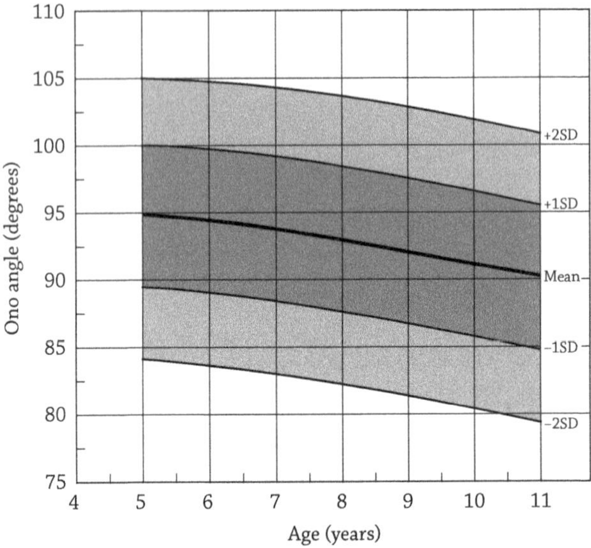

Figure 7.91. ONO angle, both sexes, 5 to 11 years. From Patton (1987), by permission.

MANDIBLE

Introduction

The mandible, or lower jaw, is the first part of the face to form, as the medial ends of the two mandibular prominences merge during the fourth week of gestation.

Agnathia, or absence of the mandible, is a developmental defect of the first branchial arch. The mandible may be missing on one side only, a condition sometimes associated with microtia or absence of the external or internal ear, or with unilateral congenital macrostomia. Micrognathia, or underdevelopment of the jaw, may be severe enough to lead to cleft palate in the Pierre–Robin sequence. This can be seen as an isolated anomaly or in conjunction with other features as part of a syndrome diagnosis. Macrognathia, or a large jaw, is otherwise termed prognathism and is best appreciated in profile. The jaw is abnormally large or jutting forward. Various measurements of the jaw can be made from radiographs. The main clinical measurement, for which a graph is provided, is the mandibular width, or bigonial distance. The shape of the jaw can vary markedly depending on the relative proportions of the ramus and body of the mandible. The jaw articulates with the skull at the temporomandibular joint. Restricted movement at that joint may produce limited mouth opening or trismus.

A median cleft of the mandible is a deep cleft resulting from failure of the mesenchymal masses of the mandibular prominences of the first branchial arch to merge completely with each other. It is extremely rare. More superficial clefts of the lower lip may also occur. Clefts of the mandible are sometimes associated with cleft lip, cleft palate, or oblique facial clefts.

A simple dimple on the chin is a common feature inherited with an autosomal dominant pattern. A more complicated H-shaped groove of the chin is associated with Freeman–Sheldon syndrome. Mental spurs are bony spurs over the most prominent part of the jaw in the midline.

The shape and size of the chin contribute to the overall facial shape. A wide chin will tend to produce a round or square face, while a narrow, pointed chin promotes the appearance of an inverted triangular face because of the relative width of the forehead and cranial vault.

Effective Mandibular Length: Cephalometric

Definition Effective length and prominence of the mandible.

Landmarks Measure from the condylion (the most posterosuperior point of the condylar outline) to the anatomic gnathion (determined by the intersection of the facial and mandibular planes) (Fig. 7.92). Typical values are shown in Figure 7.93.

Instruments Spreading calipers are used to measure this distance on a radiograph taken with "cephalostat."

Position Standard cephalometry—see introduction to Chapter 7.

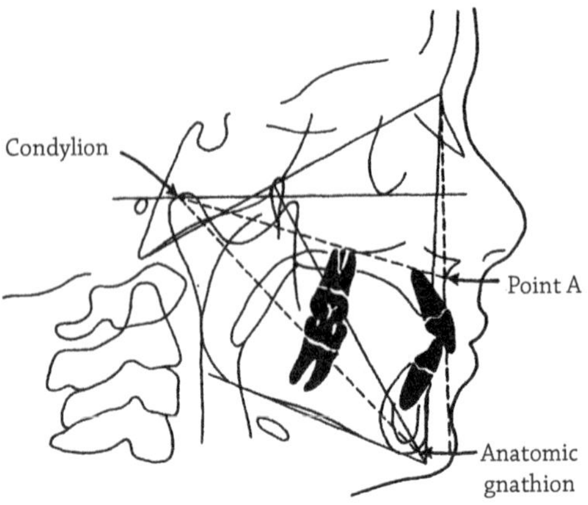

Figure 7.92. Cephalometric measurement of effective mandibular length.

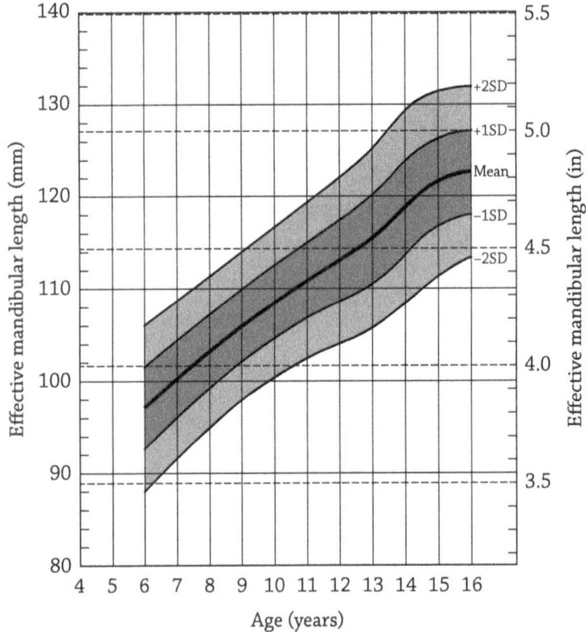

Figure 7.93. Effective mandibular length, both sexes, 6 to 16 years. From McNamara (1984), by permission.

Maxillomandibular Differential: Cephalometric

Definition This measurement is determined by subtracting the effective midfacial length from the effective mandibular length (Fig. 7.94).

Landmarks See sections on effective midfacial length and effective mandibular length for details.

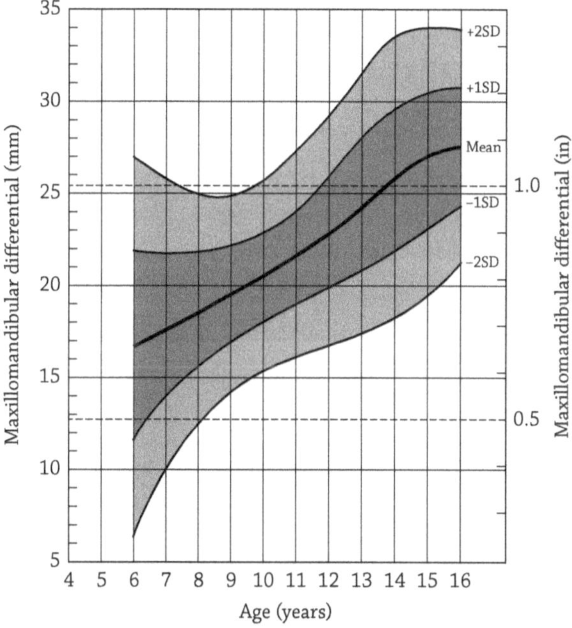

Figure 7.94. Maxillo mandibular differential, both sexes, 6 to 16 years. From McNamara (1984), by permission.

Mandible Width (Bigonial Distance)

Definition The bigonial width. The distance between the two most lateral aspects of the mandible.

Landmarks Measure from the most lateral aspect at the angle of the jaw (gonion) to the same point on the other side of the face (Fig. 7.95).

Instruments Spreading calipers.

Position The head should be held erect with the eyes facing forward.

Alternative The infant or young child may lie supine.

Remarks The mouth should be relaxed when this measurement is taken. Typical values for children age 4–16 years are shown in Figure 7.96.

Pitfalls Marked asymmetry of the mandible or malformation of the mandible may make it difficult to define the gonial points.

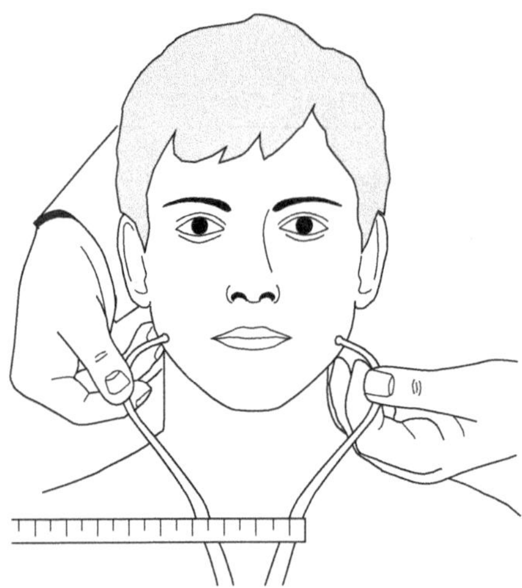

Figure 7.95. Measuring mandible width.

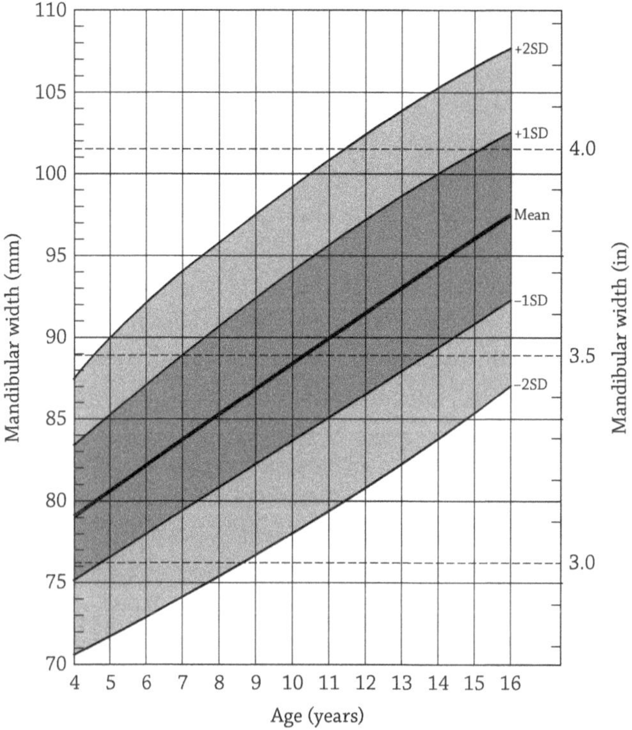

Figure 7.96. Mandibular width, both sexes, 4 to 16 years. From Farkas (1981), by permission.

THE NECK

Introduction

Most of the congenital malformations of the neck originate during transformation of the branchial apparatus into adult structures. Branchial cysts, sinuses, or fistulae may develop from parts of the second branchial groove, the cervical sinus, or the second pharyngeal pouch if they fail to regress. An ectopic thyroid gland results when the thyroid gland fails to descend completely from its site of origin in the tongue. The thyroglossal duct may persist, or remnants of it may give rise to thyroglossal duct cysts. These cysts, if infected, may form thyroglossal duct sinuses that open in the midline of the neck, in contrast to the branchial sinuses, which open more laterally, close to the borders of the sternocleidomastoid muscle.

Torticollis (wry neck) usually is attributed to injury of the sternocleidomastoid muscle during delivery; however, prenatal onset of the anomaly cannot be ruled out. Torticollis can be caused by malformations of the cervical vertebrae. The right and left sides are affected equally without any sex predilection. The incidence is 0.6 per 1000 births. The presence of unequal muscle pull on the developing cranium by torticollis may lead to unequal growth of the skull, with resultant plagiocephaly. A contralateral epicanthal fold is frequently seen. In approximately one-third of cases, torticollis is associated with congenital hip dislocation. Both can be caused by cramped circumstances in utero, for example, due to abnormal uterine anatomy, a uterine fibroid, or oligohydramnios.

Estimation of the length and width of the neck is very subjective, and normal age-related charts are not available. The neck is generally short in the neonate and begins to elongate in the older child. The width of the neck varies, increasing from a superior to an inferior aspect in general. A wide neck may be associated with marked skin folds or webs or with prominence of the trapezius muscle. Folds, webs, and a prominent trapezius may be related to prenatal onset of lymphatic obstruction. An early clue in the newborn period is the presence of excess nuchal skin and posteriorly angulated auricles with an upturned lobule. The circumference of the neck may be quantified, and the charts are available in this section.

The neck should also be inspected for branchial arch remnants such as pits, sinuses, fistulae, and tags.

Neck Circumference

Definition The distance around the neck.

Landmarks Measure around the neck in a horizontal plane at the level of the most prominent portion of the thyroid cartilage (Fig. 7.97).

Instruments Tape measure.

Position The head should be held erect (in the resting position) with the eyes facing forward.

Remarks Normal values to age 12 years are presented in Figure 7.98. The neck may be broad because of excessive prominence of the trapezius or secondary to skinfolds or webs. Both these anatomical differences can be associated with excess nuchal skin in the newborn period and with lymphatic obstruction during prenatal development.

Pitfalls In the presence of prominent folds of skin or webs at the side of the neck, the tape measure should carefully follow the surface of the skin to reflect circumference accurately. The horizontal plane at which measurement occurs should be carefully selected at the most prominent portion of the thyroid cartilage.

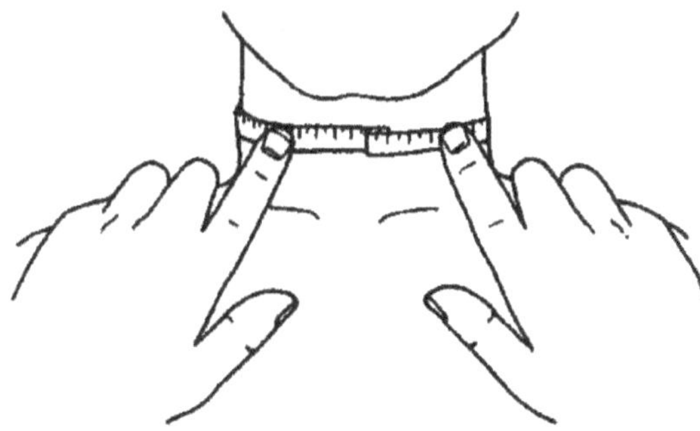

Figure 7.97. Measuring neck circumference.

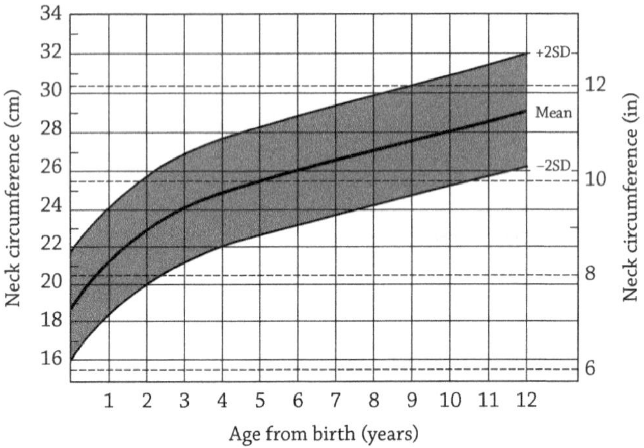

Figure 7.98. Neck circumference, both sexes, birth to 12 years. From Feingold and Bossert (1974), by permission.

BIBLIOGRAPHY

Astley, S. J., and Clarren, S. K. (1995). A fetal alcohol syndrome screening tool. *Alcoholism: Clinical and Experimental Research*, 19, 1565–1571.

Caffey, J. (1978). *J. Caffey's pediatric X ray diagnosis* (7th ed). Chicago: Year Book Publishers.

Carey, J. C., Cohen, M. M. Jr., Curry, C. J. R., Devriendt, K., Holmes, L. B., and Verloes, A. 2009. Elements of morphology: Standard terminology for the lips, mouth, and oral region. *American Journal of Medical Genetics Part A*, 149A, 77–92.

Chouke, K. S. (1929). The epicanthus or Mongolian fold in Caucasian children. *American Journal of Physical Anthropology*, 13, 255.

Cohen, M. M., and Maclean, R. (eds.) (2000). *Craniosynostosis: Diagnosis, evaluations, and management*. New York: Oxford University Press.

Currarino, G., and Silverman, F. N. (1960). Orbital hypotelorism, arhinencephaly, and trigonocephaly. *Radiology*, 74, 206–217.

Duke-Elder, S. (1963). *System of ophthalmology, Vol. 3*. St Louis: C.V. Mosby.

Faix, R. G. (1982). Fontanelle size in black and white term newborn infants. *Journal of Pediatrics*, 100, 304–306.

Farkas, L. G. (1981). *Anthropometry of the head and face in medicine*. New York: Elsevier.

Farkas, L. G., and Munro, I. R. (1987). *Anthropometric facial proportions in medicine*. Springfield, IL: Charles C. Thomas.

Feingold, M., and Bossert, W. H. (1974). Normal values for selected physical parameters: an aid to syndrome delineation. *Birth Defects: Original Article Series*, X(13), 1–15.

Garn, S. M., Smith, B. H., and LaVelle, M. (1984). Applications of pattern profile analysis to malformations of the head and face. *Radiology*, 150, 683–690.

Gerber, F. R., Taylor, F. H., deLevie, M., Drash, A. L., and Kenny, F. M. (1972). Normal standards for exophthalmometry in children 10 to 14 years of age: Relation to age, height, weight, and sexual maturation. *Journal of Pediatrics*, 81, 327–329.

Goodman, R. M., and Gorlin, R. J. (1977). *Atlas of the face in genetic disorders* (2nd ed.). St. Louis: C.V. Mosby.

Hall, B. D., Graham, J. M. Jr., Cassidy, S. B., and Opitz, J. M. (2009). Elements of morphology: Standard terminology for the periorbital region. *American Journal of Medical Genetics Part A*, 149A, 29–39.

Hansman, C. F. (1966). Growth of interorbital distance and skull thickness as observed in roentgenographic measurements. *Radiology*, 86, 87.

Hennekam, R. C. M., Cormier-Daire, V., Hall, J., Mehes, K., Patton, M., and Stevenson, R. (2009). Elements of morphology: Standard terminology for the Nose and philtrum. *American Journal of Medical Genetics Part A*, 149A, 61–76.

Hunter, A., Frias, J., Gillessen-Kaesbach, G., Hughes, H., Jones, K., and Wilson, L. (2009). Elements of morphology: Standard terminology for the ear. *American Journal of Medical Genetics Part A*, 149A, 40–60.

Iosub, S., Fuchs, M., Bingol, N., Stone, R. K., Gromisch, D. S., and Wasserman, E. (1985). Palpebral fissure length in Black and Hispanic children: correlation with head circumference. *Pediatrics*, 75, 318–320.

Laestadius, N. D., Aase, J. M., and Smith, D. W. (1969). Normal inner canthal and outer orbital dimensions. *Journal of Pediatrics*, 74, 465–468.

Lagrèze, W.A., Zobor, G. (2007). A method for noncontact measurement of corneal diameter in children. *American Journal of Ophthalmology*, 144, 141–142.

Martin, R., and Saller, K. (1962). *Lehrbuch der Anthropologie, Vol. 3.* (ed. G. Fischer), pp. 2051–2084. Stuttgart, Germany: Verlag.

McNamara, J. A., Jr. (1984). A method of cephalometric evaluation. *American Journal of Orthodontics*, 86, 449–469.

Mehes, K. (1974). Inner canthal and intermammary indices in the newborn infant. *Journal of Pediatrics*, 85, 90.

Merlob, P., Sivan, Y., and Reisner, S. H. (1984). Anthropometric measurements of the newborn infant 27 to 41 gestational weeks. *Birth Defects: Original Article Series*, 20, 7.

Moore, K. L. (1982). *The developing human* (3rd ed.). Philadelphia: W. B. Saunders.

Pashayen, H. (1973). A family with blepharo-naso-facial malformations. *American Journal of Diseases in Children*, 125, 389.

Patton, M. (1987). ONO angle. Personal communication.

Popich, G. A., and Smith, D.W. (1972). Fontanels: Range of normal size. *Journal of Pediatrics*, 80, 749–752.

Pruzansky, S. (1973). Clinical investigation of the experiments of nature. *ASHA Reports*, 8, 62–94

Ranly, D. M. (1980) *A synopsis of craniofacial growth*. New York: Prentice Hall.

Redman, R. S. (1963). Measurements of normal and reportedly malformed palatal vaults II: normal juvenile measurement. *Journal of Dental Research*, 45, 266.

Robinow, M., and Roche, A. F. (1973). Low-set ears. *American Journal of Diseases in Children*, 125, 482–483.

Saksena, S. S., Walker, G. F., Bixler, D., and Yu, P. -L. (1987). *A clinical atlas of roentgenocephalometry in norma lateralis*. New York: Alan R. Liss.

Schoenwolf, G. C., Francis-West, P. H., Brauer, P. R., and Bleyl, S. B. (2008). *Larsen's human embryology (4th ed.)*. Elsevier Health Sciences.

Shapiro, B. L., Redman, R. S., and Gorlin, R. J. (1963). Measurement of normal and reportedly malformed palatal vaults I: Normal adult measurements. *Journal of Dental Research*, 42, 1039.

Smith, D. W., and Gong, B. T. (1974). Scalp-hair patterning: Its origin and significance relative to early brain and upper facial development. *Teratology*, 9, 17–34.

Smith, D. W., and Takashima, H. (1980). Ear muscles and ear form. *Birth Defects: Original Article Series*, XVI(4), 299–302.

Thomas, I. T., Gaitantzis, Y. A., and Frias, J. L. (1987). Palepebral fissure length from 29 weeks gestation to 14 years. *Journal of Paediatrics*, III(2), 267–268. (2010). Evaluation of the accuracy of linear measurements on spiral computed tomography-derived three-dimensional images and its comparison with digital cephalometric radiography. 39(4), 216–223.

Zankl, A., Eberle, L., Molinari, L., and Schinzel, A. (2002). Growth charts for nose length, nasal protrusion and philtrum length from birth to 97 years. *American Journal of Medical Genetics*, 111, 388–391.

Chapter 8

Limbs

INTRODUCTION

Disturbance of limb growth generally leads to disproportion of the body, as the normal proportions of the body reflect changes in the relative size of the limbs at different ages.

The limb buds emerge as identifiable structures at about 4 weeks of embryonic development. Normal development depends on the interactions of developing vascular, nerve, muscle, and bony tissues. Initially, the limb is paddle shaped with a core of mesenchyme and a covering layer of epidermis. By 6 weeks, hand and foot plates can be seen and condensations of hyaline cartilage that will become bone are present (Figure 8.1). Normal limb structure is established by the end of the 8th week, and ossification begins shortly thereafter. The arms develop more rapidly than the legs and the right side slightly ahead of the left. Intrauterine movement is essential for normal development and function of limbs at birth. Normal limb length measurements at various times in gestation and in utero limb movement patterns are presented in Chapter 15.

The relative proportions of bone, skin, fat, and muscle change with age, as does the ratio of limb-to-trunk length. At birth, span is less than height and the lower segment length is much less than the upper segment. By age 10 years, the lower segment length approximately equals that of the upper segment. The limbs continue to grow disproportionately, and the lower segment becomes longer than the trunk, so that in the adult the upper-to-lower segment ratio is less than 1.0 (see Fig. 8.55). By about age 10 years in boys and 12 years

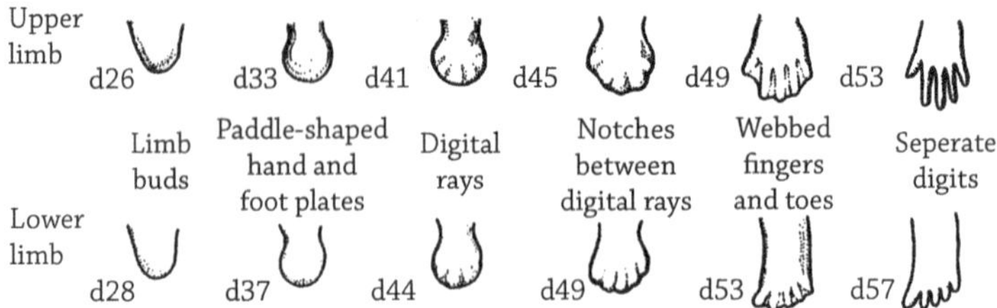

Figure 8.1. Embryologic limb development.

in girls, the span equals the height; thereafter, it exceeds height (see Fig. 8.3 and Fig. 8.57).

Many skeletal dysplasias result in disproportion of the limbs or some part of the limbs; the distal (acro), middle (meso), or proximal (rhizo) segments can be affected, either prenatally or postnatally. A variety of disorders demonstrate asymmetry of the body. One limb can be larger (hemihyperplasia or hemihypertrophy) or smaller (hemihypoplasia) than the other.

An approach to limb evaluation must include an assessment of the relative proportions of various tissues (fat, muscle, etc.) and comparison with normal age-related measurements. Bony prominences of the limbs provide good anatomical landmarks from which to measure, so that limb measurements have been well standardized. Various indices for comparison are available, but they have not been included in this text.

The inspection of limbs should answer the following questions:

1. Is the general proportion of limb-to-trunk length normal?
2. Are the limbs symmetric in length?
3. Are the limbs symmetric in circumference?
4. If one arm/leg is longer than the other, which part of the limb is longer?
5. Is there evidence of muscular or vascular anomalies?
6. Is the muscle mass symmetric?
7. Are the hands and feet symmetric in size and shape?
8. Are there contractures?

9. Are the fingers and toes symmetric in length and proportionate to the rest of the limbs?
10. Are fingernails/toenails present?
11. Do the nails have anomalies in size or shape?

The evaluation of the hands and feet includes examination of nails, skin (see Chapter 11), and flexion creases (Chapter 12).

The presence of incomplete separation of finger- or toe-rays is called syndactyly and can affect the skin only (cutaneous syndactyly) or the skin and bone (bony syndactyly).

Supernumerary digits or toes (polydactyly) can be found on the ulnar side of the hand (postaxial), the fibular side of the foot (postaxial), the radial side of the hand (preaxial), or the tibial side of the foot (preaxial); supernumerary digits can also occur between the rays (mesoaxial polydactyly). The supernumerary digits can be just an appendage of soft tissue or can contain bony parts. Radiographs will help to clarify how much of the underlying bony tissue is involved.

Terminology to describe congenital limb anomalies has been confusing. A glossary of terms to define specific anomalies is at the end of this book. Detailed information on the preferred nomenclature and illustrations are available in Biesecker et al. (2009).

SPAN

Definition Span is the distance between the fingertips of the middle fingers of each hand; the arms are stretched out horizontally from the body.

Landmarks With the arms completely extended horizontally from the body, measure between the tips of the middle fingers across the back or the front of the patient (Fig. 8.2).

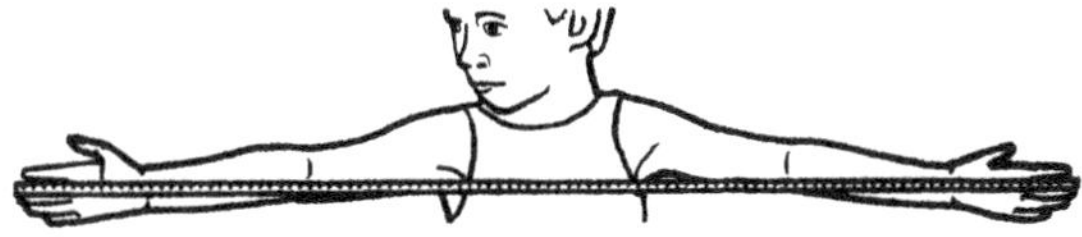

Figure 8.2. Measuring span.

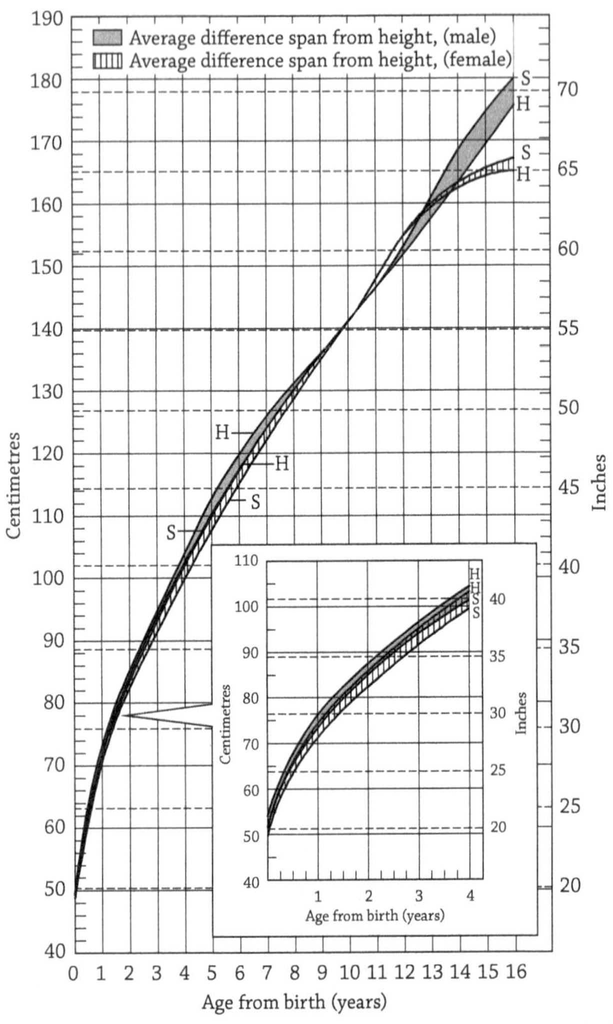

Figure 8.3. Span measured in centimeters, with average difference from height shaded, both sexes, birth to 16 years. Adapted from Belt-Niedbala et al. (1986). A normal span for age measurement is within 4.0 cm of the age-related median span.

Instruments Tape measure.

Position The patient may be standing or lying down with the arms completely extended.

Alternative Place the patient adjacent to a wall or blackboard, make marks at the tips of the middle fingers, and measure between the markings.

In the case of a squirming infant, the child may be placed prone on a bed or table, with the arms out to the sides. Measure across the back.

Remarks If the individual has a span greater than the standard 150 cm tape measure, simply bring the beginning end of the tape around and place it on the 150 cm point (be careful not to use the end of the tape) and continue the measurement, adding the additional distance to 150 cm.

In infancy and early childhood, span is less than height. By about 10 years in males and 12 years in females, span equals height; thereafter, it exceeds height.

Pitfalls The patient with contractures or limitations of full extension (as in achondroplasia) may give falsely low values unless the tape is worked along the contracture.

TOTAL UPPER LIMB (HAND AND ARM) LENGTH

Definition Length of the whole arm (the arm and hand combined).

Landmarks Measure between the acromion (the most prominent posterior lateral bony prominence of the shoulder joint) and the tip of the middle finger (Figures. 8.4, 8.5 and 8.6).

Instruments Tape measure or calipers.

Position Stand the patient erect with arms hanging loosely down at the side, parallel to the body.

Alternative In patients who cannot stand, the arms can be measured while the patient lies down with the arms parallel to the body.

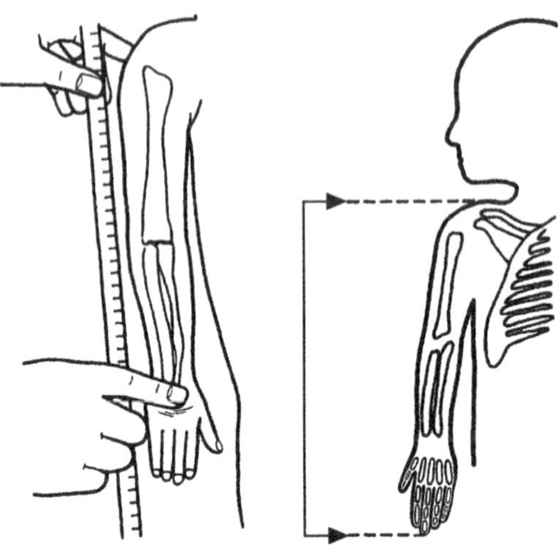

Figure 8.4. Measuring total upper limb length.

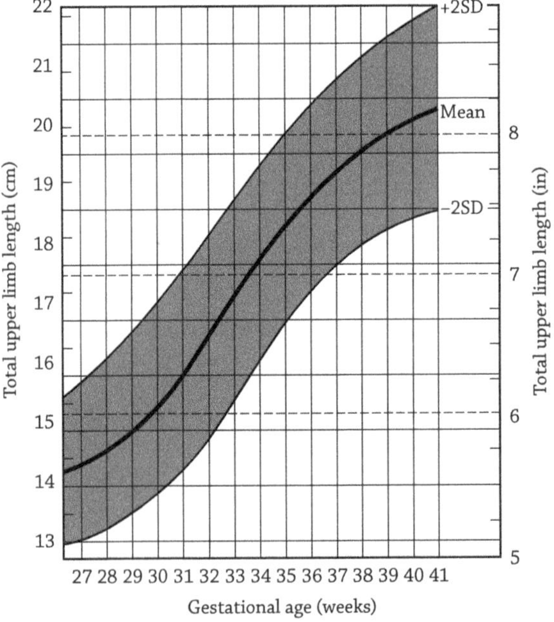

Figure 8.5. Total upper limb length at birth. From Sivan et al. (1983) and Merlob et al. (1984a), by permission.

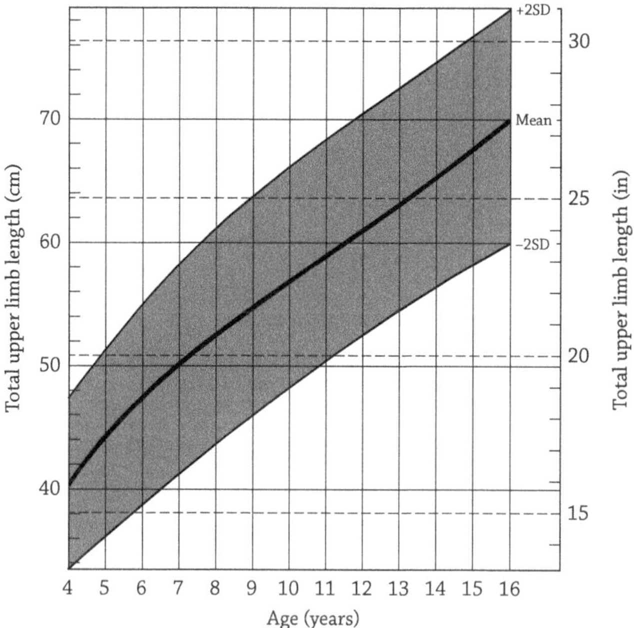

Figure 8.6. Total upper limb length, both sexes, 4 to 16 years. From Martin and Saller (1962), by permission.

Measurement of arm length by X-ray is more accurate, but the limb must be positioned properly.

Remarks The arms account for approximately 11% of the total body weight in the age group 0.5–3.0 years in boys (10% in girls) and for 13% of total body weight in the age group 3–13 years in boys (16% in girls).

In individuals with contractures, a tape measure should be worked along the limb.

UPPER ARM LENGTH

Definition Length of the upper arm or proximal (rhizomelic) segment of the arm.

Landmarks Measure from the acromion (the most prominent posterior lateral bony prominence of the shoulder joint) along the posterior lateral aspect of the arm until reaching the distal medial border of the olecranon (Fig. 8.7).

Instruments Tape measure or calipers.

Position Stand the patient erect, with arms held loosely at the side and elbows slightly bent.

Alternative The patient may lie in bed, supine, or prone, with the arms at the side of the body and elbow slightly bent. Measurement of upper arm length by radiograph is more accurate, but the limb must be positioned properly.

Remarks Typical values per upper arm length at birth and from age 4 to 16 years are presented in Figures 8.8–8.10.

Pitfalls A dislocated shoulder will give an abnormally long measurement.

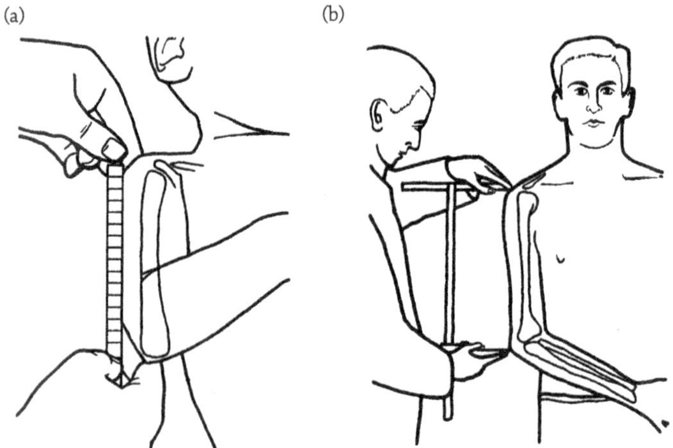

Figure 8.7. Measuring upper arm length.

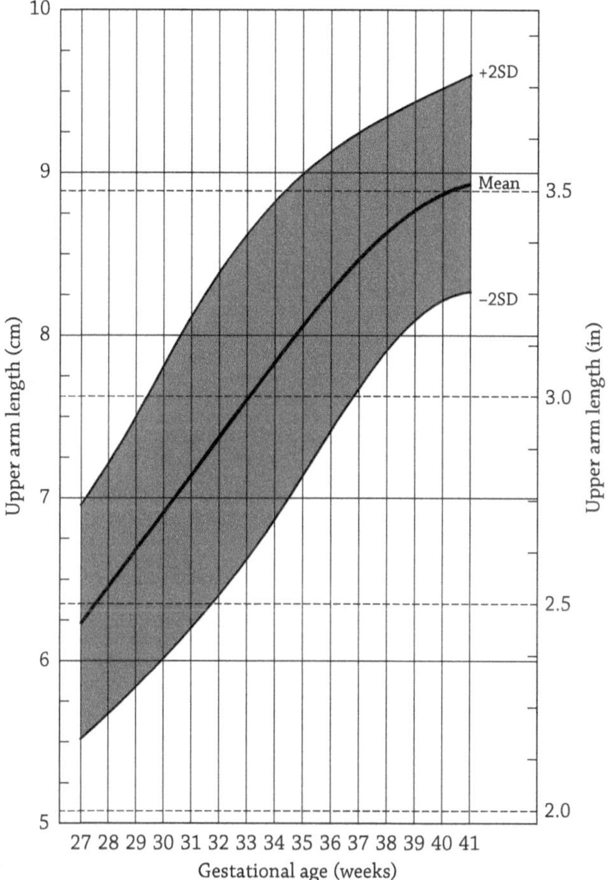

Figure 8.8. Upper arm length, both sexes, at birth. From Merlob et al. (1984a)), by permission.

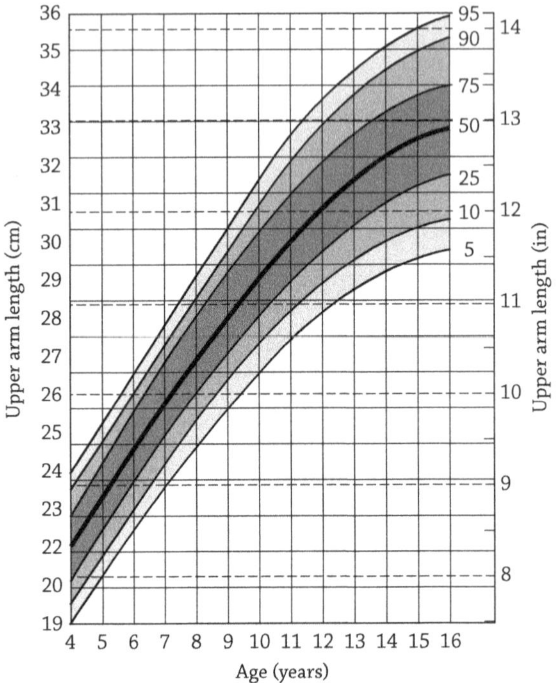

Figure 8.9. Upper arm length, males, 4 to 16 years. From Malina et al. (1973), by permission.

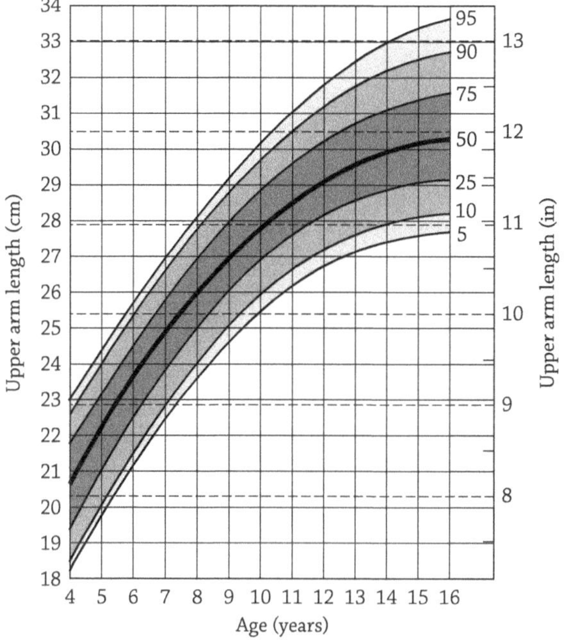

Figure 8.10. Upper arm length, females, 4 to 16 years. From Malina et al. (1973), by permission.

FOREARM LENGTH

Definition Length of the forearm or middle (mesomelic) segment of the arm.

Landmarks Measure the distance from the most prominent point of the olecranon to the distal lateral process of the radius along the lateral surface of the forearm (Fig. 8.11).

Instruments Tape measure or calipers.

Position The patient stands or sits with the upper arm hanging at the side and the elbow bent at a 90 degree angle; the arm should be held in a neutral position (not in supination or pronation), with the hand in a vertical plane.

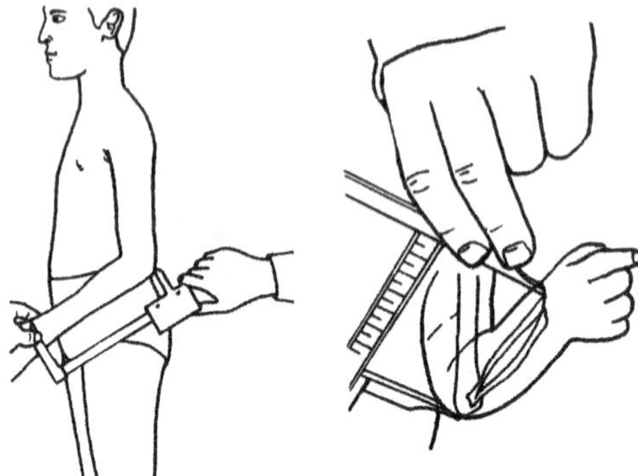

Figure 8.11. Measuring forearm length.

Alternative Measurement by radiograph is more accurate, but the arm must be positioned properly with the forearm in neutral position.

Remarks Forearm lengths are presented in Figures 8.12–8.14. Although this may seem to be an awkward measurement, standards are available from anthropological studies. These distances obviously do not represent single bone lengths, but they do allow assessment of the different segments and proportions of the arm.

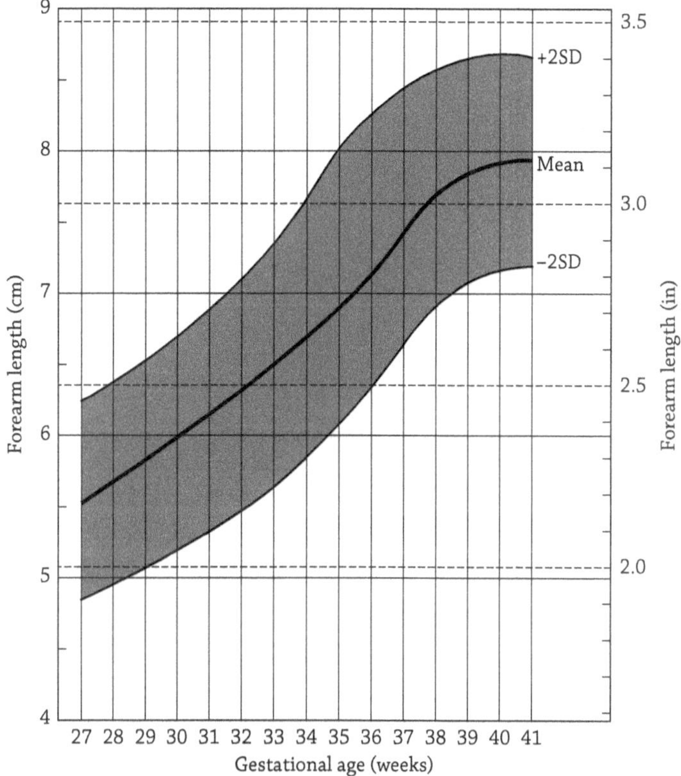

Figure 8.12. Forearm length, both sexes, at birth. From Merlob et al. (1984a), by permission.

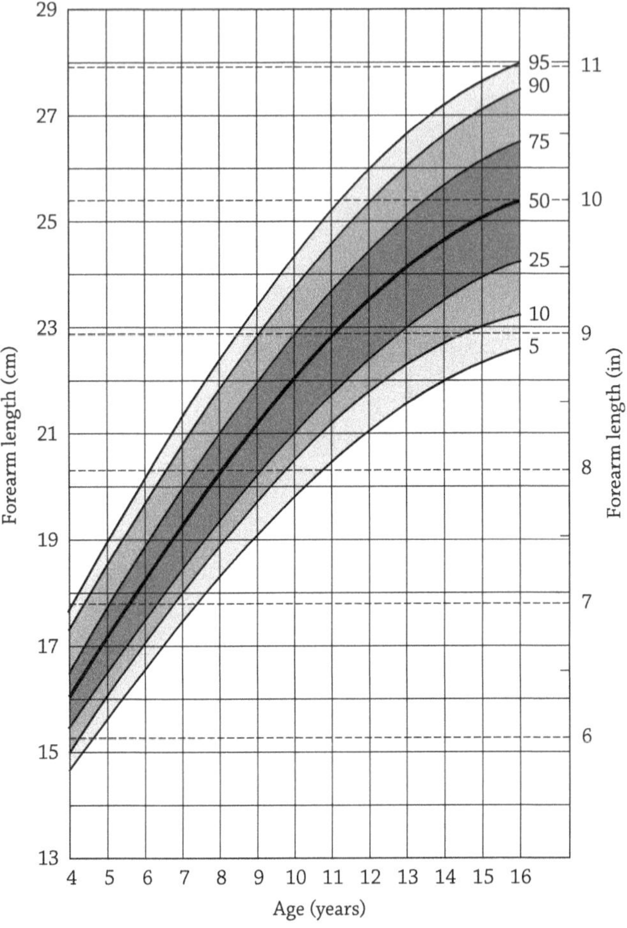

Figure 8.13. Forearm length, males, 4 to 16 years. From Roche and Malina (1983), by permission.

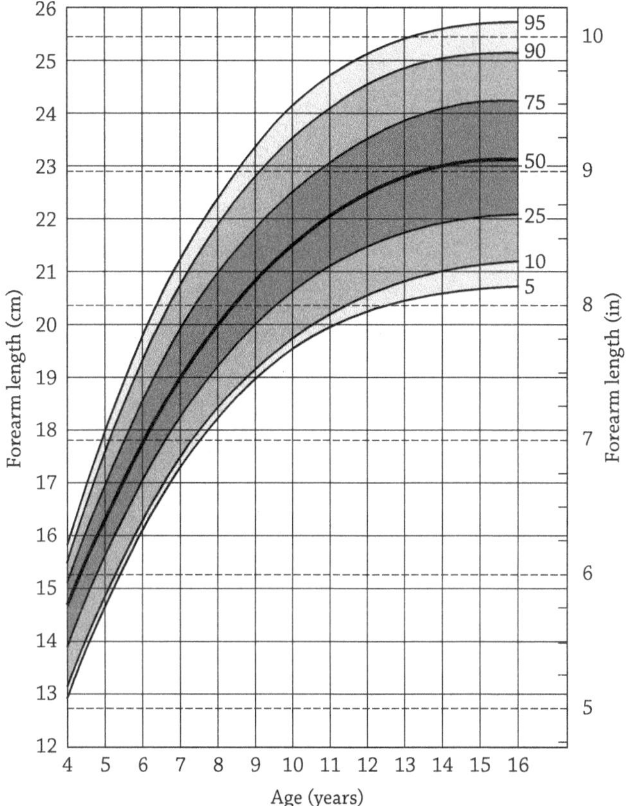

Figure 8.14. Forearm length, females, 4 to 16 years. From Roche and Malina (1983), by permission.

CARRYING ANGLE

Definition The carrying angle is the angle subtended by the forearm on the humerus (the deviation of the forearm relative to the humerus or the angle at the elbow joint).

Landmarks Draw an imaginary line (A) through the axis of the upper arm extending down to a distance equivalent to the hand. Draw a second imaginary line (B) through the axis of the forearm and hand. The angle between these two lines, at the elbow, is the carrying angle (Fig. 8.15).

Instruments A goniometer or "eyeball estimate" of the angle between the two lines.

Position Stand the patient with the shoulders hanging loosely, the palms facing anteriorly, the hands in the same plane as the body, and the arms fully extended. The elbow is extended and the forearm supinated.

Alternative The patient may lie supine with the upper arm parallel to the body and the lower arm supinated, elbow extended, and the back of the hand against the bed. Photograph the patient in one of the above positions and measure the angle from the photograph.

Remarks Normal values for carrying angle are shown in Figure 8.16. The carrying angle is usually greater in women than in men and increases slightly with age. The normal range is between 7 and 22 degrees with a mean of 14 degrees in the male and 16 degrees in the female. The carrying angle may be altered by abnormalities of the elbow joint. Sex chromosome aneuploidy often affects the carrying angle.

Pitfalls If there is limited extension of the elbow or if the arm cannot be fully supinated, the carrying angle will be difficult to assess. Radial head dislocation should not affect the carrying angle.

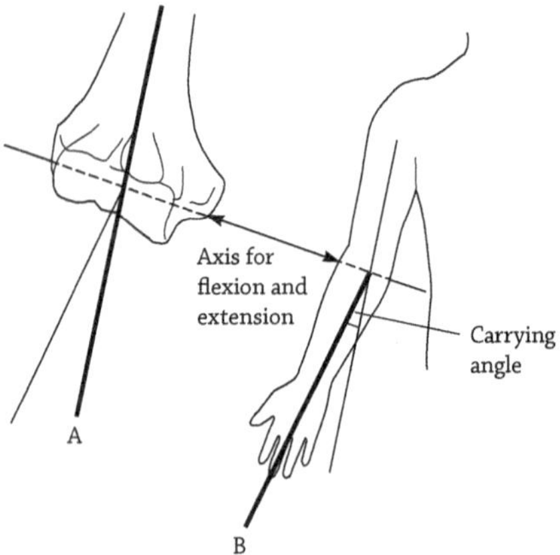

Figure 8.15. Landmarks for measurement of carrying angle.

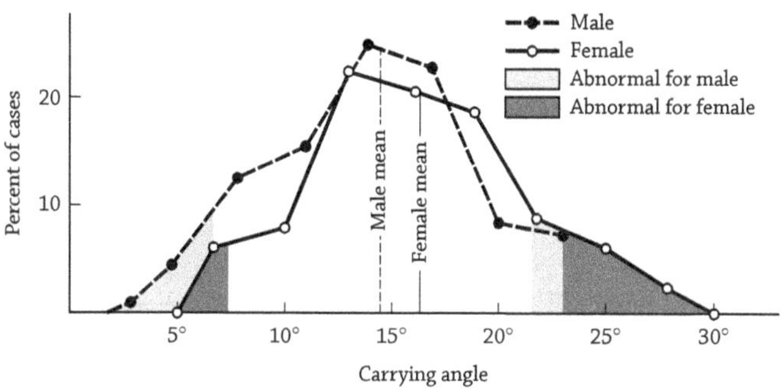

Figure 8.16. Carrying angle norms. From Atkinson and Elftman (1945), by permission.

HAND LENGTH

Definition Total length of the hand.

Landmarks Measure from the distal crease at the wrist to the tip of the middle finger (Fig. 8.17).

Instruments Tape measure, calipers, or clear ruler.

Position The wrist is held in neutral position, and the fingers are fully extended. The measurement is taken on the palmar aspect of the hand.

Alternative Draw a line around the hand and measure from an estimated point where the wrist begins.

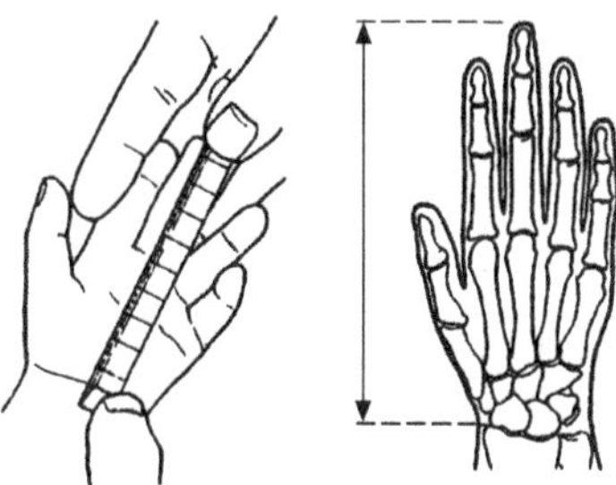

Figure 8.17. Measuring hand length.

Remarks Some patients have multiple wrist creases; choose the most distal crease.

Normal values are shown in Figures 8.18–8.20. There are no significant differences in hand length between males and females.

Pitfalls It may be necessary to evaluate various segments of the hand separately.

In individuals with contractures of the wrist or hand, the tape should be pressed along the palm of the hand, eliminating false reduction in length.

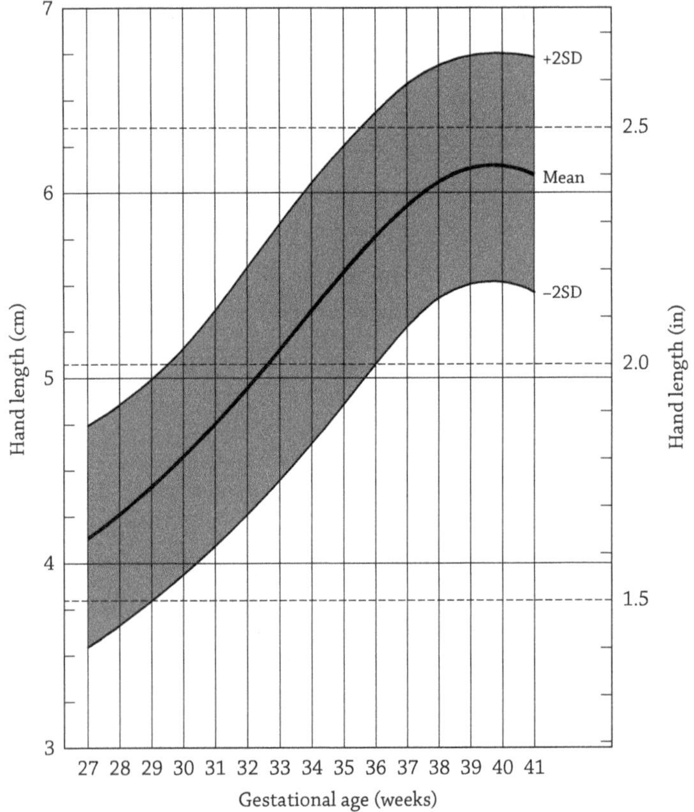

Figure 8.18. Hand length, both sexes, at birth. From Merlob et al. (1984a), by permission.

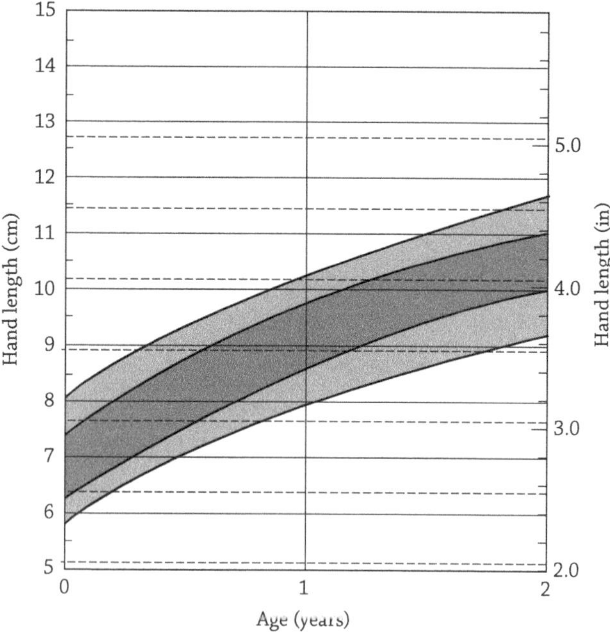

Figure 8.19. Hand length, both sexes, birth to 2 years. From Feingold and Bossert (1974), by permission.

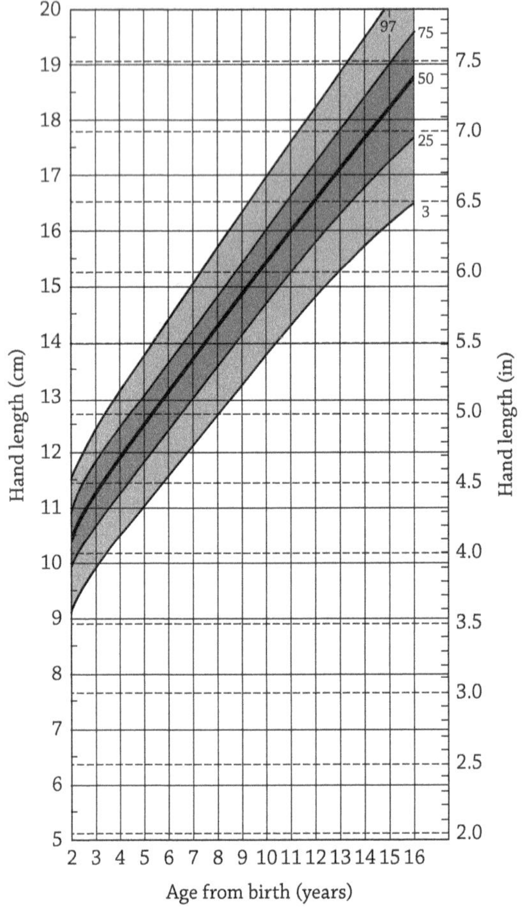

Figure 8.20. Hand length, both sexes, 2 to 16 years. From Feingold and Bossert (1974), by permission.

MIDDLE FINGER LENGTH

Definition Total length of middle finger.

Landmarks Measure from the proximal flexion crease at the base of the middle finger to the tip of the middle finger. The measurement is taken on the palmar aspect of the hand (Fig. 8.21).

Instruments Tape measure, calipers, or clear ruler.

Position The wrist is in a neutral position and the hand is fully extended.

Alternative Draw around hand and estimate where the proximal flexion crease of the middle finger would be; then measure from the paper.

Remarks The proximal finger crease on the palmar aspect of the hand is about 1–2 cm distal to the knuckle on the dorsal aspect of the hand; therefore, this measurement does not reflect the sum of the lengths of the phalanges of the middle finger. Middle finger lengths from birth to age 16 years are shown in Figures 8.22–8.24.

Pitfalls In some forms of brachydactyly, measurement of the middle finger will not reflect the lengths of the other digits. In individuals with contractures, work the tape along the finger in order to get a measurement equivalent to total finger length.

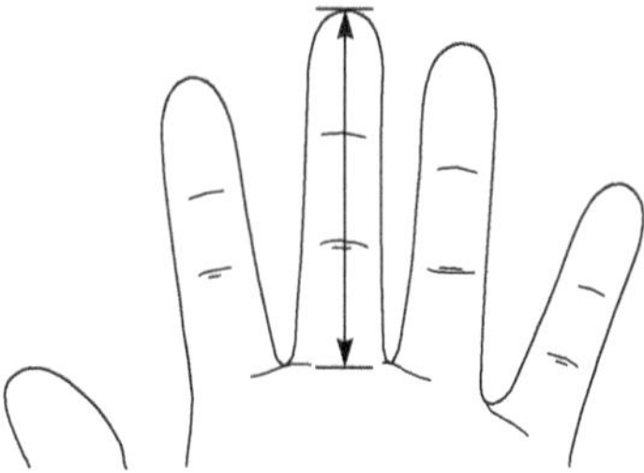

Figure 8.21. Measuring middle finger length.

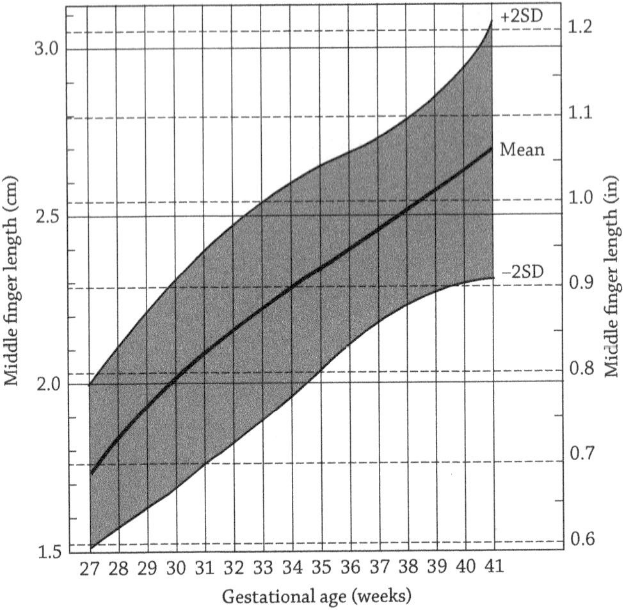

Figure 8.22. Middle finger length, both sexes, at birth. From Merlob et al. (1984c), by permission.

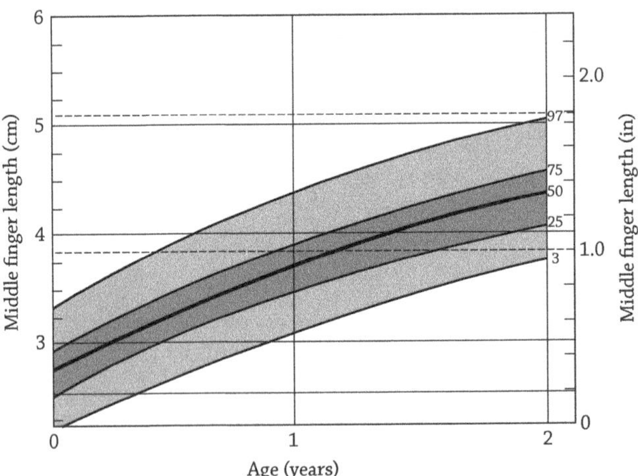

Figure 8.23(a). Middle finger length, both sexes, birth to 2 years. From Feingold and Bossert (1974), by permission.

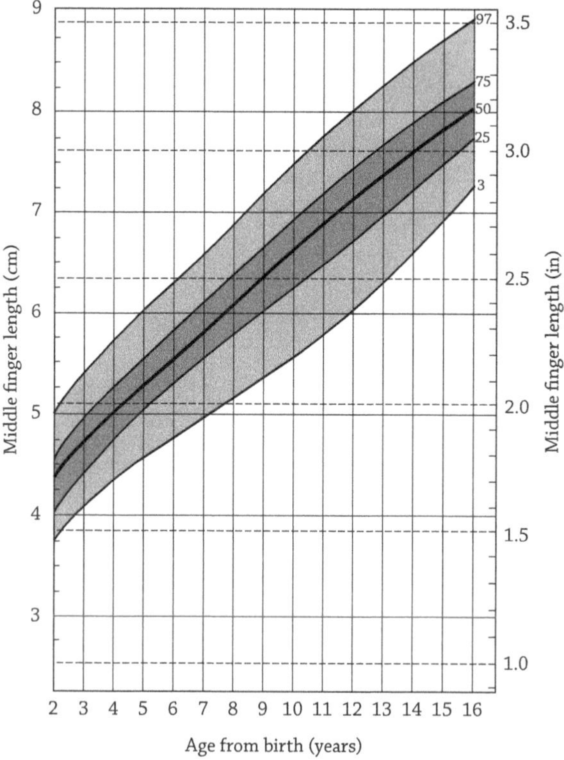

Figure 8.23(b). Middle finger length, both sexes, 2 to 16 years. From Feingold and Bossert (1974), by permission.

PALM LENGTH

Definition Total length of the palm.

Landmarks Measure between the distal flexion crease at the wrist and the proximal flexion crease of the middle finger (Fig. 8.24).

Instruments Tape measure, calipers, or clear ruler.

Position The wrist is in a neutral position and the fingers are fully extended. The measurement is taken on the palmar aspect of the hand.

Alternative Subtract the middle finger length from the total hand length. Draw around the hand and then measure the palm length from the drawing, estimating the position of the creases.

Remarks Palm lengths from birth to age 16 years are shown in Figures 8.25 and 8.26. A ratio of middle finger to total hand length (Fig. 8.27) is helpful in defining relative disproportion in the hand.

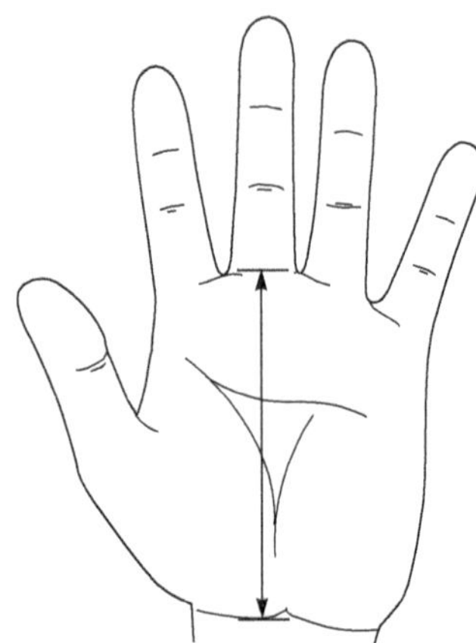

Figure 8.24. Measuring palm length.

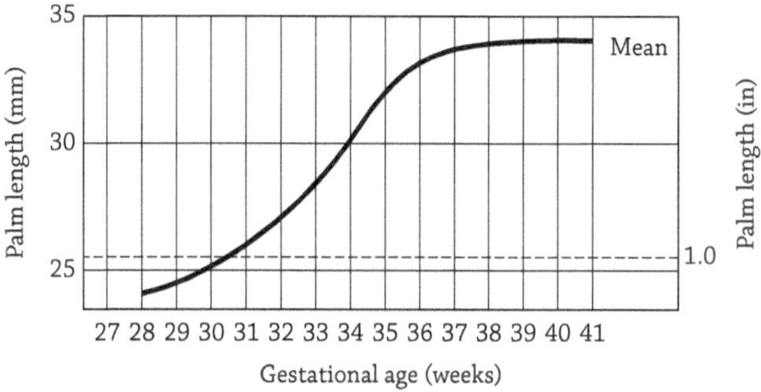

Figure 8.25. Palm length, both sexes, at birth. From Sivan et al. (1983), by permission.

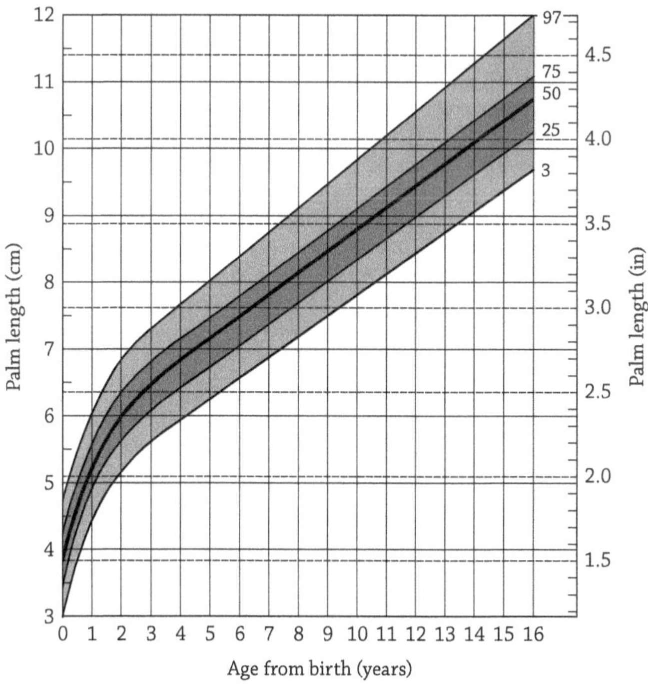

Figure 8.26. Palm length, both sexes, birth to 16 years. From Feingold and Bossert (1974), by permission.

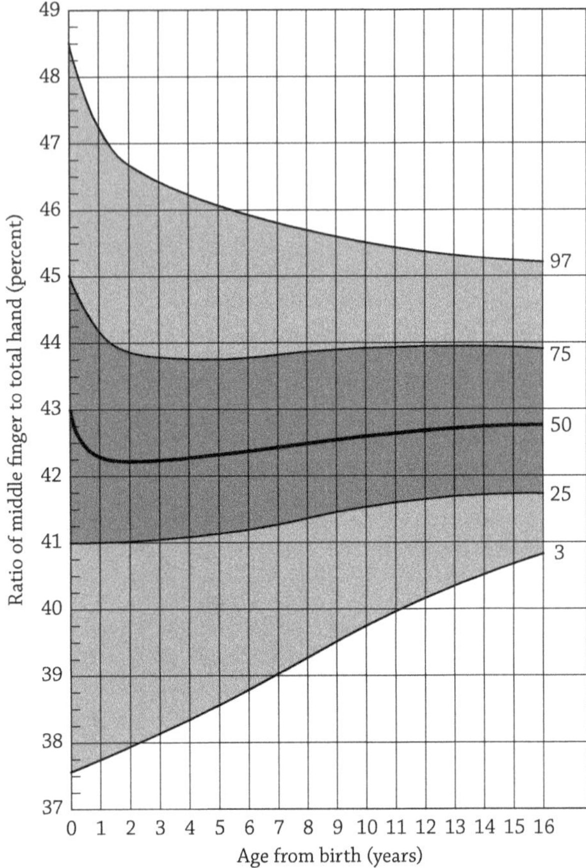

Figure 8.27. Ratio of middle finger to total hand, both sexes, birth to 16 years. From Feingold and Bossert (1974), by permission.

PALM WIDTH

Definition Width of the palm of the hand.

Landmarks Measure from the edge of the hand on one side, across the palm to the edge of the hand on the other side, at the level of the metacarpophalangeal joints, with the fingers parallel and extended (Fig. 8.28).

Instruments Tape measure, calipers, or clear ruler.

Position The wrist is in a neutral position with the fingers fully extended. The measurement can be taken on either side of the hand, but preferably it is taken across the palm.

Alternative Draw a line around the hand and measure between the markings at the level of the metacarpophalangeal joints.

Remarks Palm widths are shown separately for males and females in Figures 8.29 and 8.30. In a hyperextensible hand, care must be taken not to squash the hand excessively, since this can alter the measurement.

The ratio of hand length to hand width changes considerably during intrauterine life. The hand form becomes relatively thinner and longer by the end of intrauterine life. This tendency continues until about 5 years of age. From then on, hand length and width increase relatively proportionately (Fig. 8.31).

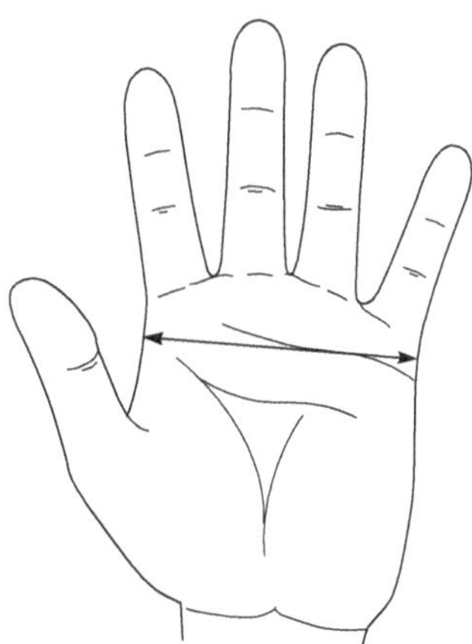

Figure 8.28. Measuring palm width.

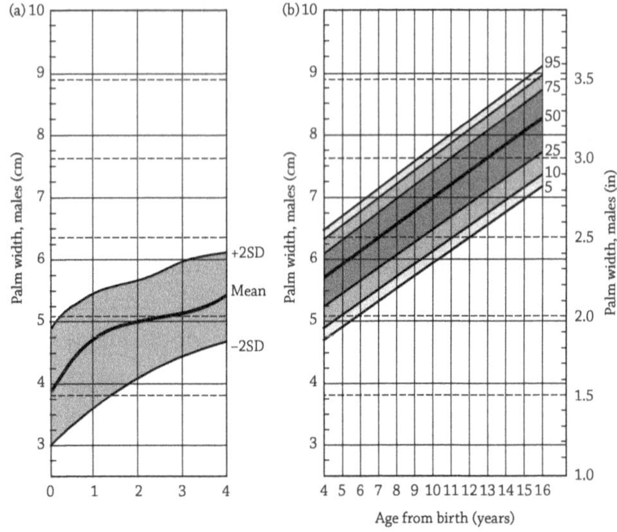

Figure 8.29. (a) Palm width, males, birth to 4 years. From Snyder et al. (1975) and Malina et al. (1973), by permission. (b) Palm width, males, 4 to 16 years. From Snyder et al. (1975) and Malina et al. (1973), by permission.

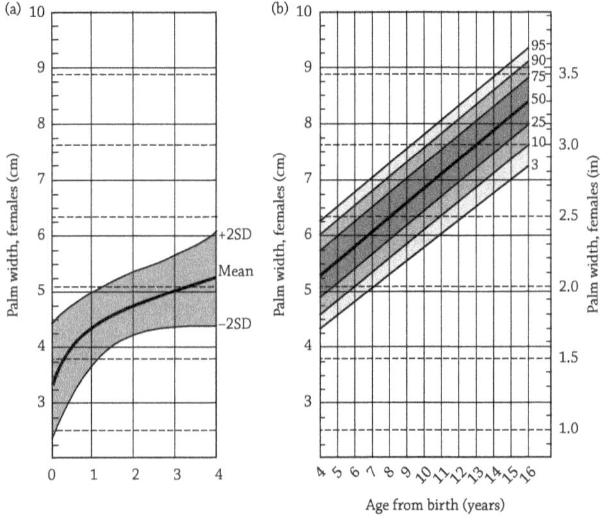

Figure 8.30. (a) Palm width, females, birth to 4 years. From Snyder et al. (1975) and Malina et al. (1973), by permission. (b) Palm width, females, 4 to 16 years. From Snyder et al. (1975) and Malina et al. (1973), by permission.

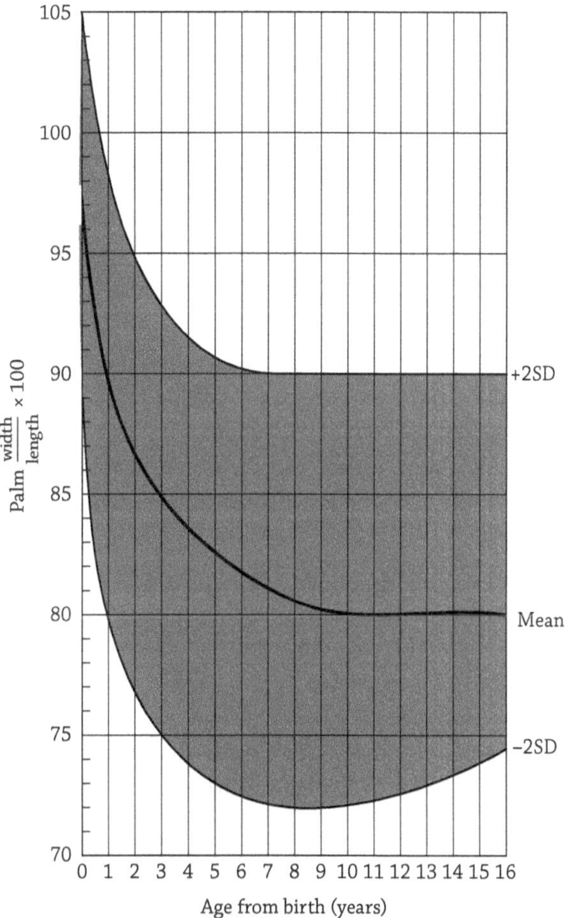

Figure 8.31. Ratio of palm width to palm length, both sexes, birth to 16 years. From Snyder et al. (1975) and Malina et al. (1973), by permission.

THUMB POSITION, PLACEMENT, AND RANGE OF MOVEMENT

Introduction

The position, placement, and range of movement of the thumb may be atypical. Photographs often delineate differences from the norm better than measurements; however, the two methods presented next have been established to describe atypical thumb position and movement.

The size of the thumb should be assessed. If the tip of the thumb is below the proximal crease at the base of the index finger when the thumb is held parallel to the hand, then the thumb is either hypoplastic or proximally placed; if the tip of the thumb is above the interphalangeal joint of the index finger, it is too long or digitalized.

Method 1. Thumb Placement Index

Definition Ratio of the distance between (1) the distance between the proximal flexion crease (A) at the base of the index finger and the distal insertion (B) of the thumb (Fig. 8.32a) and (2) the distance between the proximal crease (a) at the base of the index finger and the distal flexion crease (b) at the wrist (Fig. 8.32b).

Landmarks The first measurement (1) is taken on the lateral aspect of the index finger: Measure from the proximal crease at the base of the index finger to the basal crease of the thumb insertion. The second measurement (2) is taken from the proximal crease at the base of the index finger, on the palmar aspect, to the distal flexion crease at the wrist.

Instruments Tape measure, calipers, or clear ruler.

Position Maintain the thumb in 90 degrees abduction.

$$\text{Thumb placement index} = \frac{(1)}{(2)} = 0.51 \pm 0.04$$

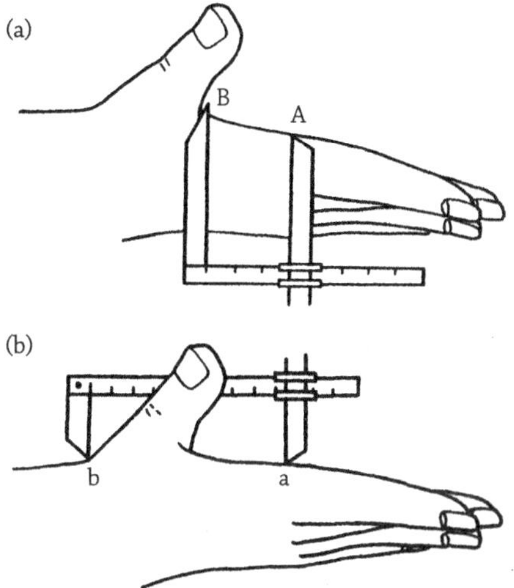

Figure 8.32(a–b). Measuring thumb placement.

Remarks If the thumb is digitalized, it may not be possible to abduct it to 90 degrees, but the creases will probably still be identifiable.

Alternative Draw around the hand with the thumb held in 90 degrees abduction and measure between the points mentioned.

Method 2. Angle of Thumb Attachment

Definition The angles of movement of the thumb (Fig. 8.33).

Landmarks With the hand at rest on a flat surface, palm up, fingers parallel, and thumb extended and abducted away from the palm as far as possible comfortably, draw an imaginary line through the main axis of the index finger and another imaginary line through the main axis of the thumb. Measure the angle made by the imaginary lines (Fig. 8.33a). Keeping the same hand position with the palm up, pick the thumb up from the flat surface and, keeping the thumb fully extended, rotate the thumb toward the palm, and measure the angle made by the thumb from the flat surface (Fig. 8.33b).

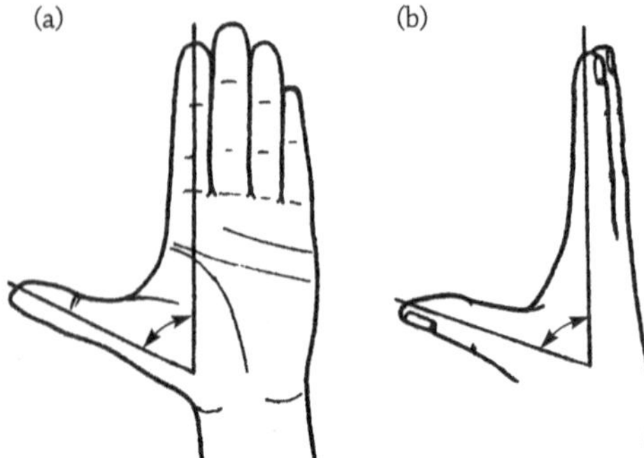

Figure 8.33(a–b). Measuring the angles of thumb attachment.

If either of the angles is greater than 90 degrees or less than 75 degrees, abnormal thumb joint movement is present.

Instruments A goniometer or "eyeball estimate" of the angle between the two lines.

Position Keep hand palm up and flat against a hard surface with fingers parallel. Keep thumb fully extended as it moves through its range of motion.

Remarks These measurements reflect thumb placement and flexibility.

TOTAL LOWER LIMB LENGTH

Definition Total length of the lower limb (including leg and foot).

Landmarks In older children and adults, the total lower limb length is measured from the greater trochanter to the plane of the sole of the foot (floor) (Fig. 8.34). Traditionally, in infants, leg length has been measured from the greater trochanter of the femur to the lateral malleolus of the ankle along the lateral aspect of the leg (total lower limb lengths are not available).

Instruments Tape measure or calipers.

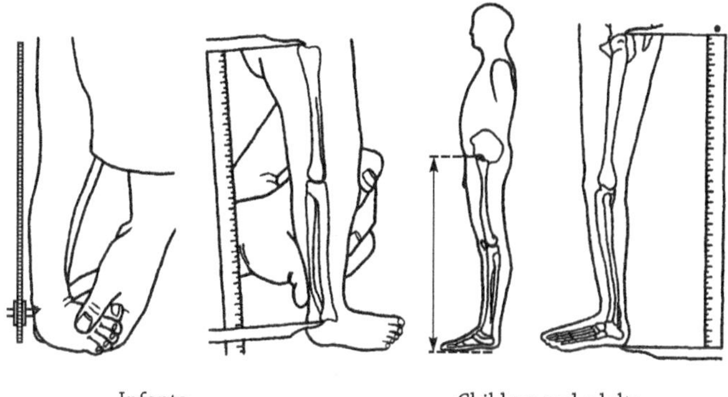

Infants Children and adults

Figure 8.34. Measuring total lower limb length.

Position Infants may be measured lying supine or prone. Older children and adults are usually measured standing upright with the legs parallel.

Alternative In children and adults, lower limb length can be calculated from total body length by subtracting upper segment or sitting height, although this is not as accurate as direct measurement.

Remarks By tradition, leg length in infants is measured only to the ankle. The newborn graphs reflect that measurement rather than total lower limb length (Fig. 8.35). Values for older children are shown in Figures 8.36 and 8.37.

In individuals with contractures or genu valgum or varum, the tape has to be worked along the leg to give an accurate estimate of total leg length.

Radiographic measurements are more precise for assessment of bone length.

The highest point of the trochanter may be difficult to find in obese individuals. It may be helpful to ask the patient to bend forward and to estimate the trochanter point.

Lower limbs account for approximately one-third of length at birth; by 5 years, the lower limbs account for one-half of height, and by adulthood, more than one-half the total height.

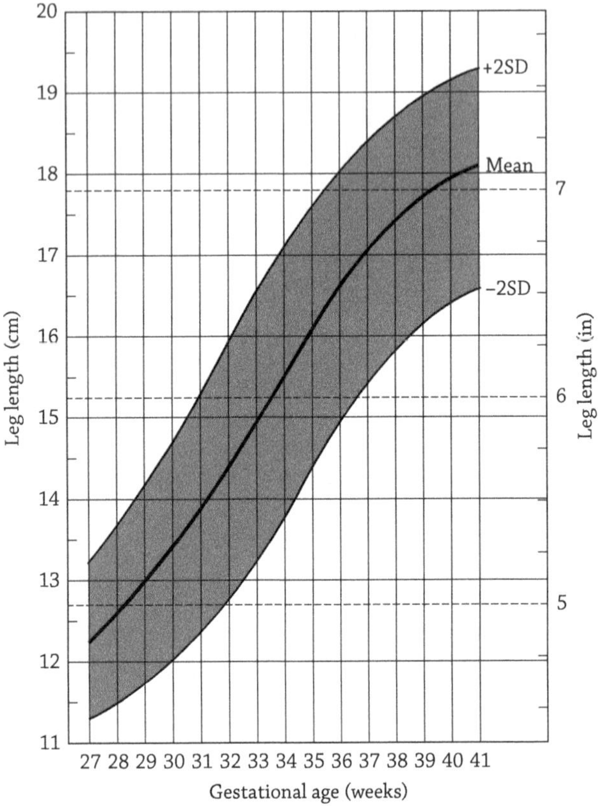

Figure 8.35. Leg length at birth. From Merlob et al. (1984b), by permission.

Pitfalls In infants, the sum of the upper and lower leg measurements, as demonstrated in this book, do not equal total limb measurement. Leg length is not equivalent to lower segment, which is measured from the pubis to the plane of the sole (i.e., floor).

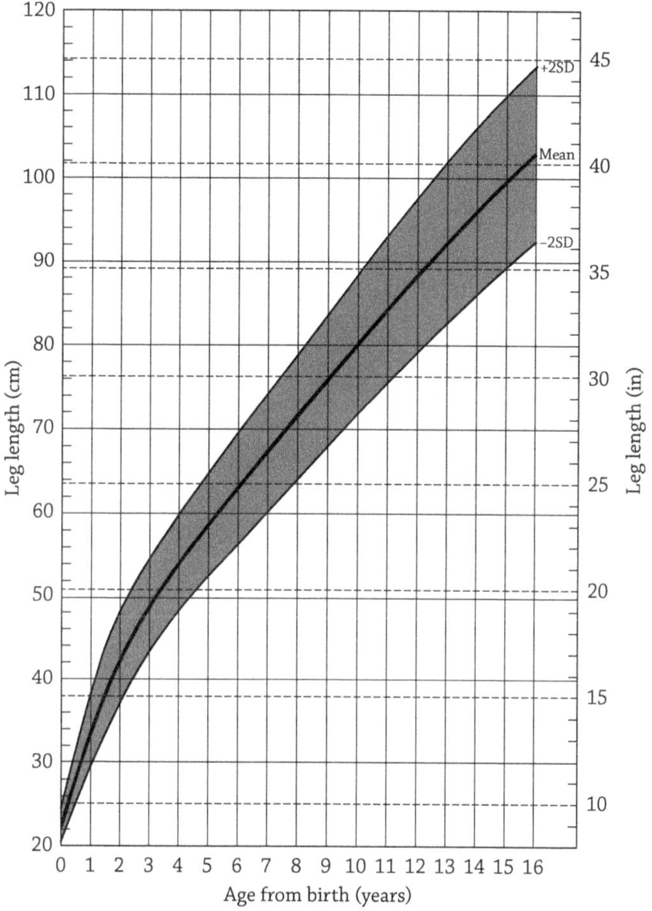

Figure 8.36. Leg length, males, birth to 16 years. From Snyder et al. (1975), by permission.

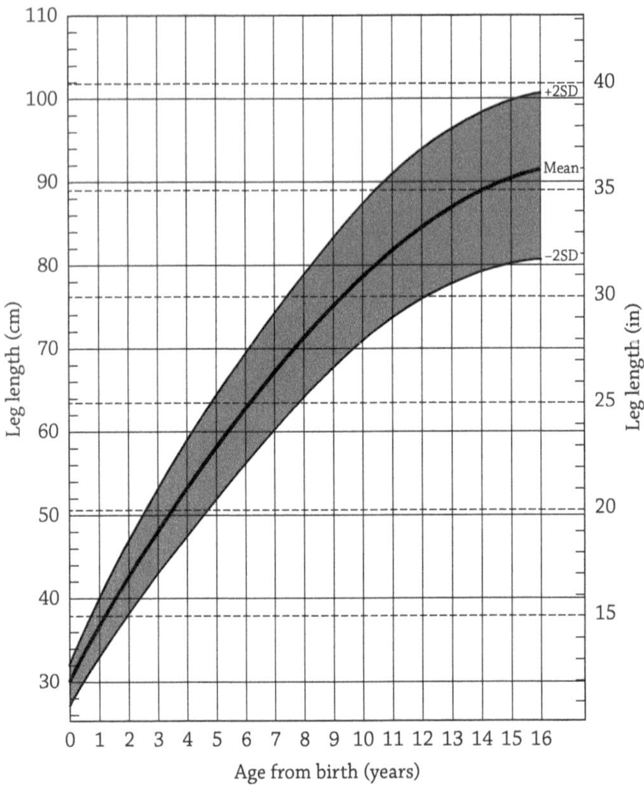

Figure 8.37. Leg length, females, birth to 16 years. From Snyder et al. (1975), by permission.

UPPER LEG (THIGH) LENGTH

Definition Total length of the upper leg.

Landmarks Measure from the greater trochanter of the femur to the proximal lateral tibial condyle along the lateral aspect of the leg (Fig. 8.38).

Instruments Tape measure or calipers.

Position Patient can stand or be lying supine.

Alternative Radiographic measurements of the femur are more precise.

Remarks When there is disproportion between the thighs, it is useful to measure circumference in addition to length for documentation. Radiographic measurements are more reliable when limb shortening or asymmetry is present. Normal values are presented in Figures 8.39 and 8.40.

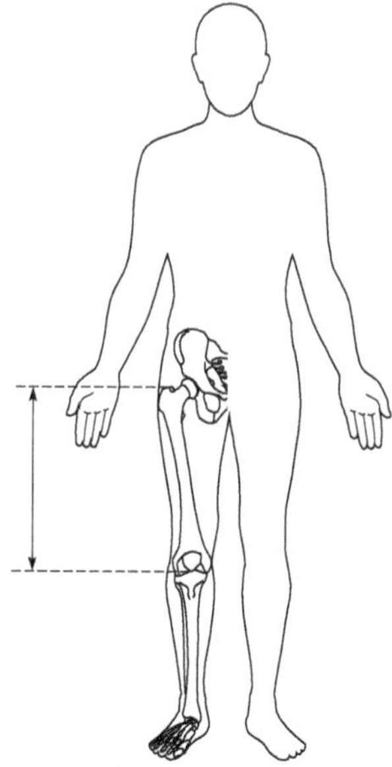

Figure 8.38. Measuring thigh length.

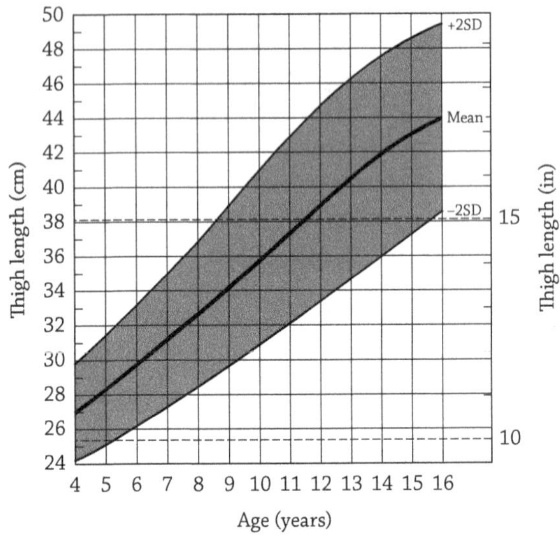

Figure 8.39. Upper leg length, males, 4 to 16 years. From Krogman (1983) and Roche and Malina (1983), by permission.

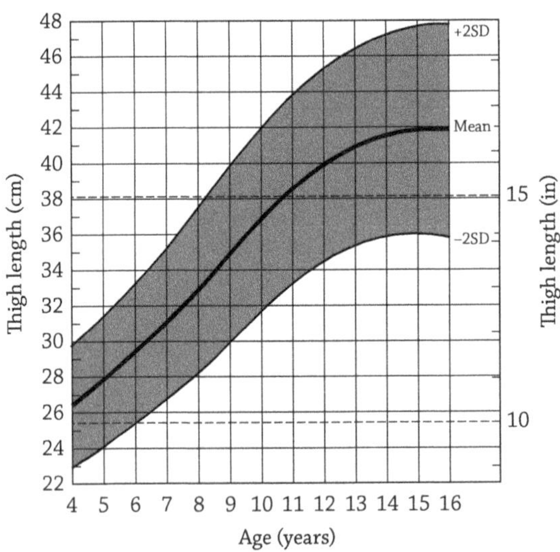

Figure 8.40. Upper leg length, females, 4 to 16 years. From Krogman (1983) and Roche and Malina (1983), by permission.

LOWER LEG (CALF) LENGTH

Definition Total length of the lower leg.

Landmarks In children and adults, measure from the proximal lateral condyle of the tibia to a plane equivalent to the sole of the foot (floor) along the lateral aspect of the leg. In infants, the measurement is made from the lateral upper condyle of the tibia to the lateral malleolus of the ankle (Fig. 8.41).

Instruments Tape measure or calipers.

Position Standing upright.

Alternative The patient may be sitting or lying down.

Remarks In individuals with contractures of the foot, it may be more accurate to use radiographs. When there is a discrepancy between the two legs, the circumference should also be measured. Normal values are shown in Figures 8.42–8.44.

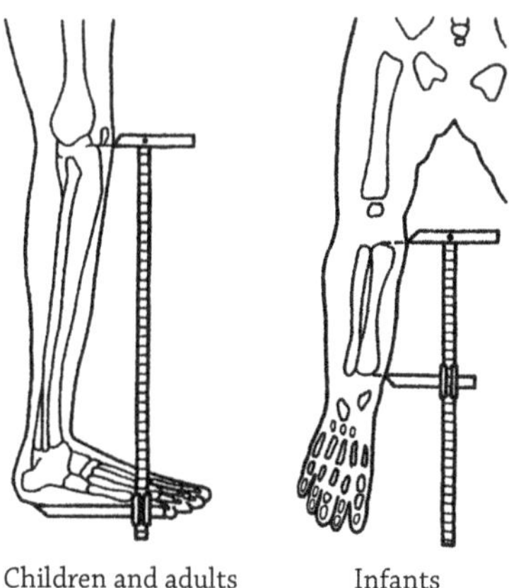

Figure 8.41. Measuring calf length.

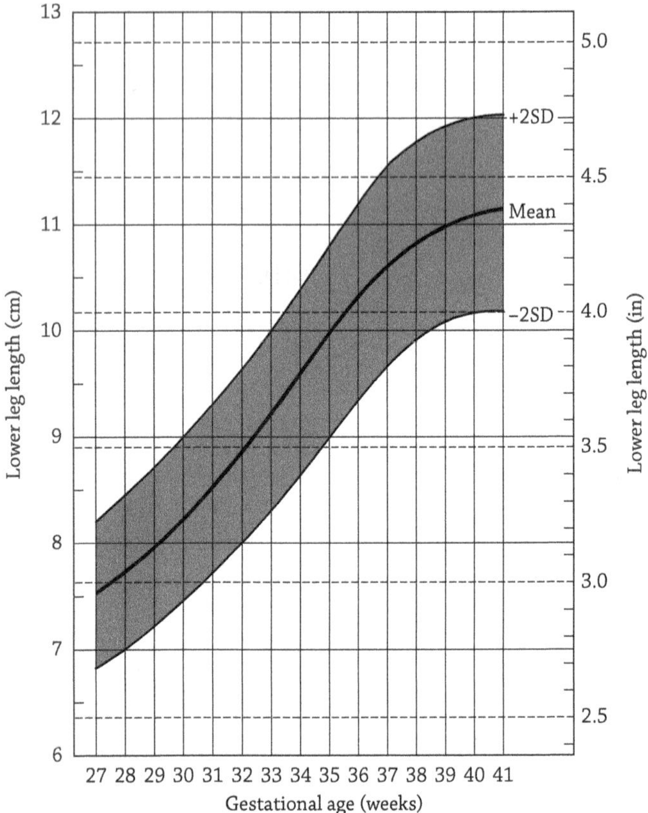

Figure 8.42. Lower leg length at birth, both sexes. From Merlob et al. (1984b), by permission.

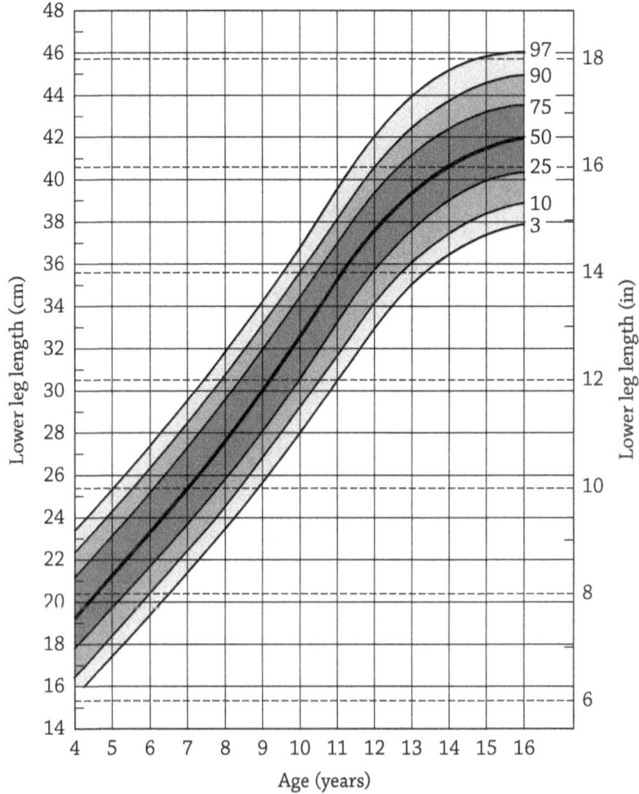

Figure 8.43. Lower leg length, males, 4 to 16 years. From Roche and Malina (1983), by permission.

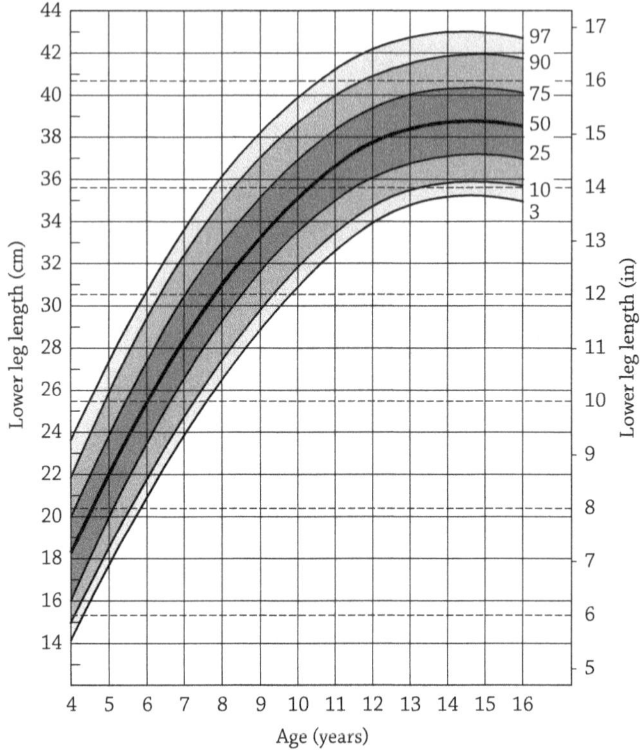

Figure 8.44. Lower leg length, females, 4 to 16 years. From Roche and Malina (1983), by permission.

FOOT LENGTH

Definition Total length of foot.

Landmarks Usually the foot length is the longest axis of the foot. It is measured from an imaginary vertical line drawn from the posterior prominence of the heel, to the tip of the longest toe, on the plantar aspect of the foot (in some people, the first toe is the longest; in other people, the second toe is the longest) (Fig. 8.45).

Instruments Tape measure or clear ruler.

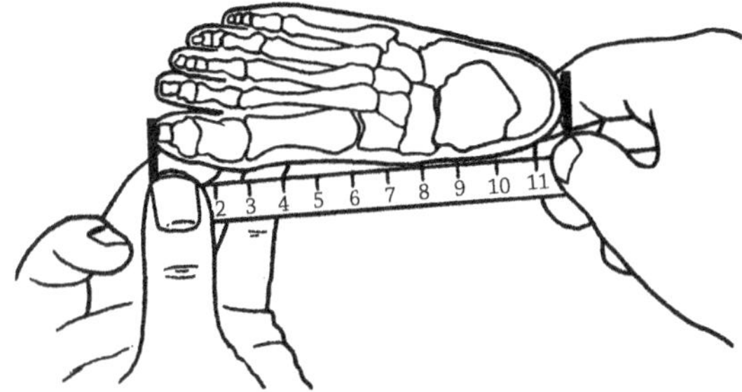

Figure 8.45. Measuring foot length.

Position The length of the foot is easily and most accurately measured by standing the individual on a tape measure.

Alternative Measurement of the foot may also be taken with the patient in a relaxed sitting position or lying down. The ankle should be perpendicular to the foot. Draw around the foot and take the measurement between the tip of the longest toe and the edge of the prominence of the heel.

Remarks In patients with contractures of the foot, the tape may be worked along the sole to give an estimate of the length. Values for foot length to age 16 years are presented in Figures 8.46–8.48.

Pitfalls In individuals with talipes or very high arches, measurements may be distorted or difficult to obtain.

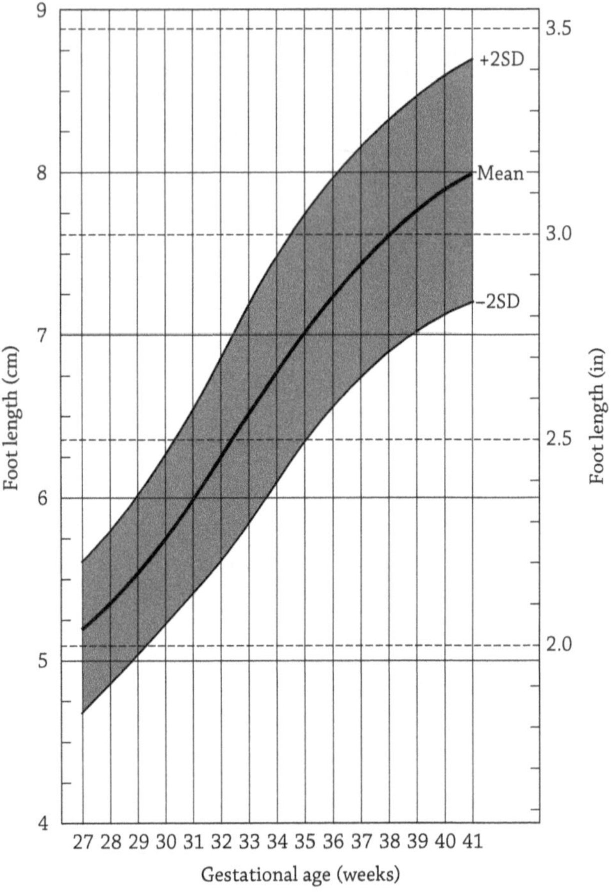

Figure 8.46. Foot length, both sexes, at birth. From Merlob et al. (1984b), by permission.

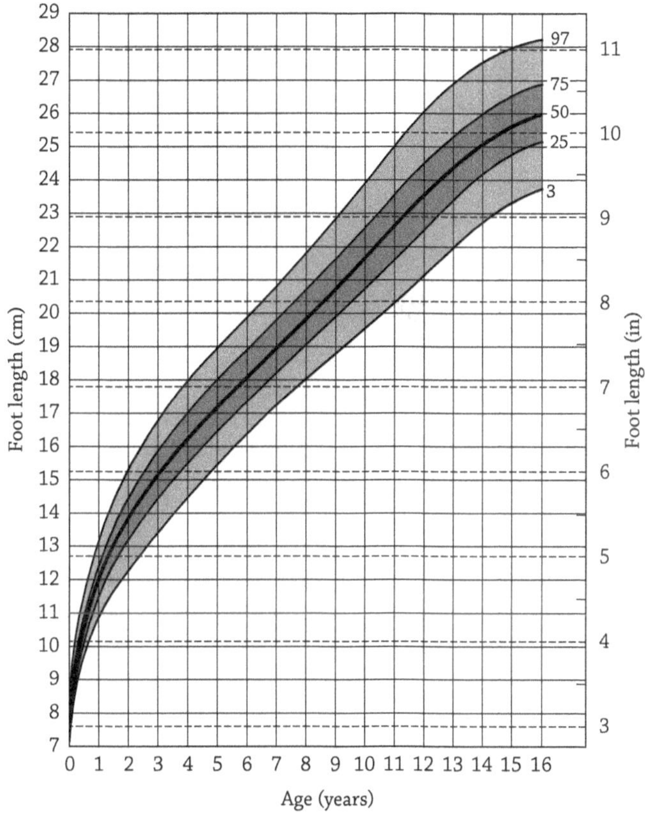

Figure 8.47. Foot length, males, birth to 16 years. From Blais et al. (1956), by permission.

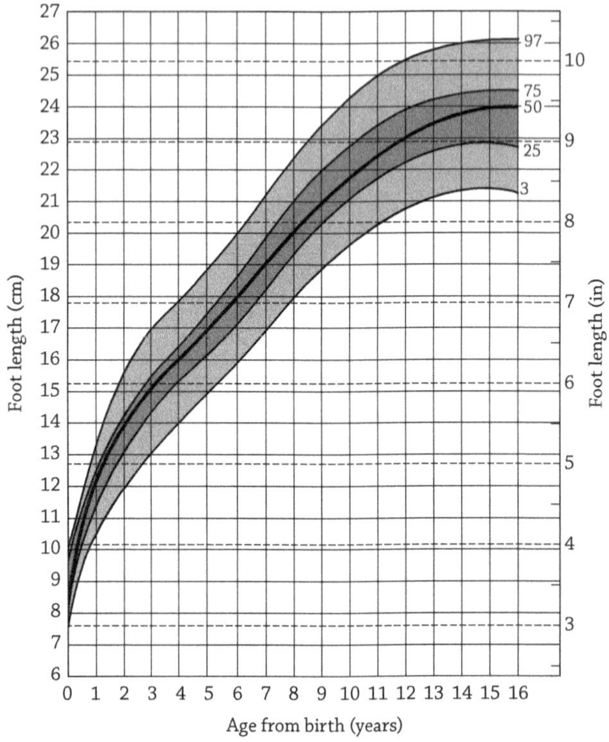

Figure 8.48. Foot length, females, birth to 16 years. From Blais et al. (1956), by permission.

FOOT WIDTH

Definition Total foot width at widest (broadest) point of the foot.

Landmarks Measure between the medial prominence of the first metatarsophalangeal (MTP) joint and the lateral prominence of the fifth MTP joint of the foot. Measure on the plantar aspect (sole) of the foot (Fig. 8.49).

Instruments Tape measure, calipers, or clear ruler.

Position Patients should be in a relaxed position, sitting, or lying down; however, foot width may be most easily measured with the individual standing on the tape measure.

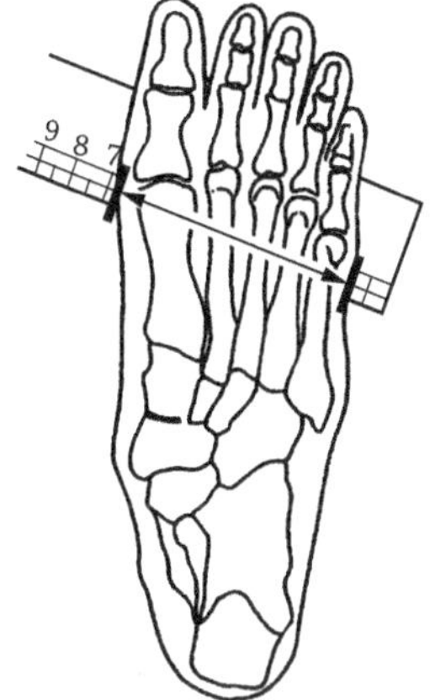

Figure 8.49. Measuring foot width.

Alternative Draw around the foot, marking the MTP joints, and measure between the markings.

Remarks Normal values for males and females age 4–16 years are presented in Figures 8.50 and 8.51.

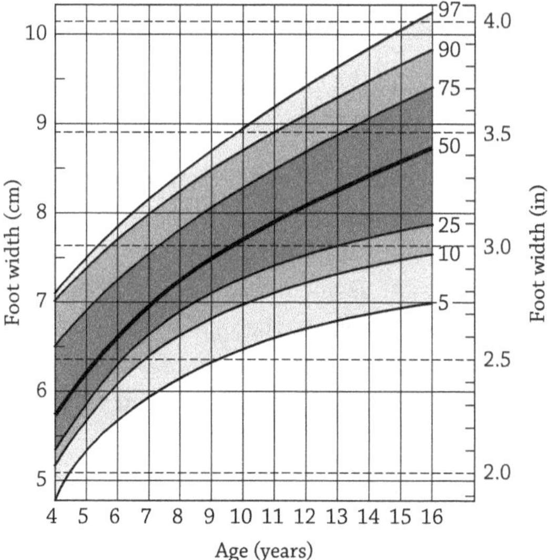

Figure 8.50. Foot width, males, 4 to 16 years. From Malina et al. (1973), by permission.

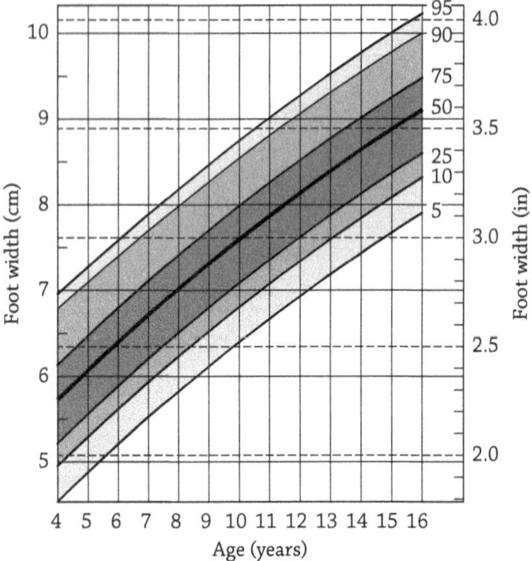

Figure 8.51. Foot width, females, 4 to 16 years. From Malina et al. (1973), by permission.

UPPER-TO-LOWER SEGMENT RATIO

Definition The ratio of the length of the upper part of the body to the length of the lower part of the body.

$$\frac{\text{Upper segment}}{\text{Lower segment}} = \frac{\text{Height} - \text{Lower segment}}{\text{Lower segment}}$$

Landmarks The lower segment is measured from the top of the middle part of the public bone to the sole of the foot (Fig. 8.52). The upper segment is measured from the top of the middle part of the pubic bone to the top of the head. Upper segment and lower segment together equal total height.

Instruments Tape measure or calipers.

Position The individual is standing upright, and the top of the pubic bone is palpated.

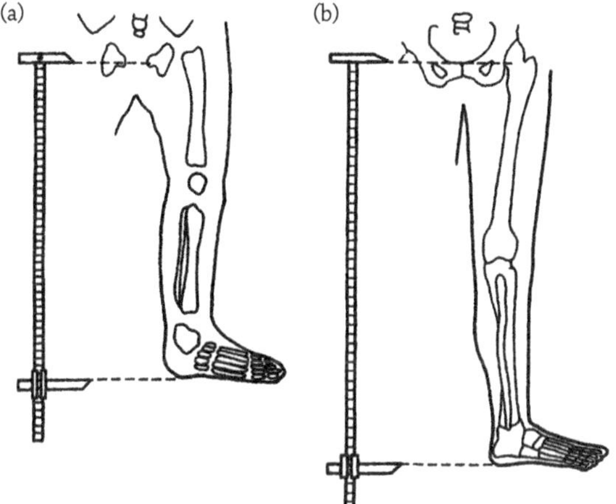

Figure 8.52. Measuring the lower segment in infants (a) and adults (b).

Remarks In infants, the upper segment approximately equals the sitting height. In older children and adults, the lower segment can be measured and subtracted from the height to establish the upper segment length. Normal values for upper and lower segment lengths to age 16 years are shown in Figures 8.53 and 8.54. The upper-to-lower segment ratio decreases progressively during childhood. Adult males have smaller upper-to-lower segment ratios than females, since they generally have relatively longer legs.

Upper-to-lower segment ratios are useful in defining different forms of disproportionate growth and in distinguishing them from immaturity or delayed growth.

There are ethnic differences in the upper-to-lower segment ratio. As a generalization, the ratio is greater than 1.0 below age 10 years, 1.0 at 10 years at age, and less than 1.0 after age 10 years (Figures. 8.55 and 8.56).

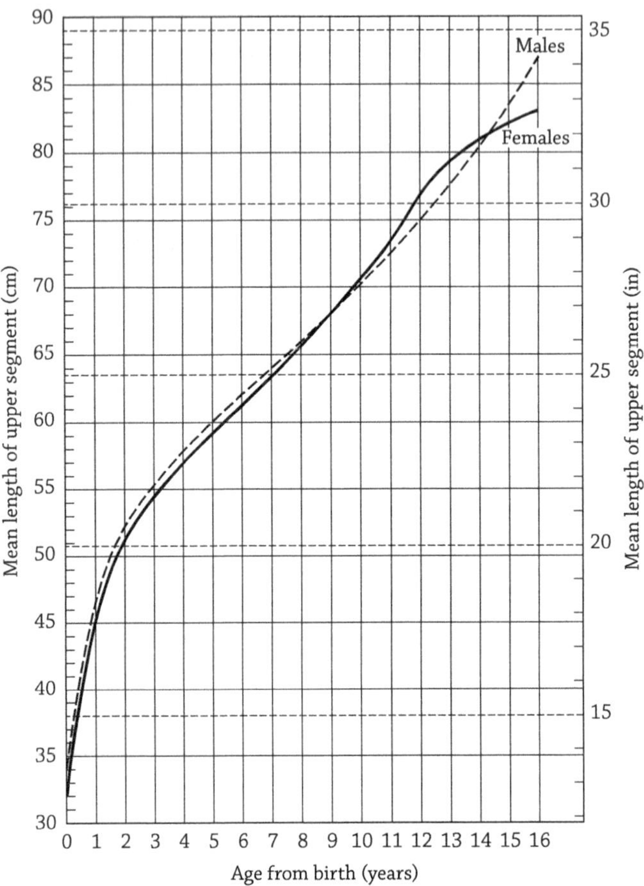

Figure 8.53. Upper segment length, both sexes, birth to 16 years. From Headings (1975), by permission.

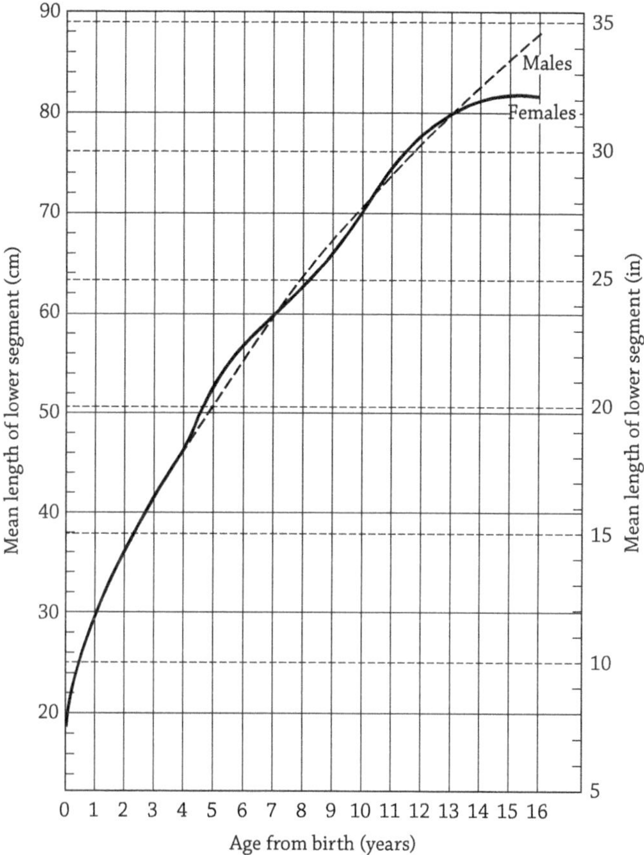

Figure 8.54. Lower segment length, both sexes, birth to 16 years. From Headings (1975), by permission.

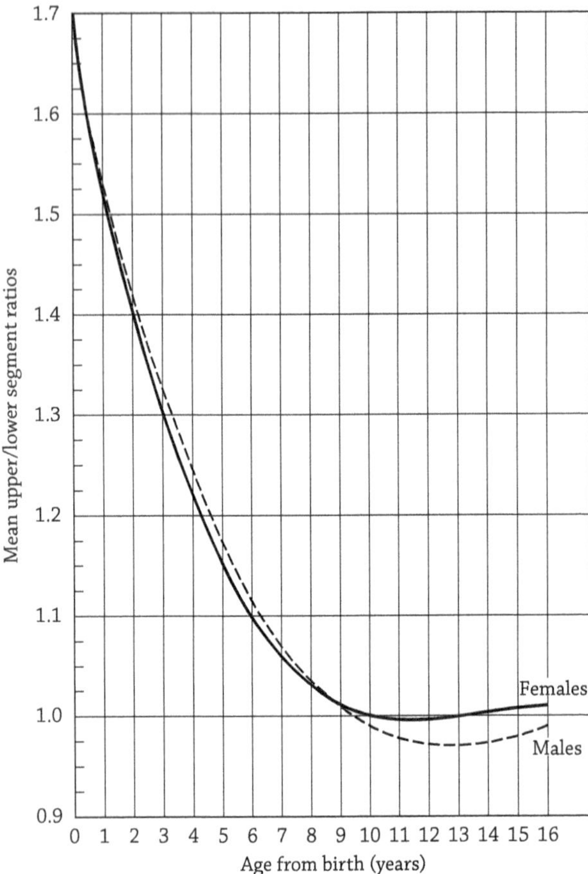

Figure 8.55. Upper-to-lower segment ratio, both sexes, birth to 16 years. From Headings (1975), by permission.

	Height (cm)		Span (cm)		Upper Segment (cm)		Lower Segment (cm)		Upper/ Lower Segment Ratio	
Age	**Male**	**Female**	**Males**	**Female**	**Male**	**Female**	**Male**	**Female**	**Male**	**Female**
Birth	51.4	50.5	48.5	48.3	32.4	31.9	19	18.6	1.69	1.73
1 m	55.8	54.4	53.7	52.1	35.1	34.2	20.8	20.3	1.67	1.69
2 m	59	57.7	56	54.5	36.8	36	22.1	21.7	1.65	1.67
3 m	61.4	60.3	58.5	57	38.4	37.7	23	22.6	1.65	1.66
4 m	63.5	62.5	61	59.3	39.5	38.6	24	23.9	1.63	1.62
5 m	65.2	64.3	62.1	61.8	40.3	39.9	24.9	24.7	1.62	1.61
6 m	67.2	66.2	64.7	63	41.6	40.7	25.6	25.5	1.61	1.60
7 m	68.9	67.6	65.9	64.3	42.4	41.4	26.5	26.2	1.61	1.58
8 m	70.2	69	67.2	65.6	43	42.2	27.2	26.8	1.58	1.58
9 m	71.4	70.2	68.4	66.6	43.7	42.7	27.7	27.5	1.58	1.56
10 m	72.7	71.4	69.5	67.9	44.2	43.1	28.5	28.3	1.55	1.53
11 m	73.7	72.6	70.7	69.2	44.5	43.8	29	28.8	1.54	1.53
12 m	75	73.7	72	70.4	45.5	44.4	29.5	29.3	1.54	1.52
15 m	78.1	77	74.5	73	47.1	46.1	31	30.9	1.52	1.50
18 m	81	79.7	78.3	76.5	48.6	47.3	32.4	32.4	1.51	1.47
21 m	83.6	82.3	80.9	79.1	49.8	48.8	33.8	33.5	1.47	1.45
24 m	86	84.9	83.2	81.6	50.7	49.8	35.3	35.1	1.44	1.42
30 m	91	89	87	85.3	53.1	51.5	37.9	37.5	1.40	1.39
36 m	95	93.2	92	89.2	54.4	53	40.6	40.2	1.33	1.32
42 m	98.5	97	95.8	93	55.9	54.4	42.6	42.6	1.31	1.29
48 m	102.2	100.5	98.7	96.7	57.2	55.7	45	44.6	1.27	1.25
54 m	105.5	103.8	102.5	101	58.3	56.8	47.2	47	1.23	1.21
5 y	108.4	107.3	105.3	103	59.4	58.2	49	49.1	1.21	1.19
5.5 y	111.5	110.3	109.1	107.5	60.1	59	51.4	51.3	1.17	1.15
6 y	114.4	113	111.8	110.1	61	59.8	53.4	53.2	1.14	1.13
6.5 y	117.3	116	114.3	112.9	61.9	61.1	55.4	54.9	1.11	1.12
7 y	120	119	117.4	116.9	62.8	62	57.2	57	1.10	1.09
7.5 y	122.4	121.6	120.3	119.7	63.2	62.6	59.2	59	1.07	1.06
8 y	124.7	124.3	123.5	122.5	64	63.6	60.7	60.7	1.06	1.05
8.5 y	127.6	126.8	126.7	125.3	65.4	64.3	62.2	62.2	1.05	1.04
9 y	129.7	129.3	129.7	128.1	65.7	65.3	64	64	1.03	1.02

(continued)

	Height (cm)		Span (cm)		Upper Segment (cm)		Lower Segment (cm)		Upper/ Lower Segment Ratio	
Age	**Male**	**Female**	**Males**	**Female**	**Male**	**Female**	**Male**	**Female**	**Male**	**Female**
9.5 y	132.9	131.8	132.7	130.9	67.3	66.2	65.6	65.6	1.02	1.01
10 y	135	134.6	135.8	133.7	67.9	67.8	67.1	66.8	1.02	1.01
10.5 y	137.5	137.4	138.5	136.5	68.6	69	69.6	68.4	1.00	1.01
11 y	140.1	140.5	141.3	140.6	69.6	70.3	70.5	70.2	0.99	1.00
11.5 y	142.5	143.5	144.2	143.2	70.5	71.5	72	72	0.99	1.00
12 y	144.9	146.5	147.2	146.2	71.7	73	73.2	73.5	0.98	0.99
12.5 y	147.2	149	150.3	148.7	72.7	74	74.5	75	0.98	0.99
13 y	149.7	151.5	153	151.8	73.9	75.3	75.8	76.2	0.98	0.99
13.5 y	151.8	153.9	155.8	154.5	74.7	76.9	77.1	77	0.97	1.00
14 y	154.1	156	157.3	155.8	75.7	77.7	78.4	78.3	0.97	0.99
14.5 y	156.5	157.3	160.1	158.6	76.9	78.2	79.6	79.1	0.97	0.99
15 y	158.4	158.8	162.9	160.1	77.8	79.2	80.6	79.6	0.97	1.00
15.5 y	160.4	159.6	164.5	161.6	78.8	79.6	81.6	80	0.97	1.00
16 y	162.3	160.5	167.3	161.6	79.8	80.3	82.5	80.2	0.97	1.00
16.5 y	164.3	161.2	168.8	163.2	80.9	80.7	83.4	80.5	0.97	1.00
17 y	166	161.8	171.6	163.2	81.6	81	84.4	80.8	0.97	1.00
17.5 y	167.8	162.2	173.1	164.7	82.4	81.2	85.2	81	0.97	1.00
18 y	169	162.5	174.3	164.7	83	81.5	86	81	0.97	1.01
18.5 y	170.3	162.5	175.9	164.7	84.1	81.5	86.2	81	0.98	1.01
19 y	171.3	162.5	177.5	164.7	84.6	81.5	86.7	81	0.98	1.01
19.5 y	171.8	162.5	179	164.7	84.8	81.5	87	81	0.98	1.01
20 y	172.5	162.5	179	164.7	85.3	81.5	87.2	81	0.98	1.01

Figure 8.56. Average height, span, upper and lower segment measurement and ratio for males and females by age Adapted from Engelbach (1932).

LIMB CIRCUMFERENCE

Definition Circumference of a particular area of a limb, usually at the widest, largest, or maximum point.

Landmarks Circumference measurements are taken at the widest or largest diameter of the limb (Fig. 8.57) or from a fixed bony point (e.g., 10 cm distal to lower edge of the patella).

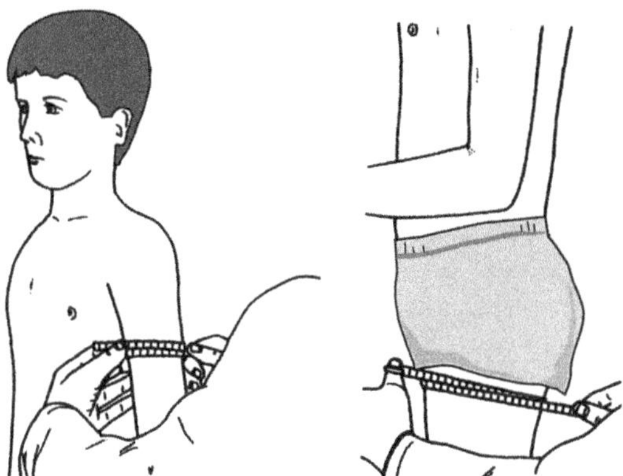

Figure 8.57. Measuring limb circumference.

In the upper arm the widest point is at the middle of the biceps, just below the insertion of the deltoid.

In the upper leg (thigh) the widest point is usually just below the gluteal crease.

In the lower leg (calf) the widest point is in the mid-upper calf muscle.

Instruments Tape measure.

Position When measuring for maximum circumference, the arm is slightly bent and the lower arm is supported so the muscle is not flexed. The tape measure is moved up and down until it reaches the widest circumference. Measurement of the leg for maximum circumference can be done with the patient either standing upright or lying down.

Pitfalls If the individual bends forward to look at the measurement, this will result in falsely low measurements.

When measuring the circumference of a limb from a fixed point, palpate the point carefully or mark it with an ink pen, then record how far up or down from it the circumference measurement is taken in order to be consistent in subsequent measurements.

Remarks Typical limb circumference values for ages 4–16 years are shown in Figure 8.58. When limb length or circumference inequalities are present, it is particularly important to measure both sides in a reproducible way, since differential growth can be anticipated.

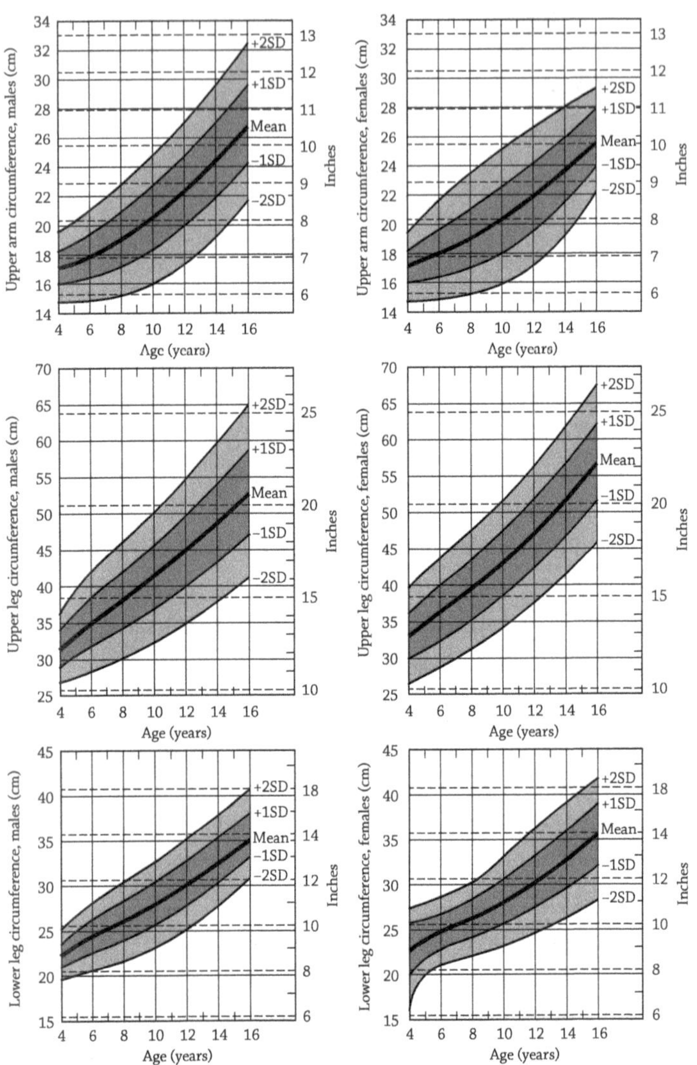

Figure 8.58. Maximum limb circumferences, both sexes, 4 to 16 years. From Maaser (1977), by permission.

RANGE OF MOVEMENT

Introduction

Normal joints allow a range of purposeful movements as well as easy shifting from one position to another. They have active and passive ranges of movement (ROM) or motion. In a healthy joint the active ROM is almost as full as the passive ROM. If there are no major apparent limitations of movement, checking four important positions will provide rough estimates of the range of movement of the major joints (Figs. 8.59–8.62).

Screening Positions

Neutral position (general)(Fig. 8.59) The patient stands upright with the legs straight and parallel. The feet are together, the arms hanging down at the sides, with elbows, wrists, and fingers extended, and the palms of the hands facing forward. The back, knees, and trunk are straight. This position excludes limitation of full extension of the hips, knees, elbows, and wrists. It also indicates that the ankles, shoulders, and back can achieve a normal resting position.

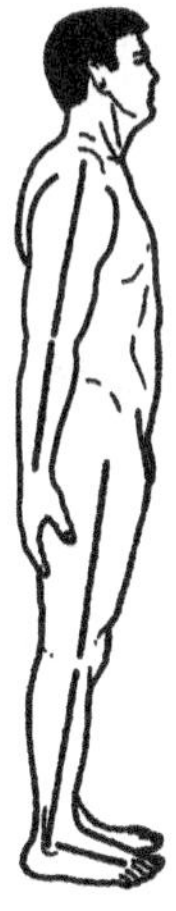

Figure 8.59. Range of movement—neutral position.

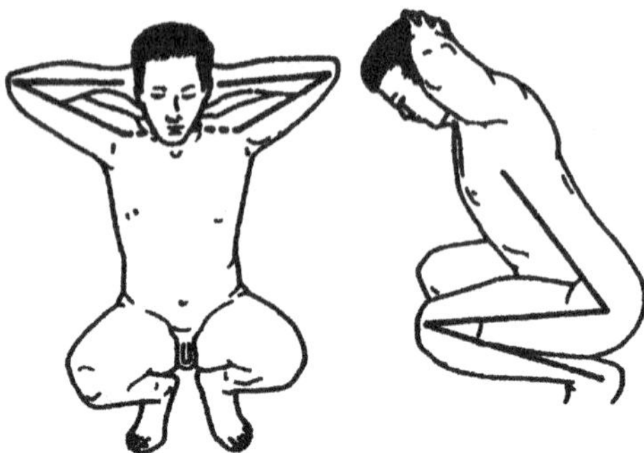

Figure 8.60. Range of motion—squatting position.

Squatting position (Fig. 8.60) The patient is asked to sit on the calves and ankles, with hands folded behind the neck. This position excludes limitation of flexion of the knees or the ankle joints. It also demonstrates limitation of abduction or external rotation of the shoulder joint, limitation of flexion in the elbow joint, and limitation of pronation of the lower arms.

Shoulder and hip stretch position (Fig. 8.61) The patient is asked to stand with the legs apart and the backs of the hands held on the lower back. This position gives an estimate of abduction of the hips, internal rotation of the joints, and back flexibility.

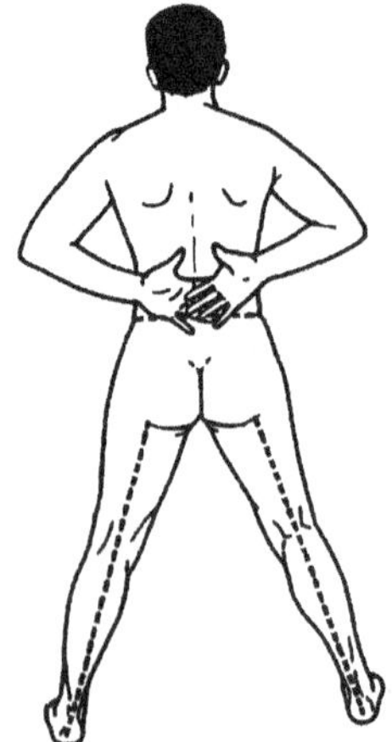

Figure 8.61. Range of movement—shoulder and hip stretch position.

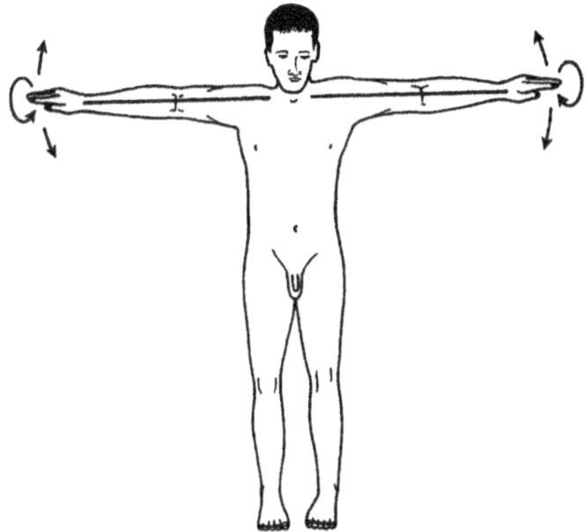

Figure 8.62. Range of movement—arm stretch position.

Arm stretch position (Fig. 8.62) The patient is asked to stand with straight legs, turning toes inward, and to stretch the arms out to the side at shoulder level with the hands stretched out as far as possible, then to separate the fingers and rotate the hand into pronation, then to make a fist and rotate the forearm into supination. This position excludes forearm, wrist, and finger limitations. The position also evaluates hip adduction and internal rotation, and shoulder rotation. If the fingers easily reach the inner palm, there is no limitation of flexion in the finger joints.

Range of Movement

Measurements of ROM for specific joints are made from the neutral reference position. Obtain this position, then measure ROM of the various specific joints (Figs. 8.63–8.68).

Instruments A goniometer for measuring angles accurately (see Fig. 8.70).

Remarks Newborns have mild limitation of ROM of most joints. Normally during infancy and childhood, the ROM increases and is 5–10 degrees greater by puberty. With aging, the ROM of all joints decreases. Hyperextensible joints are found in many conditions associated with connective tissue disorders.

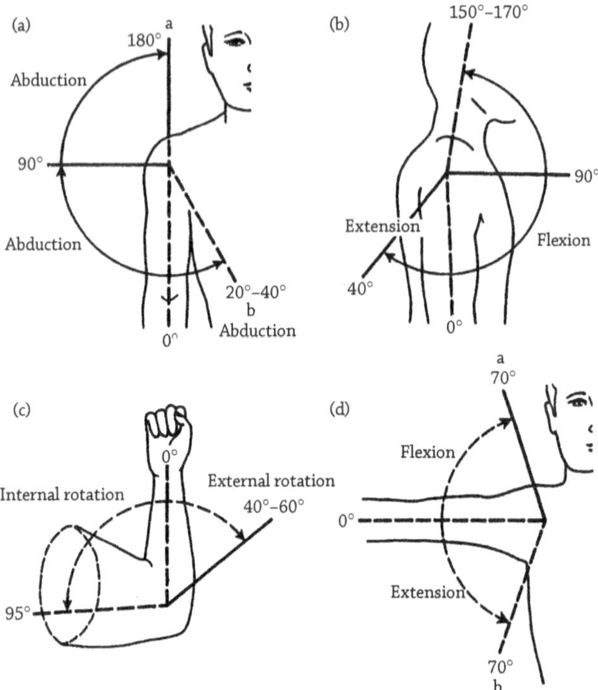

Figure 8.63. Normal range of motion of the shoulder joint.

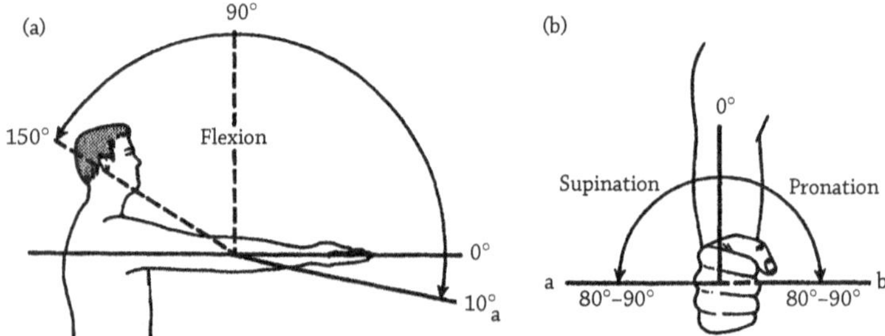

Figure 8.64. Normal range of motion of the elbow joint.

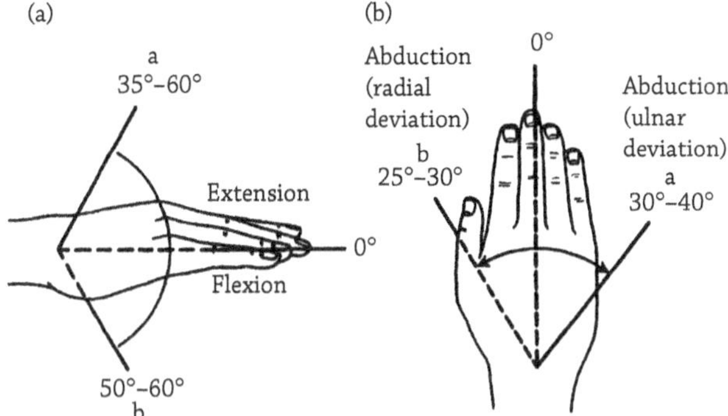

Figure 8.65. Normal range of motion of the wrist joint.

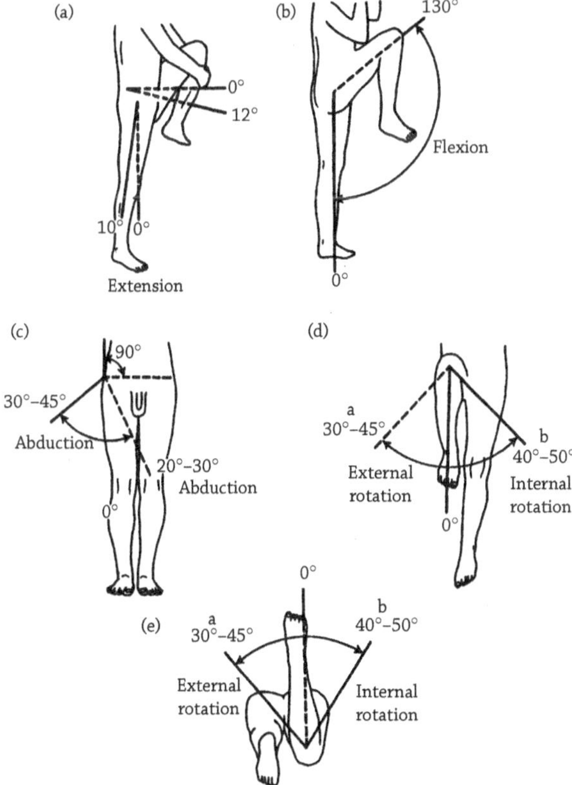

Figure 8.66. Normal range of motion of the hip joint.

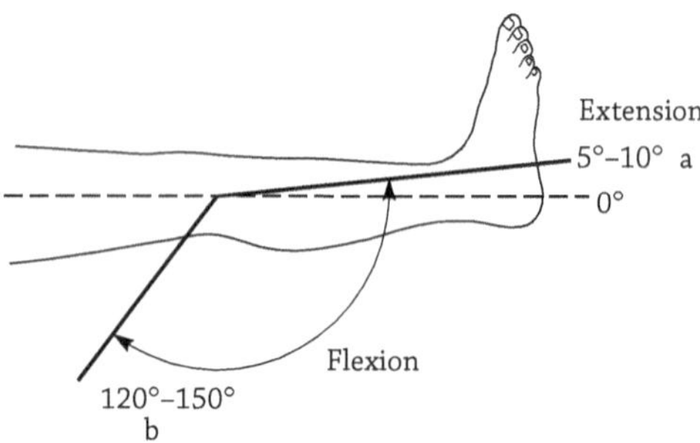

Figure 8.67. Normal range of motion of the knee joint.

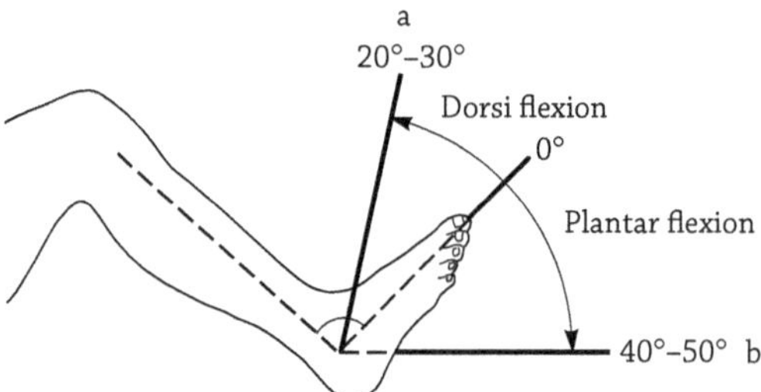

Figure 8.68. Normal range of motion of the ankle joint.

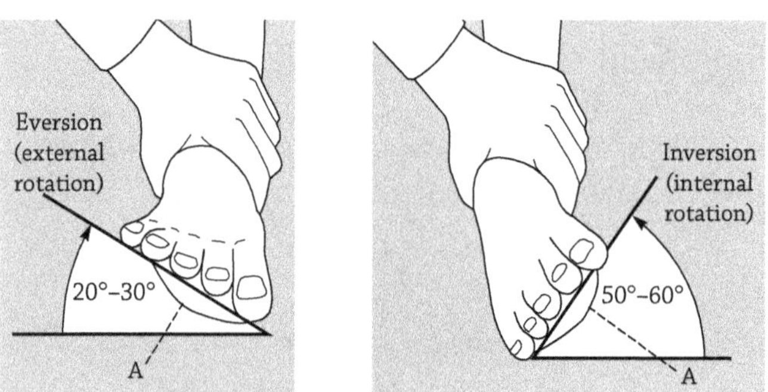

Figure 8.69. Normal range of motion of the foot.

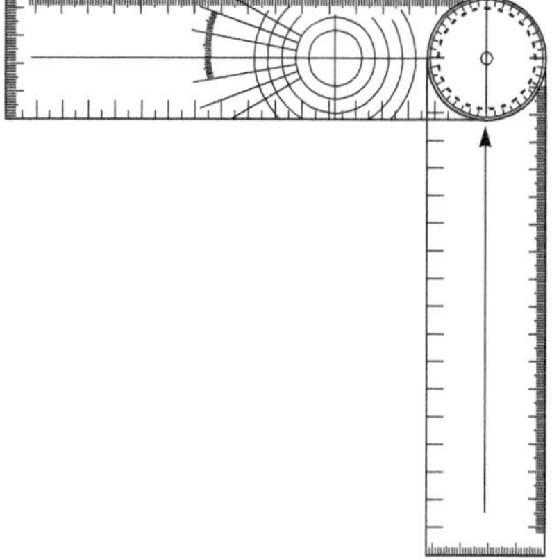

Figure 8.70. Goniometer.

HYPEREXTENSIBILITY

Definition Greater range of motion of joints than normally seen for age.

Diagnosis Determination of hypermobility in adults and adolescents can be assessed using the scale derived by Beighton et al. (1989). A score of 5/9 or greater defines hypermobility:

- Passive dorsiflexion of the little fingers beyond 90 degrees from the horizontal plane. One point for each hand.
- Passive apposition of the thumbs to the flexor aspect of the forearm. One point for each hand.
- Hyperextension of the elbows beyond 10 degrees. One point for each elbow.
- Hyperextension of the knees beyond 10 degrees. One point for each knee.
- Forward flexion of the trunk with knees fully extended so the palms of the hand rest flat on the floor. One point.

Remarks Approximately 5% of the population has hyperextensible joints. More than twice as many females as males have increased

ROM of joints. Young children and adolescents seem particularly prone to hyperextensible joints and may develop arthralgias, particularly in the knees and fingers.

BIBLIOGRAPHY

Atkinson, W. B., and Elftman, H. (1945). The carrying angle of the human arm as a secondary sex character. *Anatomical Record*, 91, 49–52.

Baughman, F. A., Higgins, J. V., Wadsworth, T. G., and Demaray, M. J. (1974). The carrying angle in sex chromosome anomalies. *Journal of the American Medical Association*, 230, 718–720.

Beals, R. K. (1976). The normal carrying angle of the elbow. *Clinical Orthopaedics and Related Research*, 119, 194–196.

Beighton, P., Grahame, R., and Bird, H. (1989). *Hypermobility of joints* (2nd ed.) London: Springer.

Belt-Niedbala, B. J., Ekvall, S., Cook, C. M., Oppenheimen, S., and Wessel, J. (1986). Linear measurement: A comparison of single arm-lengths and arm-span. *Developmental Medicine and Child Neurology*, 28, 319–324.

Biesecker, L. G., Aase, J. M., Clericuzio, C., Gurrieri, F., Temple, I. K., and Toriello, H. (2009). Elements of morphology: Standard terminology for the hands and feet. *American Journal Medical Genetics Part A*, 149A, 93–127.

Bino, F., Gwanter, H. L., and Baum, J. (1983). The hypermobility syndrome. *Pediatrics*, 72, 701–706.

Blais, M. M., Green, W. T., and Anderson, M. (1956). Length of the growing foot. *Journal of Bone and Joint Surgery*, 39A, 998–1001.

Cheng, J. C. Y., Leung, S. S. F., and Lau, J. (1996) Anthropometric measurements and body proportions among Chinese children. *Clinical Orthopaedics and Related Research*, 323, 22–23.

Engelbach, W. (1932). In *Endocrine medicine* (Vol. 1). Springfield, IL: Charles C. Thomas.

Engelbach, W. (1962). In *Growth and development of children* (4th ed.). Chicago: Year Book Medical Publishers.

Feingold, M., and Bossert, W. H. (1974). Normal values for selected physical parameters: an aid to syndrome delineation. *Birth Defects: Original Article Series*, X, 13.

Frisancho, A. R. (1981). New norms of upper limb fat and muscle areas for assessment of nutritional status. *American Journal of Clinical Nutrition*, 34, 2540–2545.

Headings, D. L. (ed.) (1975). *The Harriet Lane handbook* (7th ed.). Chicago: Year Book Medical Publishers.

Krogman, W. M. (1983). In *Manual of physical status and performance in childhood, Vol. 1B* (eds. A. F. Roche and R. M. Malina), p. 1010. New York: Plenum Press.

Maaser, R. (1977). In *Wachstum Atlas* (eds. R. Bergmann, K. Bergmann, F. Kollmann, F. Kollmann, R. Maaser, and O. Hoevels), pp. 67–71. Wiesbaden, Germany: Papillon.

Malina, R. M., Hamill, P. V. V., and Lemeshow, S. (1973). In *Manual of physical status and performance in childhood, Vol. 1B* (eds. A. F. Roche and R. M. Malina), pp. 1048–1056. New York: Plenum Press.

Martin, R., and Saller, K. (1962). *Lehrbuch der Anthropologie*. Stuttgart, Germany: Gustave Fischer.

McKusick, V. A. (1972). *Heritable disorders of connective tissue* (4th ed.). St. Louis: Mosby.

Meredith, H. V. (1955). In *Manual of physical status and performance in childhood, Vol. 1B* (eds. A. R. Roche and R. M. Malina). New York: Plenum Press.

Merlob, P., Sivan, Y., and Reisner, S. H. (1984*a*). Anthropometric measurements of the newborn infant 27 to 41 gestational weeks. *Birth Defects: Original Article Series*, 20, 7.

Merlob, P., Sivan, Y., and Reisner, S. H. (1984*b*). Lower limb standards in newborns. *American Journal of Diseases in Childhood*, 138, 140–142.

Merlob, P., Mimouni, F., Rosen, O., and Reisner, S. H. (1984*c*). Assessment of thumb placement. *Pediatrics*, 74, 299–300.

Reinken, L., Stolley, H., Droese, W., and van Oost, G. (1980). Longitudinale Koerperentwicklung gesunder Kinder. *Klinische Paediatrie*, 192, 551–558.

Roche, A. F., and Malina, R. M. (1983). *Manual of physical status and performance in childhood, Vol. 1B*, pp. 1008–1012. New York: Plenum Press.

Russe, H. O., Gerhard, J. J., and King, P. S. (1972). An atlas of examination. *Standard measurements and diagnosis in orthopedics and traumatology* (ed. O. Russe). Bern, Switzerland: Hans Huber Publishers.

Sivan, Y., Merlob, P., and Reisner, S. H. (1983). Upper limb standards in newborns. *American Journal of Diseases in Childhood*, 137, 829–832.

Snyder, R. G., Spencer, M. L., Owings, C. L., and Schneider, L. W. (1975). In *Manual of physical status and performance in childhood, Vol. 1B* (eds. A. F. Roche and R. M. Malina), pp. 999, 1105. New York: Plenum Press.

Chapter 9

Chest and Trunk

INTRODUCTION

Disturbance of growth of the chest and trunk may lead to disproportion of the body in much the same way as disproportion can be produced by disturbance of limb growth. In addition, disturbed growth of the chest may affect the relationship between the sternum and ribs (sternocostal relationship), producing a variety of pectus deformities and possibly compromising respiratory function.

The ribs develop from the mesenchymal costal processes of the thoracic vertebrae. They become cartilaginous during the embryonic period and later ossify. The original union of the costal process with the vertebra is replaced by a synovial joint. The sternum develops from a pair of mesenchymal sternal bands, which at first are widely separated, and develop ventrolaterally in the body wall, independently of the developing ribs. Chondrification occurs in these bands to form two sternal plates, one on each side of the median plane. The cranial six costal cartilages become attached to them. The plates gradually fuse craniocaudally in the median plane to form cartilaginous models of the manubrium, the sternebrae or segments of the sternal body, and the xiphoid process.

Centers of ossification appear craniocaudally before birth, except for the xiphoid process center of ossification, which appears during childhood.

The development of the vertebral column begins with a precartilaginous stage during the fourth week of gestation. Cells from the sclerotomes of the somites are found in three main areas. First, surrounding the notochord, some of the densely packed cells give rise to the intervertebral disc. The remaining densely packed cells fuse with the loosely arranged cells of the immediately caudal sclerotome to form the mesenchymal centrum of a vertebra. Thus, each centrum develops from two adjacent sclerotomes and becomes an intersegmental structure. The notochord degenerates and disappears where it is surrounded by the developing vertebral body. Between the vertebrae the notochord expands to form the gelatinous center of the intervertebral disc, called the *nucleus pulposus*. This nucleus is later surrounded by the circularly arranged fibers of the annulus fibrosus. Second, cells of the sclerotomes of the somites surround the neural tube and later form the vertebral arch. Third, cells from the sclerotomes of the somites are found in the body wall and form the costal processes, which develop into ribs in the thoracic region. During the sixth week, chondrification centers appear in each mesenchymal vertebra. Ossification begins during the embryonic period and ends at about the 25th year. Malformations of the axial skeleton include spina bifida occulta, rachischisis, accessory or fused ribs, hemivertebrae, and cleft sternum.

Abnormalities of the back may result from congenital malformations of the spine, such as hemivertebrae, or from muscular imbalance, abnormalities of the pelvis, leg length discrepancy, or unusual posture, resulting in lordosis, kyphosis, scoliosis, or a combination of these three.

The appendicular skeleton consists of the pectoral and pelvic girdles and the limb bones. Details of limb bone embryology are not presented here. The clavicle initially develops by intramembranous ossification, and it later develops growth cartilages at both ends. The clavicles begin to ossify before any other bones. Formation of the pectoral girdle and the pelvic girdle from the upper and lower limb buds, respectively, is detailed in Chapter 8.

At about 22 days of gestation, folding of the sides of the embryo produces right and left lateral folds. Each lateral body wall, or somatopleure, folds toward the midline, rolling the edges of the embryonic disk ventrally and forming a roughly cylindrical embryo. As the lateral and ventral body walls form, part of the yolk sac is incorporated into the embryo as the midgut. After folding, the region of attachment of the amnion to the embryo is reduced to the relatively narrow region—the umbilicus—on the ventral surface. Faulty closure of the lateral body folds during the fifth week produces a large defect in the anterior abdominal wall and results in most of the abdominal viscera developing outside the embryo in a transparent sac of amnion (an omphalocele). Normally, after the intestines return from the umbilical cord, the rectus muscles approach each other and the linea alba, closing the circular defect. An umbilical hernia differs from an omphalocele in that the protruding mass is covered by subcutaneous tissue and skin, rather than a sac of amnion. The hernia usually does not reach its maximum size until the end of the first month after birth. The defect through which the hernia occurs is in the linea alba.

Gastroschisis is another abdominal wall defect; it is usually sporadic and present as an isolated birth defect. Gastroschisis is a congenital fissure of the abdominal wall, possibly due to primary incomplete folding and formation of the anterior abdominal wall or secondary rupture of the wall. It does not involve the site of insertion of the umbilical cord and usually is accompanied by protrusion of the small intestine and part of the large intestine.

Much information can be obtained about prenatal development by examination of the umbilical cord. The attachment of the umbilical cord is usually near the center of the placenta, but it may be found at any point. As the amniotic sac enlarges, the amnion sheathes the umbilical cord, forming the cord's epithelial coverings. The umbilical cord usually contains two arteries and one vein surrounded by mucoid connective tissue often called Wharton's jelly. Because the umbilical vessels are longer than the cord, twisting and bending of the vessels is common. The vessels frequently form loops, producing so-called false knots that are of no significance. The umbilical cord is usually 1–2 cm in diameter and 30–90 cm in length (average 55 cm). Growth of the umbilical cord slows after the 28th week of gestation but does not stop before term. Cord length correlates positively with maternal height, pregravid weight, pregnancy weight gain, socioeconomic status, and a male fetus. The finding of a short umbilical cord suggests diminished fetal movement and may be associated with subsequent psychomotor abnormalities. A single umbilical artery is present in approximately 0.5% of placentas examined. The presence of a single umbilical artery is thought to correlate with an increased incidence of congenital anomalies. Further details of placental pathology are found in Chapter 16.

Breast development, variation, and measurements are discussed in Chapter 10.

Inspection of the chest (Figure 9.1) should answer the following questions:

1. Is it symmetric?
2. Is one side flatter than the other?
3. What is the shape of the rib cage?
4. Is there evidence of pectus excavatum or pectus carinatum?
5. Is the scapula normal in size and position?

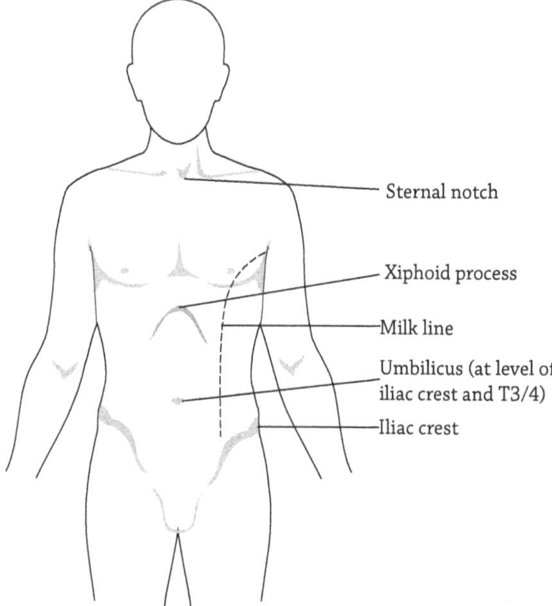

Figure 9.1. Trunk landmarks.

6. Is the scapula elevated (Sprengel deformity)?
7. Is the spine straight?
8. Is there any evidence of kyphosis, scoliosis, or lordosis?
9. Are the nipples normal?
10. Are they inverted?
11. Are accessory nipples present?
12. Is the umbilicus normal in shape and position?

Examination of the breasts is discussed in Chapter 10. Examination of the genitalia is discussed in Chapter 10. Examination of the skin is described in Chapter 11. Examination of the umbilical cord and umbilical cord length in the newborn is described in Chapter 16.

Following inspection, detailed measurements using the charts in the following pages for comparison should be performed. A glossary of terms used to define specific anomalies of the chest and trunk is included at the end of the book.

CHEST CIRCUMFERENCE

Definition Circumference of chest.

Landmarks Measure horizontally around the upper body at the level of the nipples or at the level just below the scapular angles Figure 9.2. In the postpubertal female, measure just below the breasts.

Instruments Tape measure.

Position The patient should stand upright with the arms down at the sides. The measurement should be made during mid-expiration. Infants should be measured lying supine, in mid-expiration.

Alternative Measure at the nipple line, or in adults 10 cm down from the clavicles or 5 cm down from the apex of the axilla.

Remarks Chest circumference values are presented in Figures 9.3 and 9.4. With inhalation or exhalation, the chest circumference can change. There is some value in measuring at maximum inhalation in

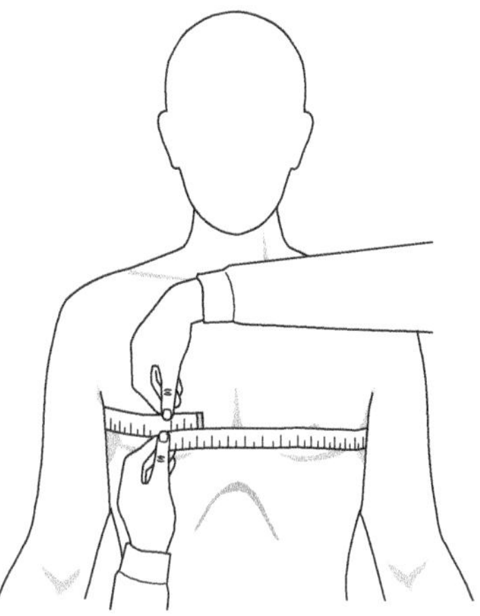

Figure 9.2. Measuring chest circumference.

conditions with contractures in order to get some sense of the lung volume.

Between 2 and 16 years of age, the chest circumference increases as much as 40 cm; a "growth spurt" occurs between 12 and 15 years of age.

Pitfalls In females, it is important to make sure that the measurement excludes the breast tissue. If the nipples are in an atypical position, for example, more caudally as may be seen in Noonan syndrome, the landmark for chest circumference needs to be related to a line 10 cm below clavicles, or at the fourth intercostal space.

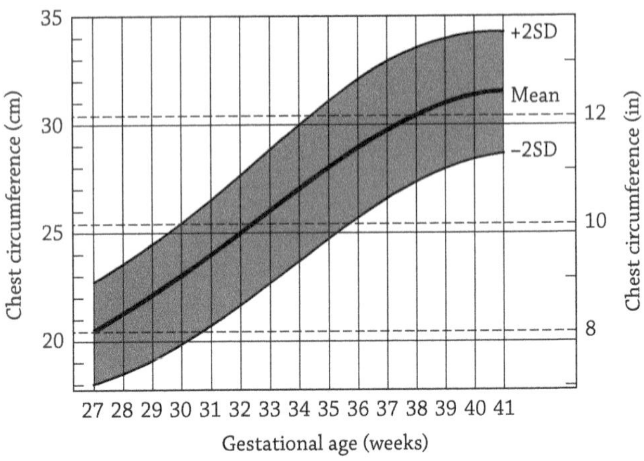

Figure 9.3. Chest circumference, both sexes, at birth. From Merlob et al. (1984), by permission.

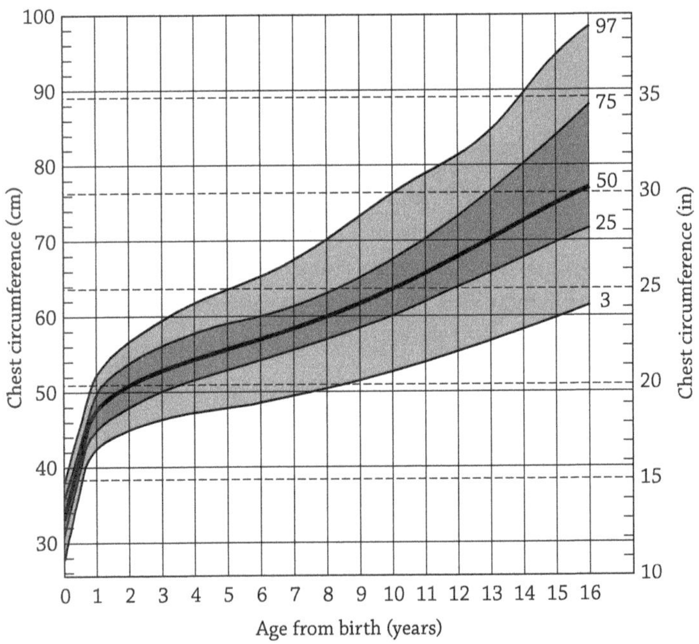

Figure 9.4. Chest circumference, both sexes, birth to 16 years. From Feingold and Bossert (1974), by permission.

INTERNIPPLE DISTANCE

Definition Distance between the centers of both nipples.

Landmarks Measure between the centers of both nipples (Fig. 9.5).

Instruments Tape measure.

Position The patient stands upright, with the arms down at the sides; measure during mid-expiration. Infants should be measured lying supine during mid-expiration.

Remarks Internipple distance cannot be measured from pictures. With inspiration and expiration the value will change, so two measurements, both taken during mid-expiration, are desirable. Values for children to age 16 years are shown in Figures 9.6 and 9.7.

Pitfalls In women with moderate to large breasts, the position of the nipples is variable, distorting this measurement.

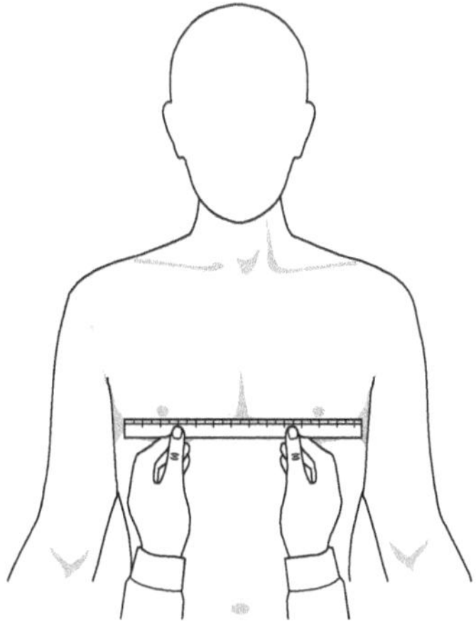

Figure 9.5. Measuring internipple distance.

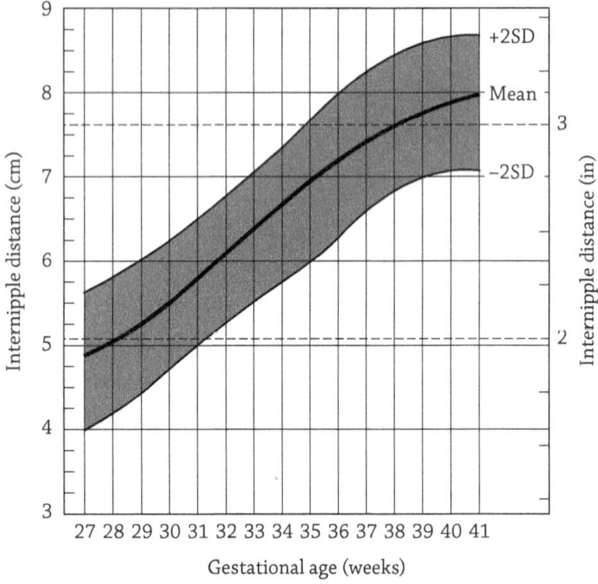

Figure 9.6. Internipple distance, both sexes, at birth. From Sivan et al. (1983), by permission.

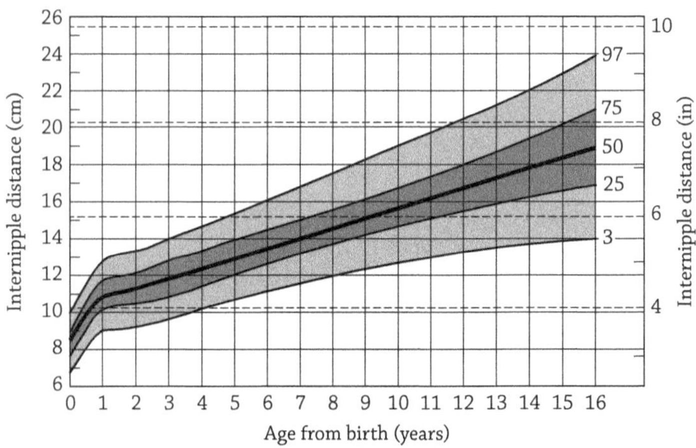

Figure 9.7. Internipple distance, both sexes, birth to 16 years. From Feingold and Bossert (1974), by permission.

THORACIC INDEX

Definition Ratio of the anteroposterior diameter of the chest to the lateral diameter (chest width) multiplied by 100.

Landmarks Anteroposterior diameter is measured (Fig. 9.8a) from the sternum, at the level of the nipples, to the vertebrae, at the same level, while at rest. Lateral diameter is measured between the midaxillary lines at the level of the nipples (Fig. 9.8b).

Instruments Calipers.

Position The patient should be standing with the arms hanging loosely at the sides; the measurement is made during mid-expiration.

Alternative If calipers are not available, the patient can be placed against a wall, facing sideways and forward for each measurement, respectively, while the boundaries of the thoracic cage, at the nipple level, are marked on the wall. The marks are then measured with a measuring tape.

Remarks Timing of respiration is important for accuracy of this measurement. Mid-expiration is the position of rest (prior to forced expiration). Ideally, each measurement should be obtained twice. Anteroposterior and lateral thoracic diameters are shown in Figure 9.9, and values for the thoracic index in Figure 9.10.

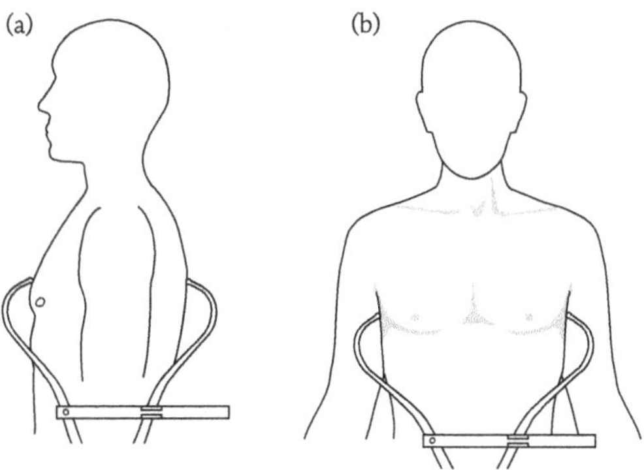

Figure 9.8. Measuring (a) anteroposterior and (b) lateral chest diameter.

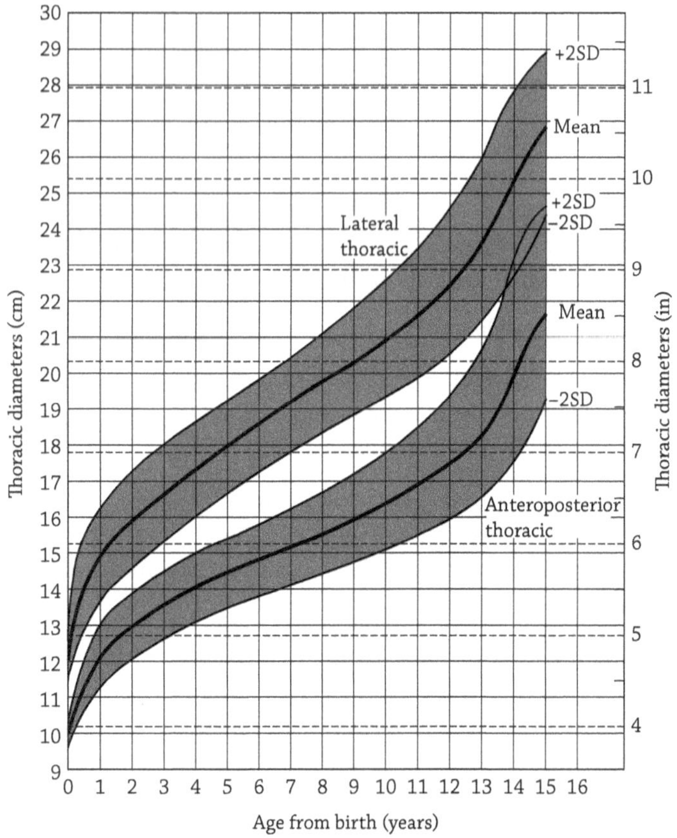

Figure 9.9. Thoracic diameters, both sexes, birth to 16 years. From Pryor (1966), by permission.

Pitfalls Variation in the chest cage's shape will distort the thoracic index. Pectus carinatum, or the barrel chest of an individual with asthma, will lead to an increased value. Pectus excavatum will reduce the value. Hypotonia will also produce a reduced anteroposterior diameter.

In women, the position of the nipples is extremely variable. This is less important in a ratio than in an absolute measurement. The fourth intercostal space can be used as an alternative landmark, or one can measure 10 cm down from the clavicles.

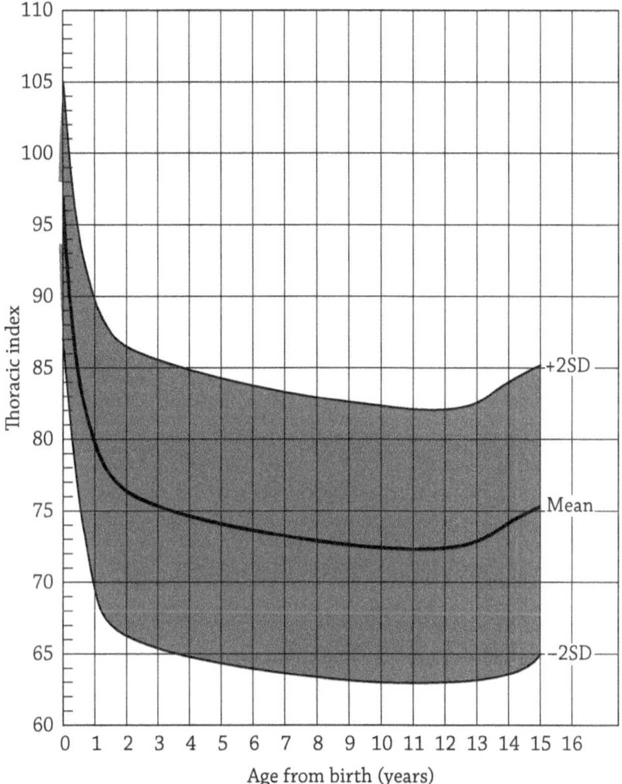

Figure 9.10. Thoracic index, both sexes, birth to 16 years. From Feingold and Bossert (1974), by permission.

STERNAL LENGTH

Definition Length of the sternum.

Landmarks Measure from the top of the manubrium to the lowest palpable edge of the sternum (Fig. 9.11).

Instruments Tape measure.

Position Patient should be standing upright. Infants should be measured lying supine.

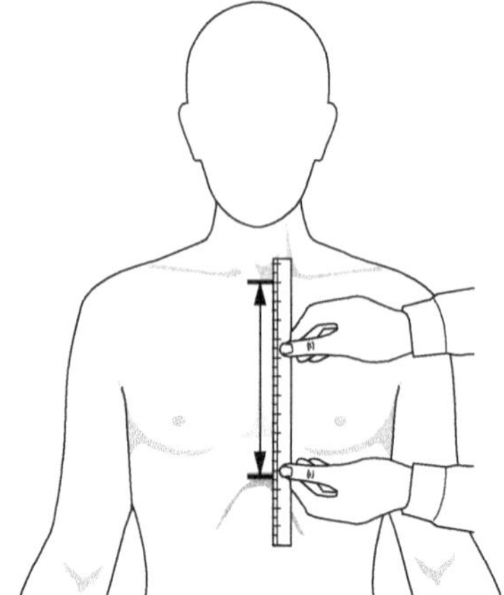

Figure 9.11. Measuring sternal length.

Alternative Patient may be recumbent.

Remarks Normal values are presented in Figures 9.12 and 9.13. Longitudinal overgrowth of the ribs produces an anterior chest deformity, either depression (pectus excavatum) or protrusion (pectus carinatum). Both defects may be present in the same patient.

Pitfalls The presence of a pectus deformity will distort the linear distance unless the tape is worked along the sternum in contact with the surface of the skin.

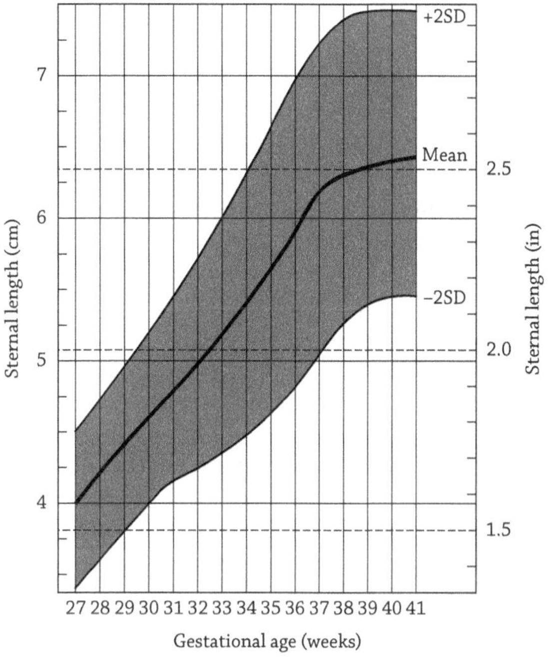

Figure 9.12. Sternal length, both sexes, at birth. From Sivan et al. (1983), by permission.

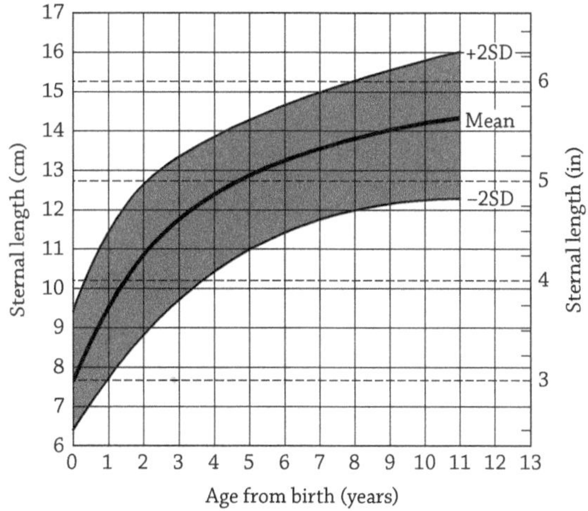

Figure 9.13. Sternal length, both sexes, birth to 13 years. From Feingold and Bossert (1974), by permission.

TORSO LENGTH

Definition Length from the top of the sternum to the top of the symphysis pubis.

Landmarks Measure from the manubrial notch to the superior border of the symphysis pubis, defined by palpation, in the midsagittal plane (Fig. 9.14).

Instruments Tape measure.

Position The patient should be standing upright, at rest, with the back straight and the shoulders back. The infant should be lying supine with legs extended.

Alternative The patient may be supine, with legs extended.

Remarks Spinal deformities, such as kyphosis or scoliosis, will reduce the torso length. Values for torso length at birth are presented in Figure 9.15.

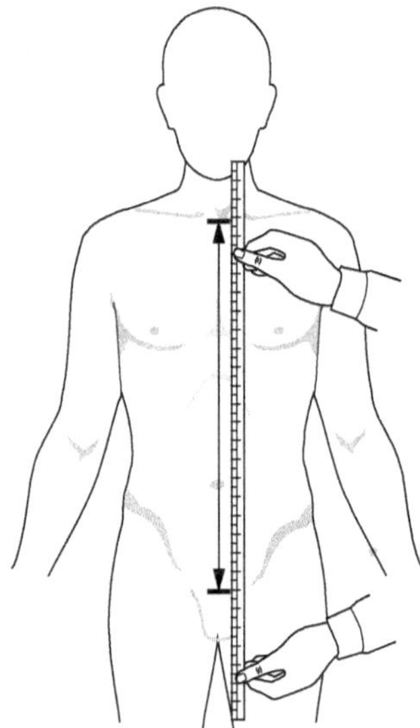

Figure 9.14. Measuring torso length.

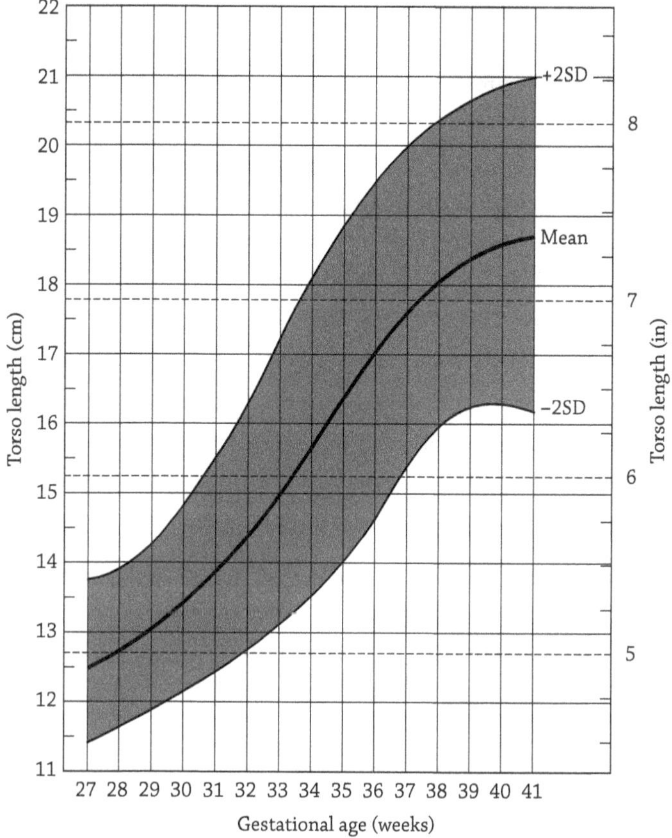

Figure 9.15. Torso length, both sexes, at birth. From Sivan et al. (1983), by permission.

Pitfalls The presence of sternal and vertebral anomalies should be disregarded in making this linear measurement. In contrast to measurement of the sternum, the tape should *not* be worked along the bony landmarks when pectus excavatum is present but should be stretched between the two points of reference.

BIACROMIAL DISTANCE

Definition Maximum distance between the right and left acromia, termed shoulder width.

Landmarks The spine of the scapula projects laterally and superiorly over the shoulder joint to form the acromion. The acromion articulates anteriorly with the clavicle. The acromion is the most lateral bony projection of the shoulder girdle and should be easily palpable. Measure between the right and left acromion across the back (Fig. 9.16).

Instruments Tape measure, or calipers.

Position The patient should stand upright, hands at the sides, with the shoulders in a neutral position. The measurement is taken from behind. The infant can be seated, or lying face down, for measurement.

Alternative The patient can sit or lie face down.

Remarks The biacromial distance, like the bi-iliac distance, is a useful measurement of trunk width. However, there is greater variation in biacrominal distance than in bi-iliac distance between the sexes. Values for males and females to age 19 years are presented in Figures 9.17 and 9.18.

Pitfalls Abnormalities of the serratus anterior muscle causing a "winged scapula," or neuromuscular disease, can result in "round" shoulders, increasing the biacromial distance. If the shoulders cannot be drawn back into a reasonable posture, the measurement should be made using calipers instead of a tape measure.

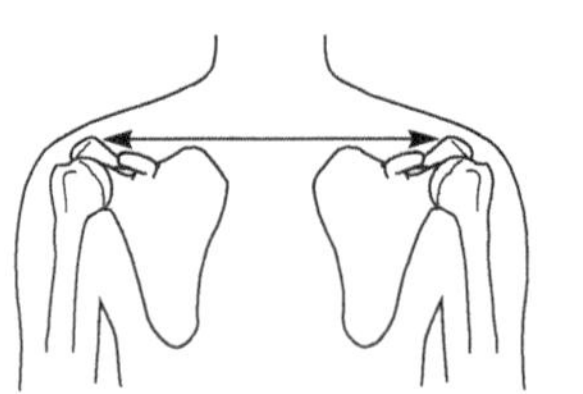

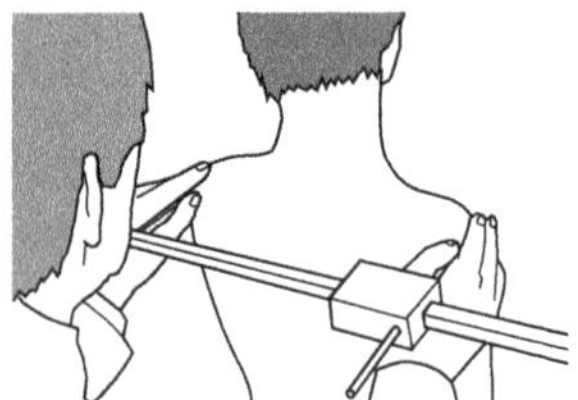

Figure 9.16. Measuring biacromial distance.

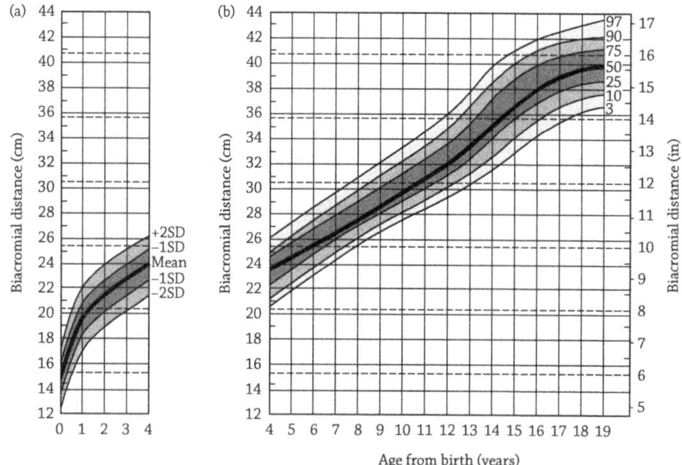

Figure 9.17. (a) Biacromial distance, males, birth to 4 years. From Maaser (1977), Demirjian and Jenicek (1983), Roche and Malina (1983), and Feingold and Bossert (1974), by permission. (b) Biacromial distance, males, 4 to 19 years. From Maaser (1977), Demirjian and Jenicek (1983), Roche and Malina (1983), and Feingold and Bossert (1974), by permission.

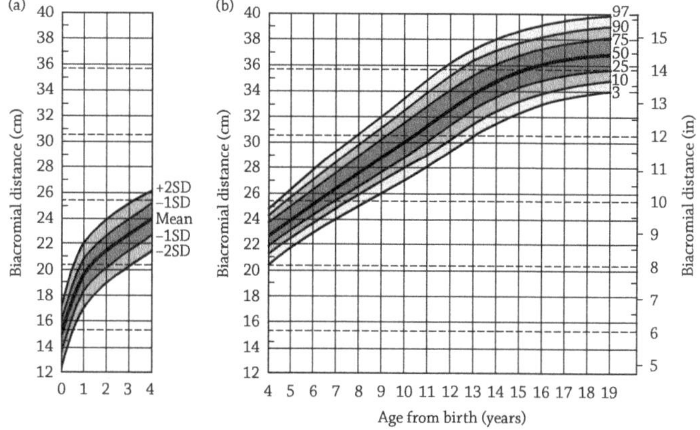

Figure 9.18. (a) Biacromial distance, females, birth to 4 years. From Maaser (1977), Demirjian and Jenicek (1983), Roche and Malina (1983), and Feingold and Bossert (1974), by permission. (b) Biacromial distance, females, 4 to 19 years. From Maaser (1977), Demirjian and Jenicek (1983), Roche and Malina (1983), and Feingold and Bossert (1974), by permission.

BI-ILIAC DISTANCE

Definition Distance between the most prominent, lateral points of the iliac crest.

Landmarks Palpate the iliac crest to define its widest flare. Measure between the right and left points, from the front, using firm pressure to get as near as possible to a skeletal measurement (Fig. 9.19).

Instruments Calipers. A tape measure may be used if calipers are unavailable, but the measurement is less accurate.

Position The patient should be standing upright. The infant should be lying supine with legs extended.

Alternative The patient may be lying supine with legs extended.

Remarks Normal values are presented in Figures 9.20 and 9.21. In the patient with a skeletal dysplasia, pelvic anatomy may be distorted and comparison with normal curves is less meaningful. The bi-iliac distance is considered the best indicator of the width of the trunk because it is not variable with posture or respiration and the landmarks are very definite. The bi-iliac distance is similar in males and females at any given age. Variation in hip width reflects soft tissue, not bony, differences between the sexes.

Pitfalls The most prominent lateral point of the iliac crest must be located precisely. If a tape measure is used, the measurement may be distorted by abdominal protrusion.

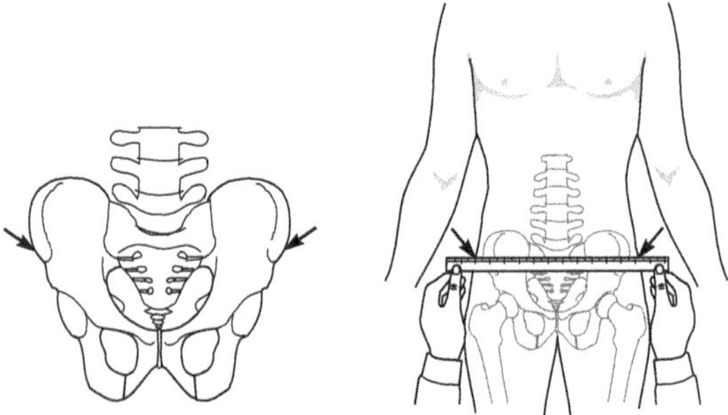

Figure 9.19. Measuring bi-iliac distance.

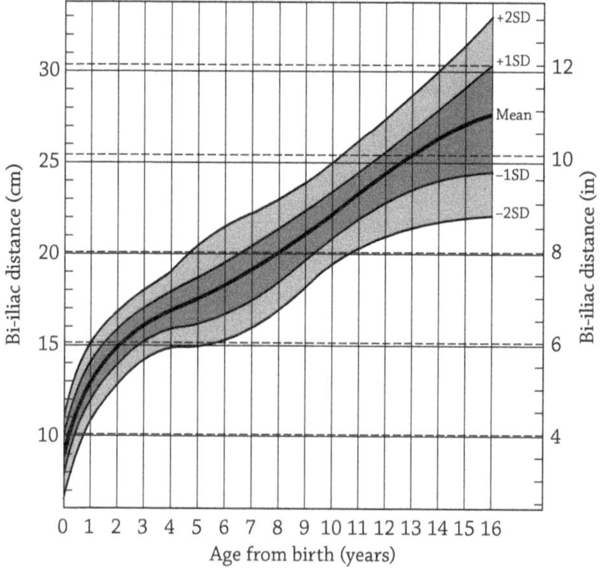

Figure 9.20. Bi-iliac distance, males, birth to 16 years. From Thelander (1966), by permission.

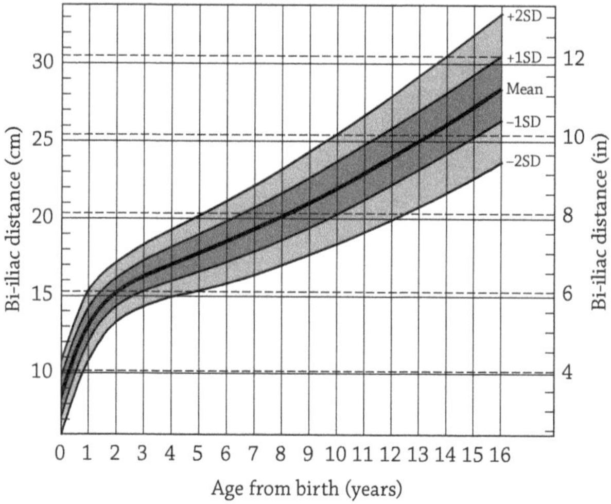

Figure 9.21. Bi-iliac distance, females, birth to 16 years. From Thelander (1966), by permission.

UMBILICAL CORD LENGTH

Definition Length of the umbilical cord.

Landmarks The umbilical cord should be measured from its attachment to the placenta to the trunk of the newborn infant.

Instruments Tape measure.

Remarks The segments attached to the baby and placenta are measured and results added. Any part that has been cut out is also measured and added to give the total cord length.

The normal anatomy of the umbilicus is shown in Figure 9.22. Normal values for umbilical cord length are shown in Figure 9.23.

Pitfalls In the presence of a supercoiled cord, once the cord is cut, it should assume its true configuration, and stretching the cord will not be necessary.

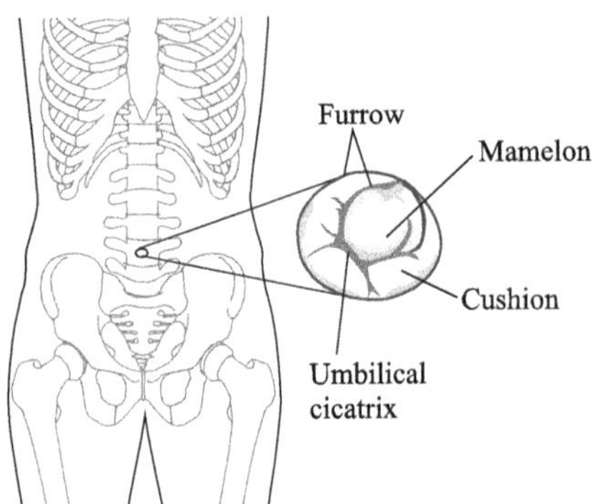

Figure 9.22. Normal anatomy of umbilicus.

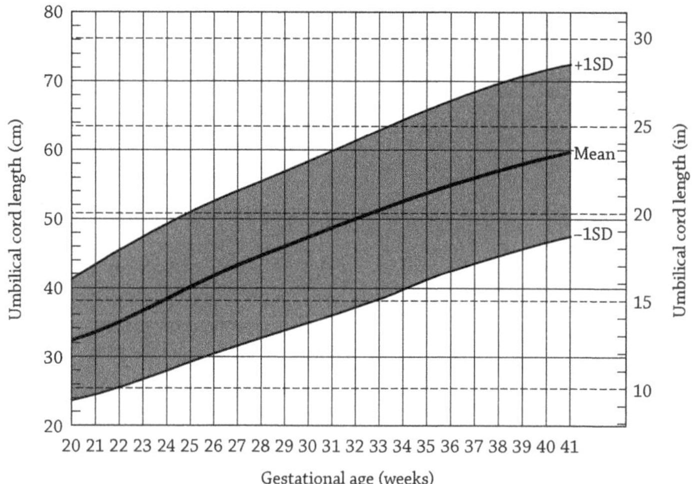

Figure 9.23. Umbilical cord length, both sexes, at birth. From Naeye (1985), by permission.

BIBLIOGRAPHY

Altshuler, G., Tsang, R. C., and Ermocilla, R. (1975). Single umbilical artery: Correlation of clinical status and umbilical cord histology. *American Journal of Diseases in Children*, 129, 697–700.

Demirjian, A., and Jenicek, M. (1983). In A. F. Rocheand R. M. Malina, *Manual of physical status and performance in childhood. Vol. 1 B. Physical status*. New York: Plenum Press.

Feingold, M., and Bossert, W. H. (1974). Normal values for selected physical parameters: an aid to syndrome delineation. *Birth Defects: Original Articles Series*, X(13), 1–15.

Maaser, R. (1977). In R. Bergmann et al. (eds.), *Wachstum: Atlas*, pp. 67–71. Wiesbaden, Germany: Papillon.

Merlob, P., Sivan, Y., and Reisner, S. H. (1984). Anthropometric measurements of the newborn infant 27 to 41 gestational weeks. *Birth Defects: Original Article Series*, 20, 7.

Moore, K. L. (1982). *The developing human* (3rd ed.). Philadelphia: W.B. Saunders.

Naeye, R. L. (1985). Umbilical cord length: Clinical significance. *Journal of Pediatrics*, 107, 278–281.

Pryor, H. B. (1966). Charts of normal body measurements and revised width weight tables in graphic form. *Journal of Pediatrics*, 68, 615.

Roche, A. F., and Malina, R. M. (1983). *Manual of physical status and performance in childhood, Vol 1 B*, pp. 1008–1012. New York: Plenum Press.

Sivan, Y., Merlob, P., and Reisner, S. H. (1983). Sternum length, torso length, and internipple distance in newborn infants. *Pediatrics*, 72, 523–525.

Thelander, H. E. (1966). Abnormal patterns of growth and development in mongolism. An anthropometric study. *Clinical Pediatrics*, 5, 493.

Chapter 10

Genitalia

INTRODUCTION

In the male, under the influence of circulating androgens, the urogenital folds fuse to form a urethra, and the penis is formed by the growth of the genital tubercle (Fig. 10.1). The labioscrotal swellings develop into the scrotum, and the testes descend into the inguinal canal at about 6 months of gestation. Shortly before birth, the testes enter the scrotum under the influence of gonadotropin stimulation. Failure of the testes to descend into the scrotum is called cryptorchidism and may be unilateral or bilateral. The internal ductal structures develop from the same primordia as the urinary tract. In the presence of androgens, the prostate gland develops from the vesicourethral canal.

In the female fetus, the clitoris (Fig. 10.1) develops from the genital tubercle; the urogenital groove remains open; the urogenital folds develop into the labia minora and the distal part of the vagina under the influence of estrogen; and the labioscrotal swellings form the labia majora.

There are many causes of aberrant sexual development, including prenatal hormonal disturbance or imbalance, absent cellular response to androgen or estrogen, chromosomal anomalies, and gene mutations.

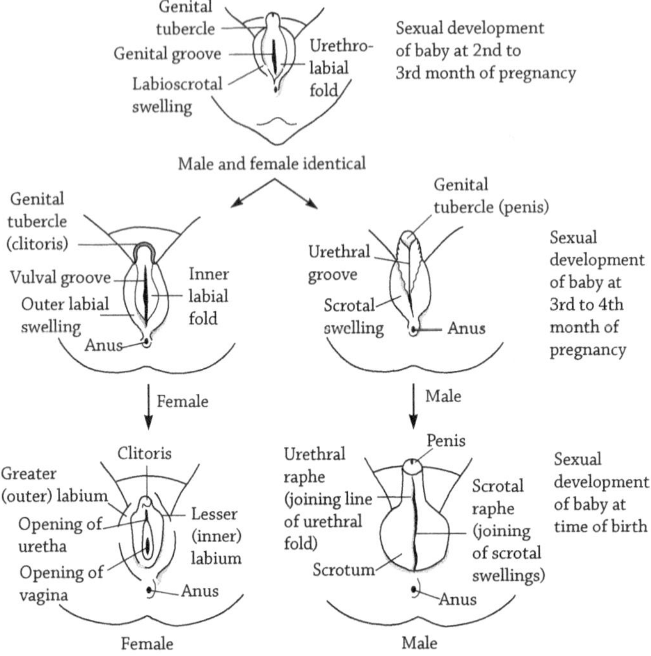

Figure 10.1. Differentiation of external genitalia in the human fetus.

PUBERTY

In the early stages of male puberty, the testicles and adrenal glands synthesize increasing amounts of androgens, which stimulate the growth of the penis and scrotum; initiate the appearance of pubic, axillary, facial, and body hair; lead to the development of apocrine sweat glands; accelerate growth and maturation of the skeleton; and increase the muscle mass. Testicular growth antedates penile growth by 6 to 12 months. Enlarging testicular volume and the subsequent testicular sensitivity to pressure are the first signs of puberty in males.

In female puberty, estrogens produced by the ovary stimulate growth of the breast, uterus, fallopian tubes, and vagina. Androgens produced by the adrenal gland stimulate the growth of pubic and axillary hair, linear growth, and skeletal maturation. Apocrine sweating is usually the first sign of puberty in females.

STAGES OF PUBERTY (TANNER STAGES)

To assess how far an individual has progressed through puberty, a rating scale that describes the successive stages of growth of the genitalia and pubic hair in boys and breast development and pubic hair development in girls, was introduced by Tanner (Fig. 10.2). The stage of development in the individual is compared with visual standards, which are referred to as G-1 to G-5 for male genitalia development, B-1 to B-5 for breast development, and PH-1 to PH-5 for pubic hair development. The sequence and timing of stages is illustrated in Figure 10.3.

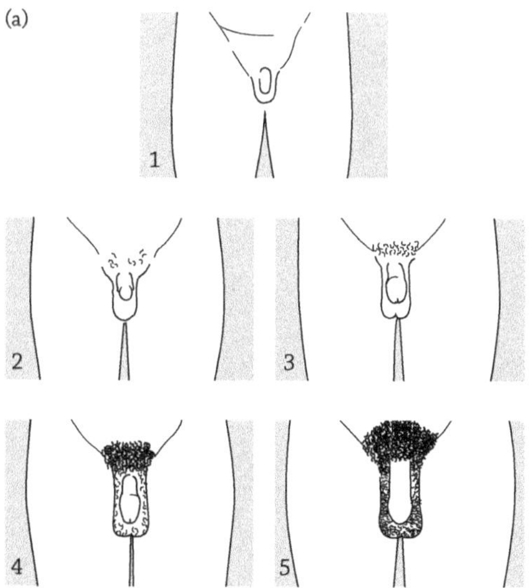

Figure 10.2(a). Male genital development (G-1 to G-5) and pubic hair (PH-1 to PH-5). Tanner stages. From Tanner (1975), by permission.

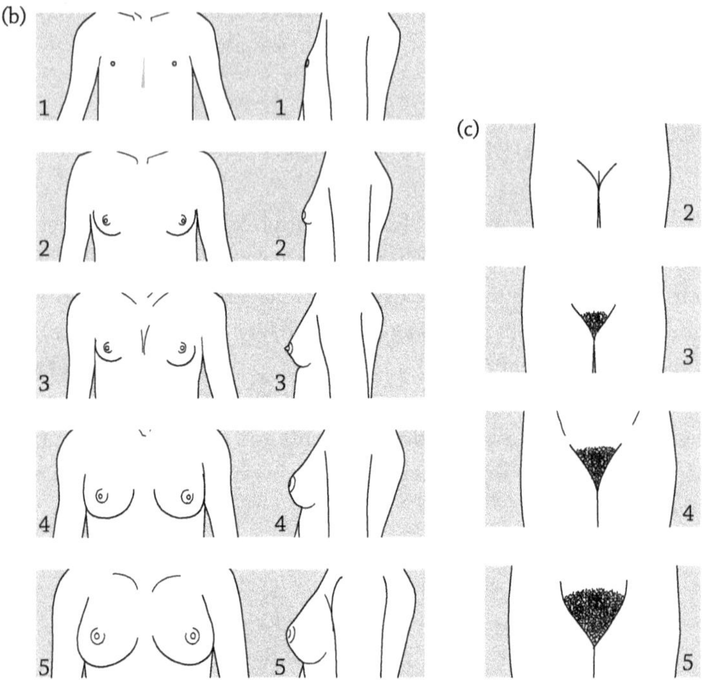

Figure 10.2(b,c). (b) Female breast development (B-1–B-5) and (c) pubic hair (PH-2 to PH-5). Tanner stages. From Tanner (1975), by permission.

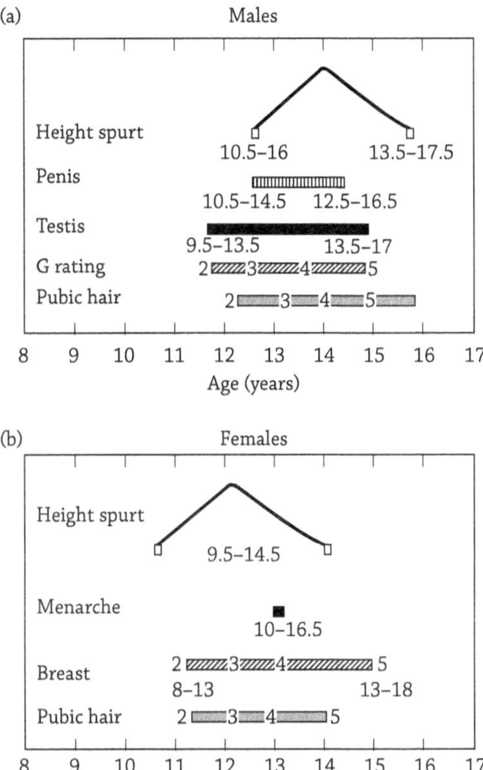

Figure 10.3(a,b). Sequence and timing of Tanner stages of puberty in (a) males and (b) females. From Tanner (1975), by permission.

			Time between stages (years)		
				Percentile	
	Mean age of stage onset ± 2 SD (year)	Stage	Mean	5th	95th
Males					
G-2	11.6 ± 2.1	G2–G3	1.1	0.4	2.2
G-3	12.9 ± 2.1	PH2–PH3	0.5	0.1	1.0
PH-2	13.4 ± 2.2	G3–G4	0.8	0.2	1.6
G-4	13.8 ± 2.0	PH3–PH4	0.4	0.3	0.5
PH-3	13.9 ± 2.1	G4–G5	1.0	0.4	1.9
PH-4	14.4 ± 2.2	PH4–PH5	0.7	0.2	1.5
G-5	14.9 ± 2.2	G2–G5	3.0	1.9	4.7
PH-5	15.2 ± 2.1	PH2–PH5	1.6	0.8	2.7
Females					
B-2	11.2 ± 2.2	B2–B3	0.9	0.2	1.0
PH-2	11.7 ± 2.4	PH2–PH3	0.6	0.2	1.3
B-3	12.2 ± 2.1	B3–B4	0.9	0.1	2.2
PH-3	12.4 ± 2.2	PH3–PH4	0.5	0.2	0.9
PH-4	12.9 ± 2.1	B4–B5	2.0	0.1	6.8
B-4	13.1 ± 2.3	PH4–PH5	1.3	0.6	2.4
PH-5	14.4 ± 2.2	B2–B5	4.0	1.5	9.0
B-5	15.3 ± 3.5	PH2–PH5	2.5	1.4	3.1

Figure 10.3(c). Means and standard deviations in the timing of stages of puberty. From Barnes (1975) by permission.

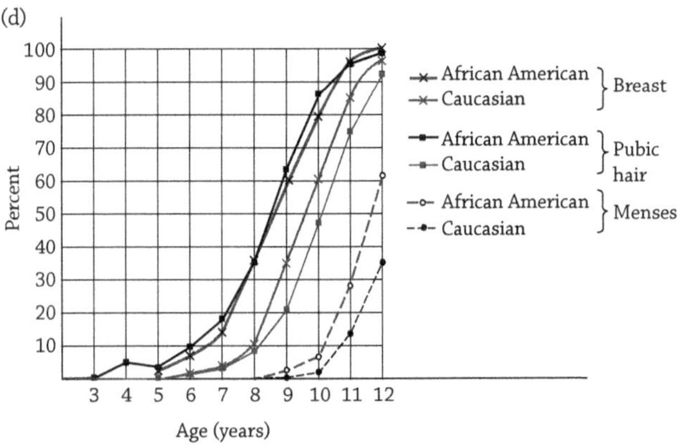

Figure 10.3(d). Racial differences in female pubertal development. Prevalence of breast development at Tanner stage 2 or greater by age and race; prevalence of pubic hair development at Tanner stage 2 or greater by age and race; and prevalence of menses by age and race. Adapted from Hermann-Giddens et al. (1997).

PENILE LENGTH

Definition The length of the gently stretched penis from the base of the tip.

Landmarks Measure from the base of the penis (pubic ramus) to the tip of the glans with the penis gently stretched. The glans of the penis may need to be palpated through the foreskin in individuals who are not circumcised. Alternatively, the foreskin can be retracted (Fig. 10.4).

Instruments A straight-edged clear plastic ruler, a tape measure, or blunt calipers.

Position Any comfortable position.

Remarks The penis may appear small if there is a ventral insertion of the scrotum (shawl scrotum or webbing of the penis). This anomaly is believed to be due to failure of the scrotal swelling to shift caudally in fetal life. This penis is buried within the scrotal fold but can be palpated and is usually of normal size.

Pitfalls If the fat pad at the base of the penis is not depressed so that the ruler touches the pubic ramus, a falsely short penile length will be perceived. If the penis is not gently stretched as a measurement is taken, the length of the penis may be as much as 2 cm shorter (Figures 10.5 and 10.6).

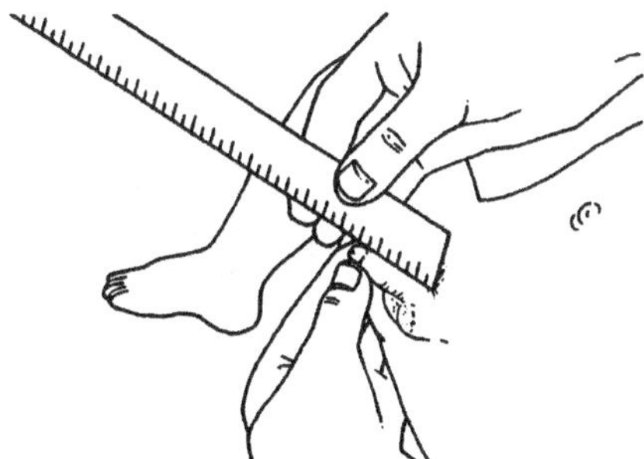

Figure 10.4. Measurement of penile length.

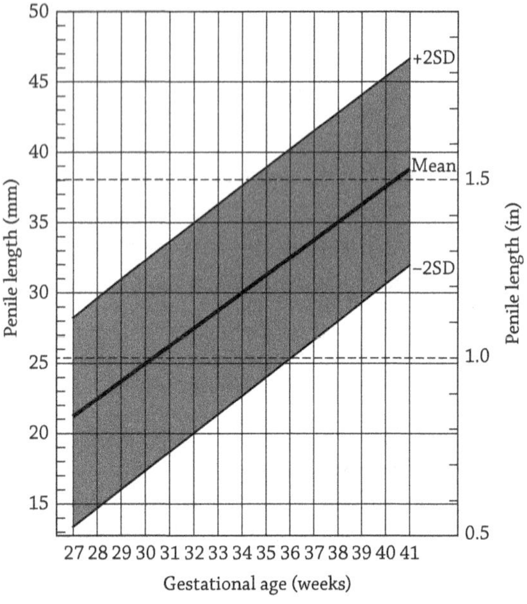

Figure 10.5. Penile length, 28–41 gestational weeks. From Feldmann and Smith (1975), by permission.

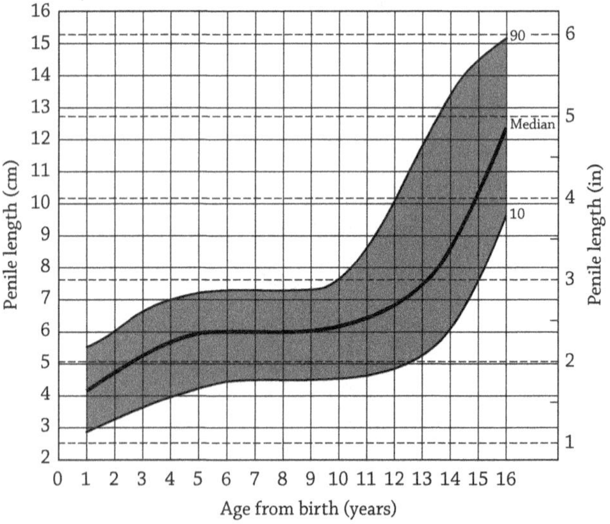

Figure 10.6. Penile length, 1 to 16 years. From Schonfeld (1943), by permission.

HYPOSPADIAS

Usually the urethra leaves the penile shaft at the tip of the glans of the penis. Hypospadias is an abnormal placement of the outlet of the urethra on the penis shaft. The location of the urethral outlet can be best seen by pulling the ventral skin of the penis outward. Classification of hypospadias is shown in Figure 10.7 and includes glandular, penile (along the shaft), penoscrotal (at the junction of the penis and scrotum), and perineal (the urethra opening on the perineum) outlet of the urethra. If the urethra opens on the dorsal side of the penis, this is called *epispadias* and again may have different degrees of severity.

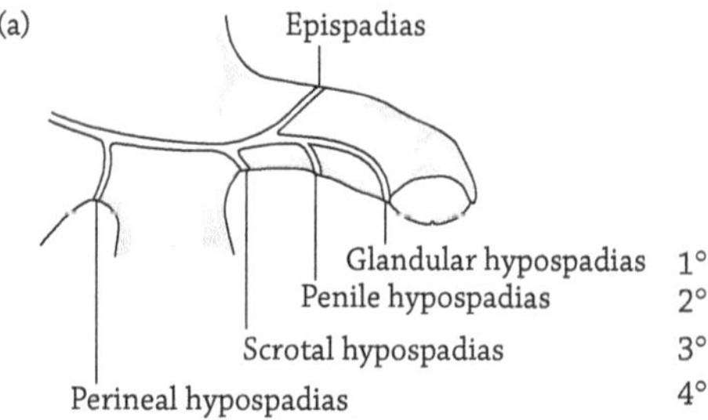

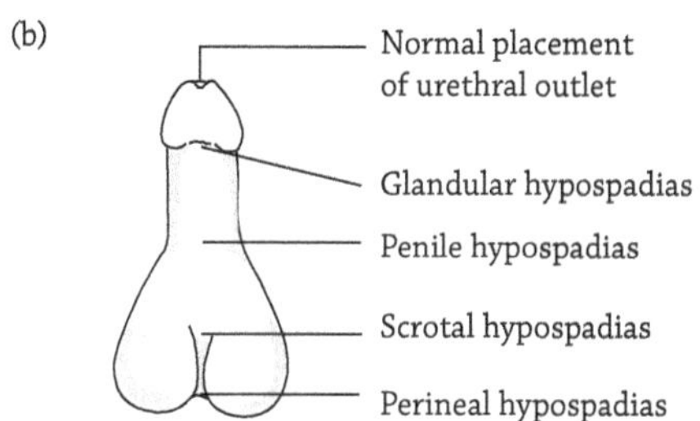

Figure 10.7. Types of hypospadias. From Alken and Soekeland (1976), by permission.

TESTICULAR VOLUME

Definition The volume of the testes.

Landmarks The length and width of the testis can be measured along a vertical axis between the upper and lower pole of the testis and at the broadest width.

Position The individual should be standing upright or lying supine.

Instruments The size of the elliptical shaped testis is most easily estimated by palpation and comparison with standardized, graded ellipsoid models of different volume sizes (Fig. 10.8). Since Prader developed and standardized these volume models, they are often referred to as "Prader beads." Several alternative methods for testis measurement are available, including blunt calipers, a tape measure, or straight ruler, or the measurement may be made using ultrasonography.

Remarks Comparative palpation with the orchidometer of Prader is a quick and fairly accurate way to estimate testicular size (Fig. 10.9). The volume in milliliters is clearly printed on each of the elliptical models. At young ages, intermediate volume size models can be

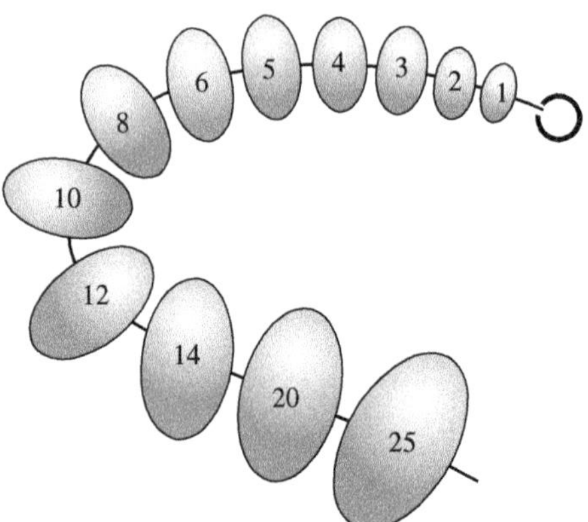

Figure 10.8. Prader orchidometer.

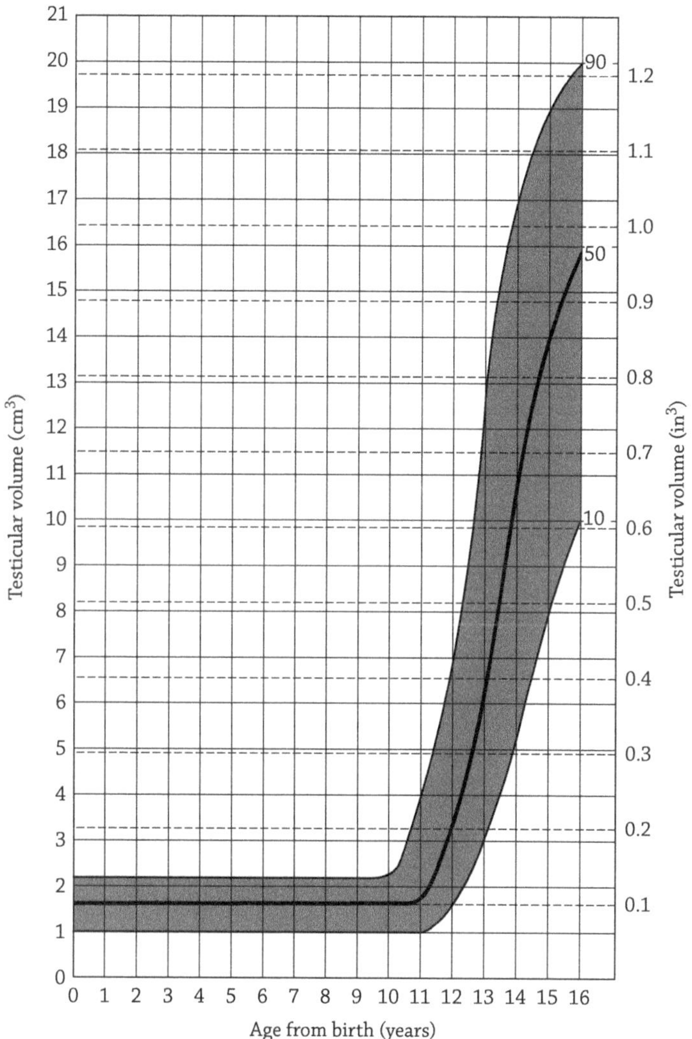

Figure 10.9. Testicular volume, birth to 16 years. From Zachmann et al. (1974) and Goodman and Gorlin (1983), by permission.

obtained (0.5, 1.5, and 2.5 mL size), and very large volume size models have also been developed for macroorchidism.

The use of a tape measure or a straight ruler to determine the longest and widest diameters is less accurate. When these linear measurements are used, the testicular volume must be calculated from comparison with age-matched normals. The calculation is made using the formula for ellipsoid volume:

$$\text{Testicular volume} = 0.71 \times \text{length}^2 \times \text{width}$$

If volumes are calculated or estimated, they should not be compared with the curves based on the measurements obtained from the orchidometer of Prader, because the calculation usually gives larger estimates of testicular volume. Only one method should be used to follow any individual patient over time and for comparison with other normal standards such as bone age (Fig. 10.10).

Testicular volumes for Japanese and Swiss males are compared in Figure 10.11.

Ultrasound measurements of testicular length and width have been utilized and seem to give the greatest accuracy and consistency of testicular volume.

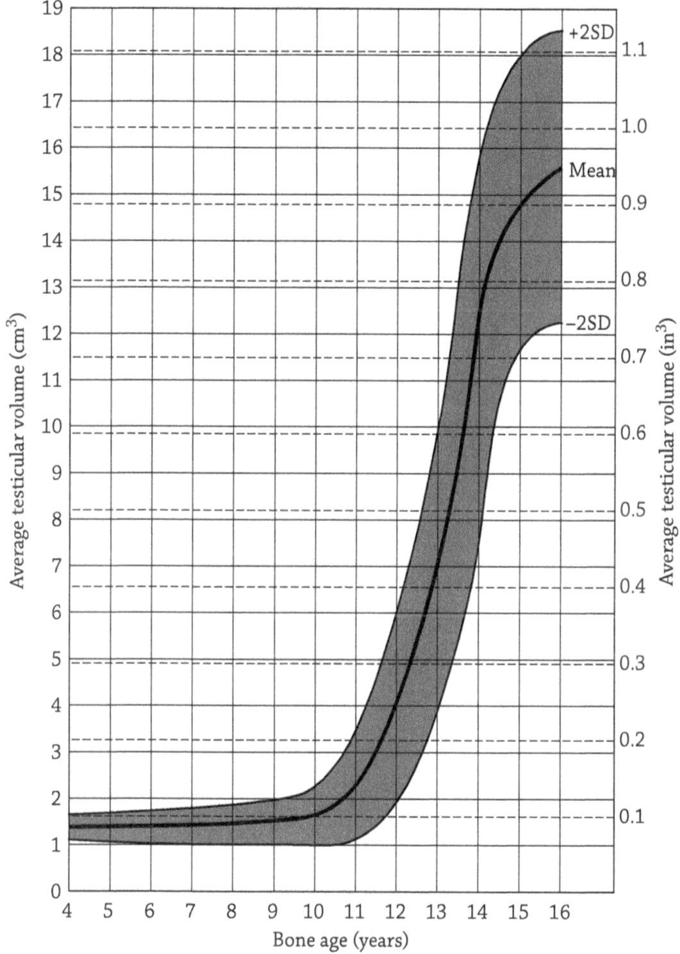

Figure 10.10. Testicular volume from bone age, 4 to 16 years. From Waaler et al. (1974), by permission.

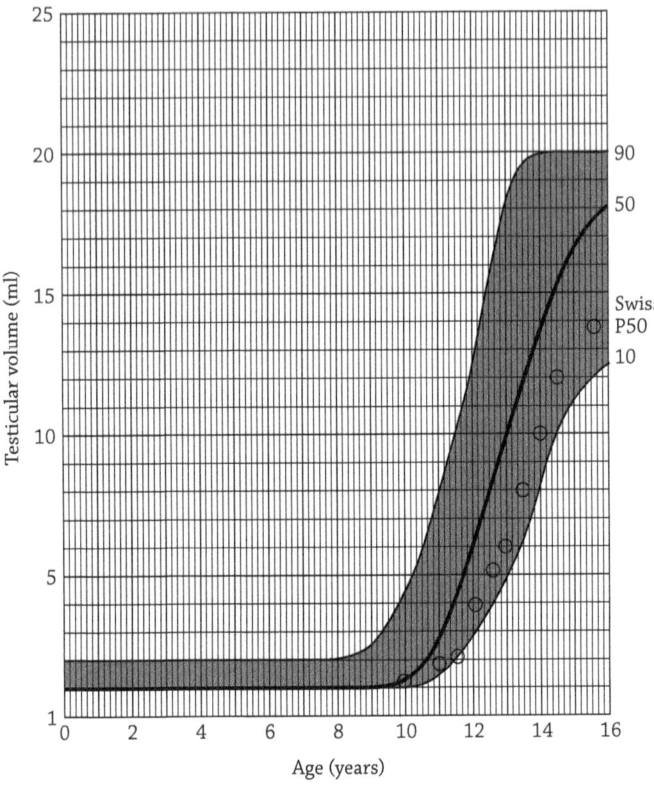

Figure 10.11. Testicular volume of Japanese males, birth to 16 years, compared to Swiss 50th percentile. From Zachmann et al. (1974); adapted from Matsuo et al. (2000).

TESTICULAR DESCENT

Definition Position of the testicle in its descent from the inguinal canal into the scrotum.

Landmarks The base of the penis and the superior margin of the testicle are identified. The testicle is gently retracted away from the body. The distance from the base of the penis to the superior margin of the testicle is measured.

Position This measurement is best taken when the patient is resting in the supine position.

Instrument A plastic ruler or a tape measure may be used.

Remarks Values for testicular descent are shown in relation to age in Figure 10.12a and by Tanner stage in Figure 10.12b.

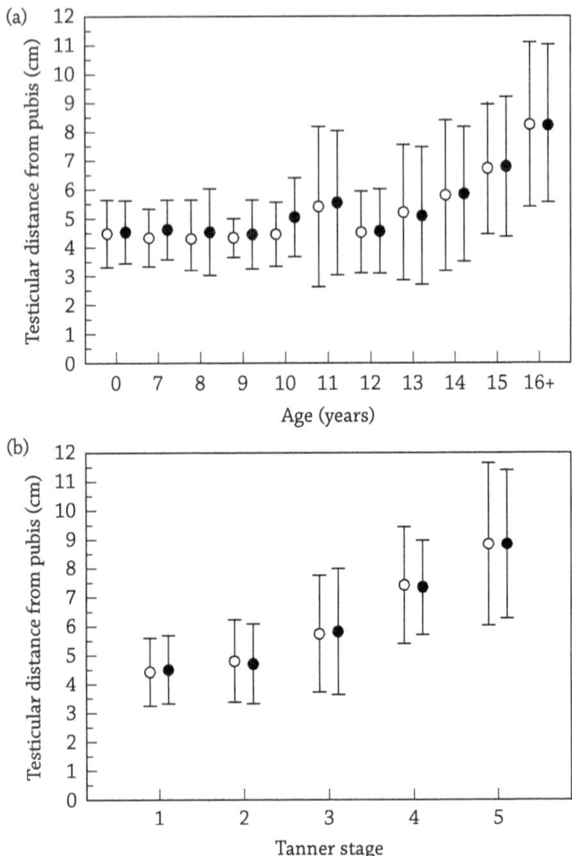

Figure 10.12. Testicular descent measurement by age (a) and by Tanner stage (b); symbol indicates mean measurement, and vertical line indicates two standard deviations from the mean. Open circles, right testicle; filled circles, left testicle. Adapted from Sack et al. (1993).

ANAL PLACEMENT

Definition The position of the anus in relation to the vaginal introitus or beginning of scrotal tissue.

Landmarks The distance between the posterior aspect of the introitus of the vagina (fourchette) in the female, or the end of scrotalized skin in the male, and the anterior border of the anal opening is measured.

Position The small infant should be in a supine position with the hips and knees held flexed, allowing the gluteal folds to open. A child or older individual can bend forward at the hips or be prone with the legs drawn up toward the abdomen, opening the perineal area for measurement.

Remarks Normal measurements are presented in Figures 10.13 and 10.14. In the male an abnormality in anal placement usually presents as an anus that is anteriorly placed on the perineum, or as a skin-covered anus; in the female it is generally as a persistent fistula between the rectum and vagina or as an aberrant placement of the anus, with no space or too little space between the anus and the vaginal introitus.

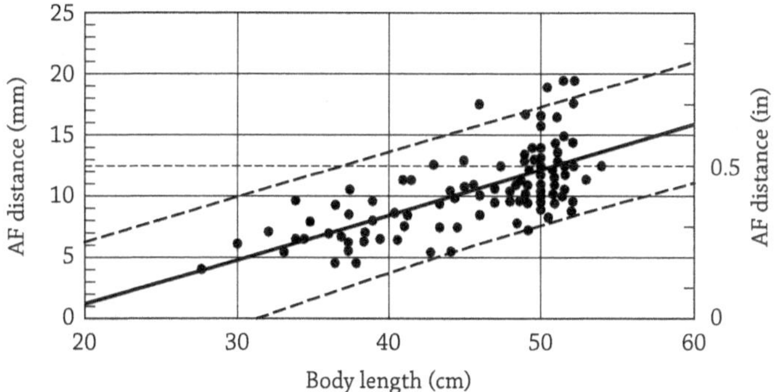

Figure 10.13. Anus-to-fourchette (AF) distance, related to body length in newborns, both sexes. From Callegari et al. (1987), by permission.

	Anus–fourchette (AF) (mm)	Fourchette–clitoris (FC) (mm)	Anus–clitoris (AC) (mm)	AF/AC	FC/AC
Infants ($n = 115$)	10.9 ± 3.5	19.4 ± 4.3	29.6 ± 6.3	0.37 ± 0.07	0.67 ± 0.07
Adults ($n = 10$)	30.1 ± 7.5	54.2 ± 11.1	84.0 ± 13.9	0.36 ± 0.07	0.64 ± 0.05

Figure 10.14. Clinical measurements. Values represent mean ± SD. From Callegari et al. (1987) by permission

ANAL DIAMETER

A serious anal stenosis can be excluded by determining the anal diameter. This is done either by placing a gloved little finger into the anal opening or by the use of graduated sounding instruments (Hegar sounds). In the newborn, there is a correlation between anal diameter and weight (Fig. 10.15).

Incomplete development and separation of the cloaca into the urogenital sinus and the rectum will result in various anorectal anomalies. An international classification of anorectal anomalies is available (Fig. 10.16) that helps to relate the embryologic aberration with the clinical appearance and presentation of the anomaly.

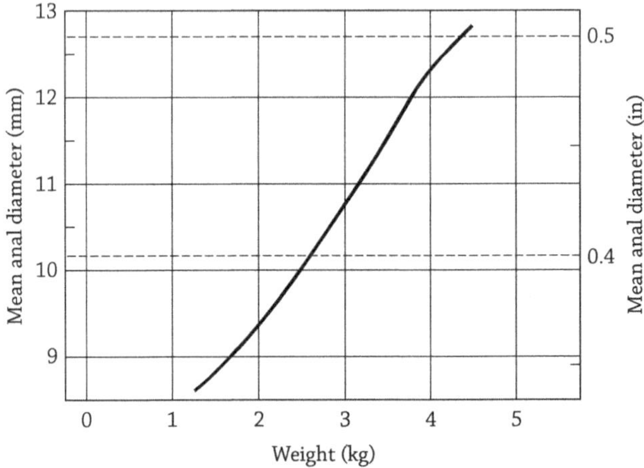

Figure 10.15. Mean anal diameter. From Haddad and Corkery (1985), by permission.

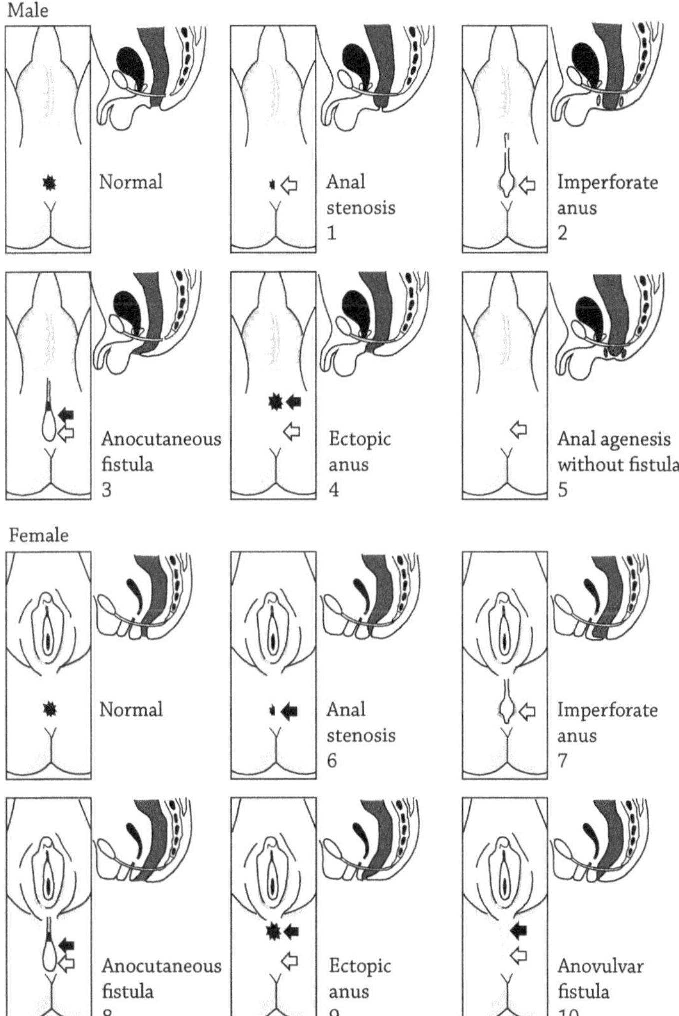

Figure 10.16. Anal anomalies. From Santulli et al. (1970), by permission.

BREAST AND NIPPLE SIZE AND SHAPE

Introduction

The female breast undergoes physiological changes with age, starting with an infantile form, in which the areola and papilla of the nipple are visible, but flat. In the next stage, during early adolescence, a slight prominence of the nipple area ("pouting") can be observed, which is followed by primary development of breast tissue with continued prominence of the areola. During puberty, the epithelial and fibrous tissues of the mammary gland proliferate under the influence of estrogens, and the stroma, fat, and connective tissues develop, while the ducts grow. In the sexually developed female breast the nipple is integrated into the rounded shape of the adult breast.

The mammary gland consists of 15–20 lobes that radiate from the nipple. The ducts of the lobes unite and form a single excretory duct, which ends in the nipple. The size of the breast varies with age, nutritional state, and the number of pregnancies, as well as with ethnic and genetic background. It is difficult to establish a normal size. An average adult female breast size of 400 mL (range 120– 600 mL) has been calculated for nonpregnant northern European women of normal weight using a Plexiglas cylinder to measure breast volume.

Landmarks The female breast can be measured in a vertical diameter (length), measuring lateral to the breast along the trunk wall from the lower insertion along the base of the breast to the point of upper insertion, where a slight curve away from the thorax wall can be found (Fig. 10.17).

The prominence or protrusion of the breast is measured from the middle of the base of the breast on the chest wall to the point of elevation of the areola insertion (Fig. 10.17). Since the size of the nipple varies, it is not included in the measurement.

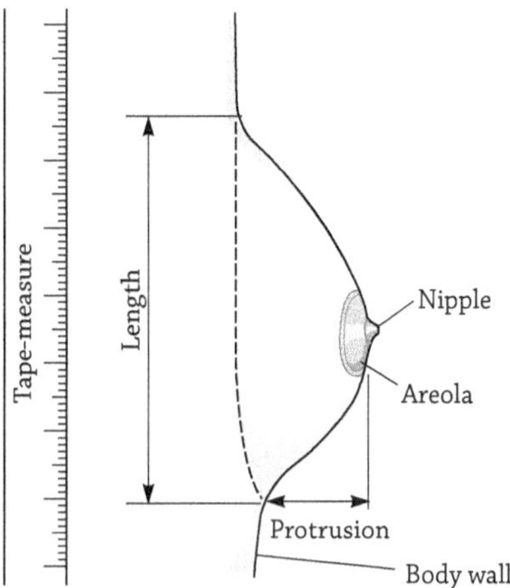

Figure 10.17. Measurement of breast size.

MEASUREMENT OF BREAST VOLUME

A variety of methods may be used to define the breast volume:

1. weighing the breast on a scale, which can be done with pendulous breasts;
2. using a water-filled container placed over the breast and into which the breast is placed. Since the volume of water in the container is known, the breast size can be calculated from the amount of water displaced;
3. making a cast of the breast, and the volume of the breast is measured from the cast;
4. measuring the breast size with a special breast-measuring cylinder of Plexiglas with a fitted domed piston and a scale, from which the breast size can be read.

Instruments Calipers, tape measure, solid ruler, or, for breast volume, a Plexiglas cylinder with a domed piston.

Position The individual should stand or sit with the arms hanging loosely. The measurements with a tape measure or calipers are taken from along the side of the breast.

If a cylinder is used to assess breast volume, the breast is placed in the cylinder, and the position of the piston is read off the scale.

Remarks There are a variety of normal shapes of the female breast. Usually the left breast is slightly larger than the right. Asymmetric development (anisomastia) and overgrowth of breast tissue (macromastia) can be part of specific syndromes.

A small amount of breast development is often present in the newborn due to maternal hormones. It is usually not pathological. Mild breast development in males frequently occurs around puberty.

PTOSIS OF THE BREAST

Ptosis of the breast means drooping of the breast, so that in an upright position, the lower surface of the breast is below the lower insertion on the thorax (submammary fold) and the skin of the breast is in direct contact with the skin of the thorax. Ptosis of the breast occurs with aging and after nursing and multiple pregnancies. To measure ptosis of the breast, the woman is seated and a tape measure is placed from the middle of the clavicle down to the nipple. Alternatively, an imaginary horizontal line can be drawn between the nipples and the distance from the top of the manubrium to the nipple line measured. The normal position of the nipple is 21–23 cm from the top of the manubrium.

Areola Measurements

Areola measurements include diameter and prominence from the breast tissue. The diameter of the nipple is very variable, as is the diameter of the areola. On average, the adult female areola measures 3–4 cm in diameter.

Instruments The nipple diameter can be measured with a plastic template circular cutouts, calipers, or a transparent ruler.

Remarks Significant differences in nipple diameter can be noted between stages B1 to B5 of breast development during puberty. Nipple size can be a useful measurement in girls with primary amenorrhoea. Girls with a large nipple diameter (greater than 0.7 cm) can be considered to have undergone hormonal stimulation.

Abnormalities of the nipple include extra or accessory nipples along the "milk line," absent or hypoplastic nipples (as in Poland anomaly, where part of the pectoral muscle and limb may also be missing), polythelia (more than one nipple on a breast), and inverted nipples (the tip of the nipple is directed inward and does not protrude from the areola). Hypoplasia or absence of the nipple and/or the mammary gland may be seen in ectodermal dysplasia.

BIBLIOGRAPHY

Alken, C. E., and Soekeland, J. (1976). *Urologie* (7th ed). Stuttgart, Germany: Georg Thieme Veriag.

Barnes, H. V. V. (1975). Physical growth and development during puberty. *Medical Clinics of North America*, 59, 1305–1316.

Callegari, C., Everett, S., Ross, M., and Brasel, J. A. (1987). Anogenital ratio: Measure of fetal virilization in premature and full-term newborn infants. *Journal of Pediatrics*, 11, 240–243.

Feldmann, K. W., and Smith, D. W. (1975). Fetal phallic growth and penile standards for newborn male infants. *Journal of Pediatrics*, 86, 395–398.

Goodman, R. M., and Gorlin, R. J. (1983). *The malformed infant and child.* Oxford, England: Oxford University Press.

Haddad, M. E., and Corkery, J. J. (1985). The anus in the newborn. *Pediatrics*, 76, 927–928.

Herman-Giddens, M. E., Slora, E. J., Wasserman, R. C., Bourdon, C. J., Bhapkar, M. V., Koch, G. G., and Hasemeier, C. M.(1997). Secondary sexual characteristics and menses in young girls seen in office practice: A study from the Pediatric Research in Office Settings Network. *Pediatrics*, 99, 505–512.

Matsuo, N., Anzo, M., Sato, S., Ogata, T., and Kamimaki, T. (2000). Testicular volume in Japanese boys up to the age of 15 years. *European Journal of Pediatrics*, 159, 843–845.

Prader, A. (1966). Die Hodengroesse. Beurteilung und klinische Bedeutung. *Triangel*, 7, 240–243.

Sack, J., Reichman, B., and Fix, A.(1993). Normative values for testicular descent from infancy to adulthood. *Hormone Research*, 39, 118–121.

Santulli, T. V., Kiesewetter, W. B., and Bill, A. H. (1970). Anorectal anomalies: A suggested international classification. *Journal of Pediatric Surgery*, 5, 281–287.

Schonfeld, W. A. (1943). Primary and secondary sexual characteristics. *American Journal of Disease in Children*, 65, 535–542.

Tanner, J. M. (1975). Growth and endocrinology of the adolescent. In *Endocrine and genetic disease in childhood* (2nd ed.) (ed. A. Gardner). Philadelphia: W.B. Saunders.

Waaler, P. E., Thorsen, T., Stoa, K. F., and Aarskog, D. (1974). Studies in male puberty. *Acta Paediatrica Scandinavica*, *249*, 1–36.

Zachmann, M., Prader, A., Kind, H. P., Haeflinger, H., and Budliger, H. (1974). Testicular volume during adolescence. *Helvetica Paediatrica Acta*, 29, 61–72.

Chapter 11

Skin and Hair

INTRODUCTION

The skin consists of two main layers: the superficial epidermis and the underlying dermis. At about 3 weeks of gestation, the epidermis consists of a single layer, while in the 4- to 6-week-old fetus, two layers can be distinguished: the superficial periderm and the basal, proliferative stratum germinativum. The periderm keratinizes and desquamates, giving rise to cells in the amniotic fluid and the vernix caseosa (the white cheese-like substance that covers the fetal skin until near term). By 8 to 11 weeks of gestation, proliferation of the stratum germinativum has produced several intermediate layers of epidermis, and at birth, all the layers normally seen in adult epidermis, including a keratinized layer and the pigmentary cells (melanocytes), are present.

At about 11 weeks of gestation, mesenchymal cells in the dermis begin to produce collagen and elastin fibers. When the epidermal ridges grow into the dermis at 11 to 12 weeks and begin to form the ridges and grooves that will produce dermatoglyphics, the dermis projects up into the epidermis to form the dermal papillae that will contain capillary loops and sensory nerve endings. A network of blood vessels forms in the fetal skin; some of these vessels are transitory and normally disappear.

The completely developed skin has three layers: the epidermis, the dermis, and the subcutis or subcutaneous, which is loose subcutaneous tissue. The surface of the epidermis is keratinized and covers an area of approximately 1.5 to 2 m^2, weighing 0.5 kg in an adult. There is variation in epidermal thickness, depending on the body area. The skin is thinner, for example, around the eyes and lips, and it is thicker in the palmar and plantar areas. On average, the skin is 0.1 cm thick. The dermis is separated from the epidermis by a basal membrane. The dermis consists of collagen, elastin, and reticular fibers, as well as a variety of cell types and a matrix with many complex carbohydrates. The subcutis connects the skin with underlying tissue and consists of a loose organization of fibers and septa. It contains a variable amount of fat, known as the panniculus adiposus. Skin turgor relates to the amount of subcutaneous fat. Thinning of the panniculus adiposus will result in an increased number of skin creases.

The surface of the skin is complex and varies in different body areas. Small lines can be found in the skin surface that criss-cross the body surface. These lines are thought to be the result of the configuration of the dermal papillae, which reach up to the epidermis, the underlying collagen bundles, and the pull of muscles underneath the skin. Some regions of the skin are oilier than others, reflecting the presence of a variable number of sebaceous glands. Other areas are covered with numerous vellus hairs, like the superior helices of the ears, or the upper lip in females. Skin texture also depends on the number, function, and size of the sweat glands. Skin can be firm, soft, rough, moist, dry, or oily. The texture of skin changes with age, resulting in uneven atrophy and hyperplasia, development of yellowish thickened plaques and subcutaneous nodules, areas of erythema, telangiectasia, and brown macular irregular pigmented lesions. With aging, there are progressive degenerative changes in collagen and the collagen is replaced by elastic fibers. Thinning of the overlying epidermis also occurs with aging.

EXTENSIBILITY OF SKIN

The extensibility of the skin varies with age and is greatest in older people. There are also differences between the sexes, apparently dependent on hormonal variations. Female skin is more extensible at all ages. There is variable extensibility in different parts of the body—the neck and elbow skin is looser than the skin on the forearms and hips. Extensibility depends on the collagen content of the skin. There are ways to precisely measure the extensibility of skin that involve attaching a weight onto a piece of skin and measuring how far it stretches.

For clinical purposes, a subjective estimate of skin extensibility is usually sufficient. An easy way to estimate extensibility of skin is to pinch the outer side of the upper arm, holding the skin between the thumb and index finger, then lightly pulling it upward. If the skin stretches more than 1 cm, hyperextensibility should be suspected.

PATTERNS REFLECTED BY THE SKIN

Because the human embryo is originally segmental, various structures reflect a segmental pattern that can be appreciated on the surface of the body.

The melanin-producing cells are of neural crest origin and apparently migrate embryologically in a predictable pattern. This pattern was first described by Blaschko. When pigmented streaks reflecting that migration are seen, they are called "Blaschko lines" (Fig. 11.1). Disorders of pigmentation and mosaicism for two or more genetically different cell lines can be associated with the presence of these lines.

The sensory innervation of the skin is structured segmentally, according to the dermatomes (Fig. 11.2a,b). Some skin disorders, such as herpes zoster, may reflect this dermatome distribution. It is extremely useful to know the sensory nerve distribution of specific nerves when trying to pinpoint a neurological disorder. The distribution of motor nerves is also segmented but follows a different distribution than the sensory distribution.

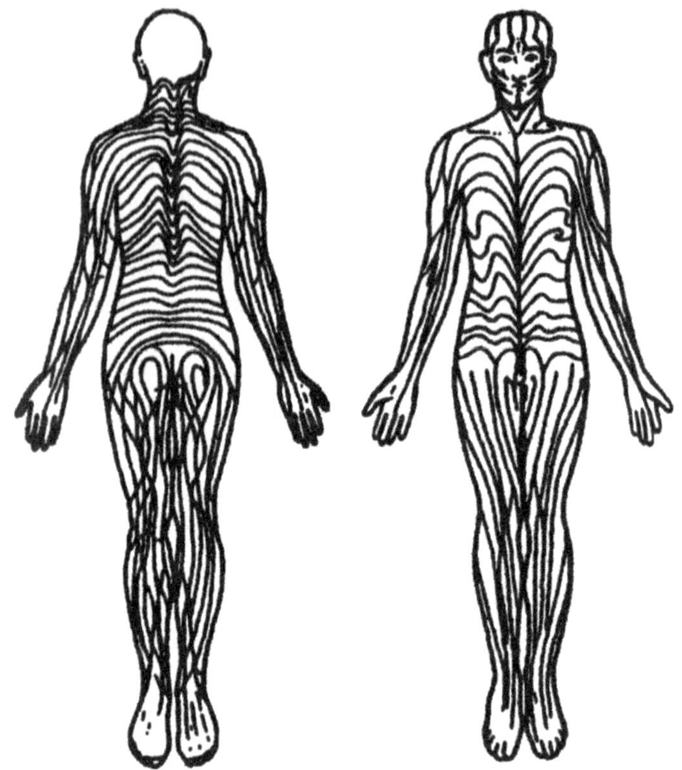

Figure 11.1. Blaschko lines.

SKIN COLOR

Origin and Distribution

Melanin is the black or brown pigment that is responsible for the color of the skin, hair, and local variation in pigmentation. It is produced only by the melanocytes. Melanocytes derive embryologically from melanoblasts. They migrate from the inner neural crest to the dermoepidermal junction. Mature melanocytes are essentially confined to the basal layers of the epidermis. In dark-skinned ethnic groups, pigment activity can be observed from the fourth fetal month.

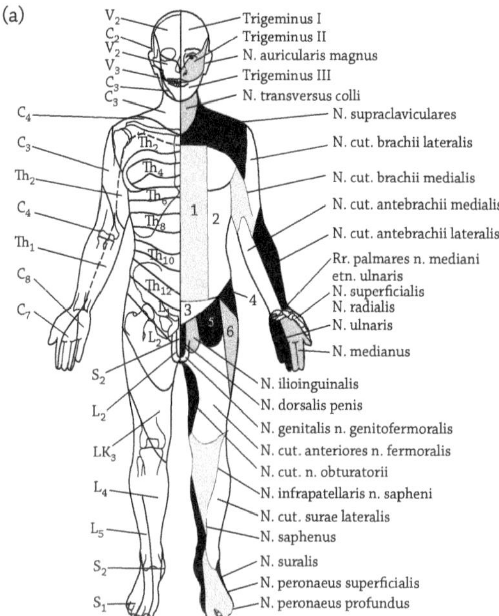

Figure 11.2(a). Sensory innervation of the skin.

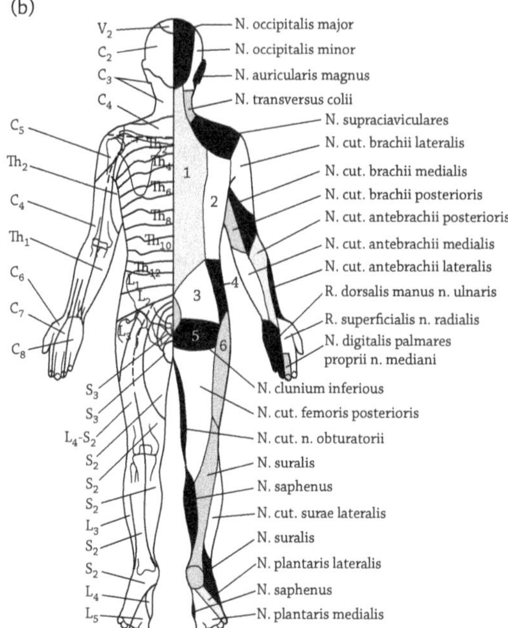

Figure 11.2(b). Sensory innervation of the skin.

The color of the skin depends on both the amount and distribution of the melanin in the epidermis (and occasionally in the dermis) and the vascularization of the skin. Additional factors that influence the skin color include hormones, such as melanocyte-stimulating hormone and the sex steroids, and exogenous factors, such as heat, injury, and exposure to ultraviolet light. Skin color can range from pale-yellow to gray-black. There are characteristic regional variations in skin color common to all ethnic groups (e.g., palms are lighter than the rest of the hands; skin color around the eyes is usually darker) as well as specific ethnic differences, such as pigment-free mucous membranes in Europeans.

Describing Skin Color

In describing skin color, it is essential to name the body area of observation (ventral, dorsal, chest, palms, etc.). Usually the skin is lighter on the ventral part of the body compared to the dorsum. In addition, the appearance of areas exposed to the sun versus protected areas should be described, together with the differences between them. A skin color table may be helpful for special situations (see Bibliography).

Remarks For documentation of skin color, a color photograph is useful. The color of tooth enamel, nails, iris, body hair, and scalp hair, as well as skin, should be recorded. The skin around the nipple, especially after pregnancy, may be darker due to hormonal influences. Genital skin and areas of apocrine sweating are usually darker. Pigment changes can occur in specific diseases, such as Addison's disease (a bronze skin color) or albinism (skin and hair pigment may be reduced or absent).

Pitfalls

Skin color can be artificially altered and pigmented by make-up, dirt, and different forms of tattooing. Artificial light may give unusual tones or hues to the natural colors.

BIRTHMARKS

Definition Various regionally limited, congenital alterations of skin pigmentation or skin color are referred to as birthmarks. They may not be observed at birth, but usually they are obvious by several months of age. They can be due to the presence of an increased number of superficial lymph or blood vessels, increased pigment in the epidermis, aberrant tissue present in the skin, or pigment variation in the dermis.

Local Variations in Pigmentation

Café au lait macule Macular area of increased pigment

- *Size*, a few millimeters to many centimeters
- *Frequency*, 5% of the population
- *Localization*, all body areas
- *Origin*, local melanocyte activity
- *Remarks*, may be a sign of neurofibromatosis type I (NF1) if more than six café au lait spots greater than 0.5 cm before puberty or 1.5 cm after puberty are present

Blue nevus Bluish macular area, also known as dermal melanosis

- *Size*, usually larger than 5 cm
- *Synonym*, previously known as Mongolian spot; the blue color is an optical effect of deep-seated melanin
- *Frequency*, 9.6% in Caucasians, 95.5% in African Americans, 81% in Asians
- *Localization*, primarily over the sacrum and the gluteal region
- *Origin*, ectopic melanocytes in the dermis
- *Remarks*, no pathological significance; can be present from the fifth gestational month and usually disappears during childhood because of the loss of dermal pigment

Depigmentation Macular area of reduced pigment:

- *Frequency*, 1% of the population
- *Localization*, can affect small, circumscribed body areas or with a patchy distribution
- *Origin*, lack of functional melanocytes
- *Remarks*, multiple small, leaf-shaped depigmented areas may be a sign of tuberous sclerosis

Mole Circumscribed area of dark pigment:

- *Synonym*, lentigo, compound nevus
- *Frequency*, very common
- *Localization*, all body parts, usually present at birth but may occur later
- *Color*, varies from dark brown to black
- *Shape*, may be flat, elevated, verrucoid, dome-shaped
- *Origin*, proliferation of melanocytes

Capillary Hemangioma

Local variation of vasculature Pink macular area, commonly on the nape of the neck, eyelids, glabella, and mid-forehead in newborns:

- *Synonyms*, nevus simplex, erythema nuchae, angel's kiss, salmon patch, stork bite
- *Size*, very small fleck to several centimeters
- *Frequency*, very common; may be obvious at birth or appear within the first few days; persists throughout life but becomes less obvious with age
- *Origin*, dermal capillaries or telangiectases, representing fetal circulatory patterns in the skin
- *Remarks*, may be a sign of capillary malformation syndromes, such as megalencephaly-capillary malformation syndrome (previously known as macrocephaly-capillary malformation syndrome) or capillary malformation-arteriovenous malformation syndrome

Elevated vascular nevus Elevated irregular lesion of solid red color:

- *Synonym*, strawberry nevus, cavernous hemangioma, capillary hemangioma
- *Frequency*, 10% of the population
- *Localization*, single or multiple, all body areas
- *Origin*, enlarged or dilated vessels of the skin (nevus vascularis). Thrombosis may occur inside the nevus, which may resolve spontaneously, but rarely it may require therapeutic intervention, especially if a vital function or vision is disturbed.
- *Remarks*, usually not present at birth, but appear in the first few months of life, enlarging during the first year and then most often resolving spontaneously.

Port wine nevus Large, dark angioma; may start as pink-colored macule that later becomes purple and may be raised; at first they may be smooth but can become irregular later.

- *Synonym*, nevus flammeus
- *Frequency*, 0.3% of the population
- *Localization*, any area of the body, but usually anterior or lateral, not posterior; most frequently unilateral and rarely crosses the midline
- *Origin*, dilated mature capillaries of the dermis
- *Remarks*, can be a sign of Sturge–Weber syndrome if in the distribution of the first branch of the trigeminal nerve; does not resolve spontaneously.

Telangiectasia Prominent blood vessel on the surface of the skin.

- *Origin*, results from a widening of the capillaries
- *Localization*, the main location is on the nose, the upper lip, conjunctiva, and the cheeks
- *Remarks*, the number increases with age; it can be seen in the ataxia–telangiectasia syndrome and in hereditary hemorrhagic telangiectasia

Lymphangioma Overgrowth of lymphatic vessels.

- *Synonym*, cystic hygroma
- *Localization*, mostly found in the neck area, less commonly affects the tongue area
- *Origin*, results from abnormal lymphatic vessels
- *Remarks*, can lead to an excess of skin in the neck area when it occurs prenatally and subsequently resolves

Other Anomalies of the Skin

Nevus sebaceous Raised waxy patch, often linear.

- *Synonym*, Jadassohn nevus
- *Origin*, organoid nevus of the epidermis with a preponderance of sebaceous glands
- *Frequency*, 0.2% of the population
- *Localization*, frequently on scalp or head
- *Remarks*, may be associated with developmental disabilities and seizures; may be present in Proteus syndrome

Cutis aplasia Area of absence of skin.

- *Frequency*, rare, less than 0.1%
- *Localization*, usually in the midline at the vertex of the scalp
- *Origin*, Gene mutations can cause aplasia cutis as part of a syndrome; early prenatal exposure to methimazole or carbimazole can also cause cutis aplasia of the scalp
- *Remarks*, frequent in trisomy 13 and Adams-Oliver syndrome

Dimple Area in which the skin is attached to underlying structures.

- *Localization*, frequently over knuckles and on cheeks; occasionally at ankles, knees and elbows; rarely over buttocks or sacrum
- *Origin*, occurs in areas where there is unusually close proximity between bone, joints, or muscle and the skin during fetal life

Congenital alopecia Patch of skin without hair growth.

- *Localization*, may occur anywhere on the scalp or body
- *Origin*, absence or loss of hair follicles may result from failure of hair follicles to develop or from follicles that produce a decreased amount of hair.

GLANDS OF THE SKIN

Introduction

There are two kinds of glands in the skin: the sebaceous glands and the sweat glands (Fig. 11.3). Most sebaceous glands develop along the side of a developing epithelial root sheath of a hair follicle. In the child and adult, they produce oil for the skin.

Two kinds of sweat glands occur: eccrine and apocrine. The eccrine sweat glands are found almost all over the body, whereas the apocrine sweat glands are situated primarily in the axillary area, the pubic area, around the nipple, and to a lesser extent, around the nose, in the outer ear canal and on the eyelids.

Quantification of the Number of Sweat Glands

There are normally about 2 million sweat glands on the surface of the skin. To assess the number of sweat glands on the skin surface, several different techniques exist. Most ignore the apocrine sweat glands.

Chemical method A solution of *o*-phthaldialdehyde can be put on the skin. The chemical produces a black color if sweat is excreted, designating the sweat pores.

Stereomicroscopy Using a 7× objective of a stereomicroscope, the sweat pores on the epidermal ridges of the fingertips can be quantitated by recording the number of pores along 0.5 cm of a dermal

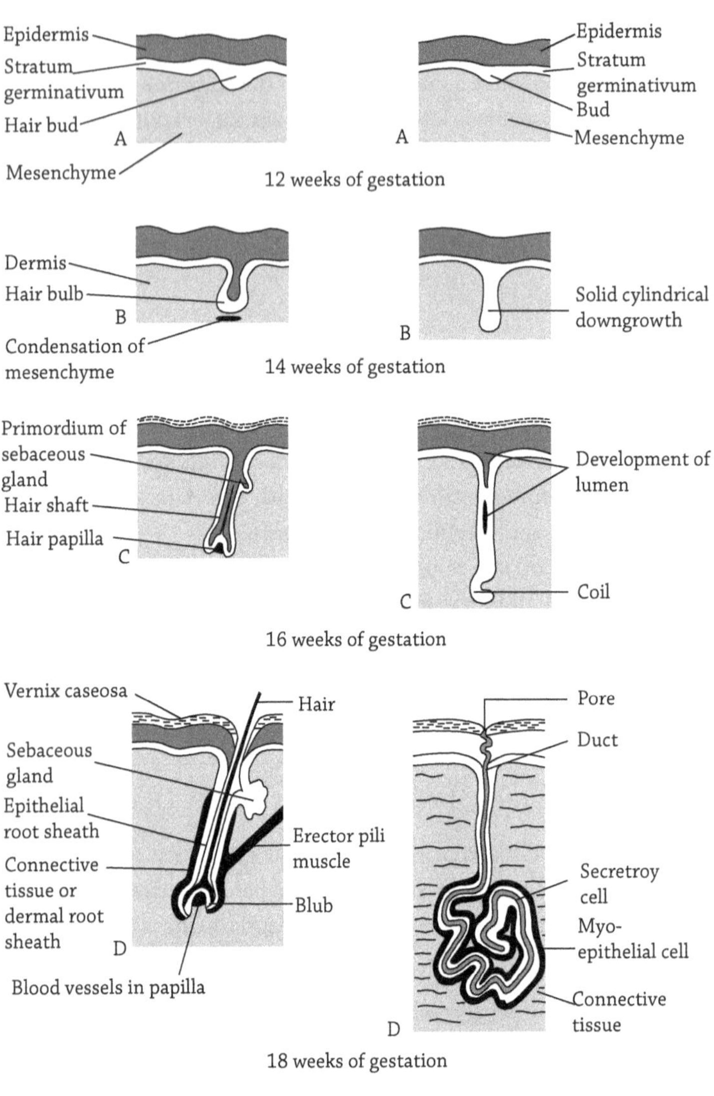

Figure 11.3. Development of sweat glands and sebaceous glands and the hair shaft. From Moore (1982), by permission.

Skin area	No.
Forehead	113 (>60 years, 83)
Dorsum of hand	130 (>60 years, 89)
Shoulder	35 (>60 years, 27)
Upper arm	36 (>60 years, 36)
Elbow, flexion side	751
Palmar	373
Breast	155–250
Backside	57
Fingertips	32 (2–3 weeks)
	23 (18–30 years)
	<20 (60–84 years)

Figure 11.4. Average number of sweat pores in skin body area (per cm^2) From Fiedler (1969) and Frias and Smith (1968), by permission.

ridge. A transparent plastic template with an open square of 0.5 cm per side is used. The count should be performed on 10 ridges from 10 different fingers (Fig. 11.4).

Electron microscopy A more accurate way to quantitate sweat glands is to determine the number of glands seen on electron microscopic examination of a skin biopsy.

Alternative Another method is to count the sweat pores on a fingerprint using a microscope or other high magnification device (Fig. 11.4).

Remarks Different numbers of sweat glands occur in various parts of the body and decrease with age (Fig. 11.4). On average, before 20 years of age, there are 177 sweat pores/cm^2, whereas at 80 years of age there are only 101 sweat pores/cm^2.

In many forms of ectodermal dysplasia, the glands of the skin do not form or do not function in a typical way. Normally, a single sweat gland secretes 0.003–0.01 ng/mm per day. In the course of a day, the skin may secret 800 mL of sweat. Sweating is important for thermal regulation, and without normal numbers of sweat glands, an individual may become hyperthermic in hot weather.

HAIR

Introduction

The total amount of body hair is difficult to estimate. The head alone has approximately 100,000 hairs. There are three phases in the life cycle of the hair that need to be distinguished:

1. the growing stage, called *anagen*;
2. the involution stage, called *catagen*;
3. the resting stage, called *telogen*.

Many factors, including general health, climate, drugs, hormones, and genetic programming, affect the growth of hair. The rate of hair growth varies in different body regions (Fig. 11.5). On average, human hair grows 0.37 mm daily. In males, the scalp hair grows slower and the body hair grows faster than in females. Androgen increases the hair growth on the trunk and plays a role in male-pattern balding; however, the exact mechanism is not fully understood. Seventy to 100 scalp hairs are shed daily in the normal telogen phase. In the ageing process, the hair also loses color because melanin fails to be synthesized in the hair matrix.

	Hair growth (mm)			
Age (years)	Frontal	Whorl	Occipital	Temporal
5	0.25	0.27	0.40	0.31
25	0.44	0.35	0.39	0.39
30	0.35	0.39	0.41	0.37
60	0.27	0.28	0.28	0.23

Figure 11.5. Daily hair growth in different body areas. From Martin and Saller (1962), by permission.

Embryology and Hair Types

Hair is first recognizable at the eyebrow, upper lip, and chin areas at about the 20th week of gestation. The first hair, called lanugo, is fine and colorless, and is usually lost during the perinatal period. It will be replaced by coarser hair, the vellus. This persists over most body areas, except the axillary and pubic region, where it is replaced at puberty by coarse terminal hair. In males, similar terminal hair appears on the chest and the face.

All the hair follicles are present in the fetus. The distribution of hair in later life is mainly due to the difference in growth at the skin surface. Hair color, texture, and distribution need to be examined and recorded, particularly when an ectodermal dyplasia is suspected. The pattern of hair follicle distribution is discussed in Chapter 12.

Hair Color

Hair color depends on the degree of pigmentation. It can vary in different body areas and thus it is useful to record the color of eyebrow and eyelash hair in addition to that of the scalp and beard.

The hair color can be recorded by describing the shades of color. Examples are black, black-brown, dark-brown, red-brown, light-brown, dark-blond, fair, light, red, and albino. It can also be compared with hair color tables, as used by anthropologists (see Bibliography). Hair color can be altered by dyeing. The hair color charts for various hair dyes are also useful for recording the color.

Hair Texture

The texture of the hair can vary greatly between individuals, even from the same ethnic group (Fig. 11.6). The twisting of a single hair shows great variability along its shaft. Physiologically significant differences in hair structure from various body areas also exist. Body hair is usually curlier than scalp hair. Curly hair is flatter in cross-section

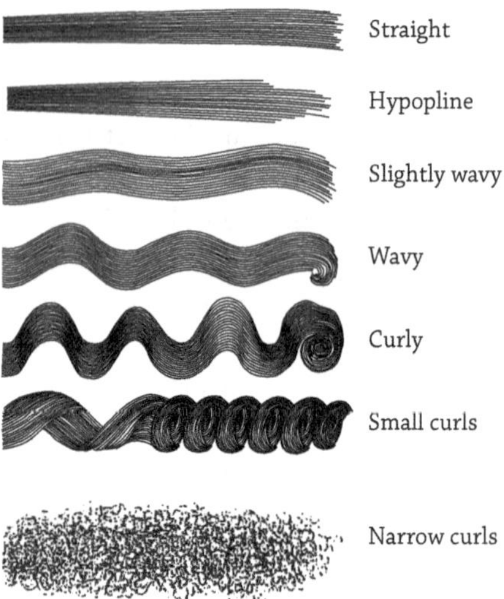

Figure 11.6. Normal forms of hair texture. From Martin and Saller (1962), by permission.

compared with straight hair, which is round. The major designations for hair texture include straight, wavy, curly, or narrow curls, but they can be further described as fine, coarse, wiry, stiff, or flexible. Structural anomalies of the hair can best be seen with the microscope (see Bibliography).

Balding

Balding occurs as part of the physiological process of aging. Timing of male baldness depends on the influence of androgens, age, and genetic predisposition. It usually starts in the frontoparietal area and this distribution is called "male-pattern" balding.

Female baldness usually occurs later, and the loss of hair is diffuse rather than starting with frontoparietal recession. Female balding is due to random atrophy of follicles and is associated with a decrease in circulating estrogen.

Alopecia

There are various pathological forms of hair loss; the most common is alopecia (see earlier), which is a premature loss of hair. It can be diffuse or circumscribed and can involve areas of the scalp or the whole body. It can also be transient or permanent.

Remarks Distinct, circumscribed areas of bilateral parietal-occipital alopecia are seen in association with a rare hindbrain malformation, rhombencephalosynapsis.

NAILS

Embryology and Normal Structure

The nails begin to develop at the distal end of the digits at about 10 weeks of gestation. They appear as thickened areas of the epidermis (Fig. 11.7). These nail fields are surrounded by a fold of the epidermis, the nail fold. Cells from the proximal part (the nail bed) of the nail fold grow over the nail field and become keratinized, forming the nail or nail plate. New nail growth is produced by the nail bed in the proximal part of the nail field. The nail bed can be seen in some individuals as a white crescent at the base of the nail. The developing nail is covered by an epidermal layer called the eponychium that later degenerates except at the base of the nail, where it is called the cuticle. The fingernail plate grows to reach the fingertip at about 32 weeks of gestation. The toenail plate reaches the tip of the toe at 36 weeks. The size of the nail field is influenced by the size of the underlying distal phalanx.

In the newborn, the mean width of the index fingernail is 5.0 ± 0 mm and the length is 3.5 ± 0.3 mm.

With aging, the convexity of the nail plate increases, and the nail plate thickens and may develop ridges. These changes can sometimes be confused with a nail infection. The rate of nail growth is more rapid in warm climate, while nail growth slows down with infections and age.

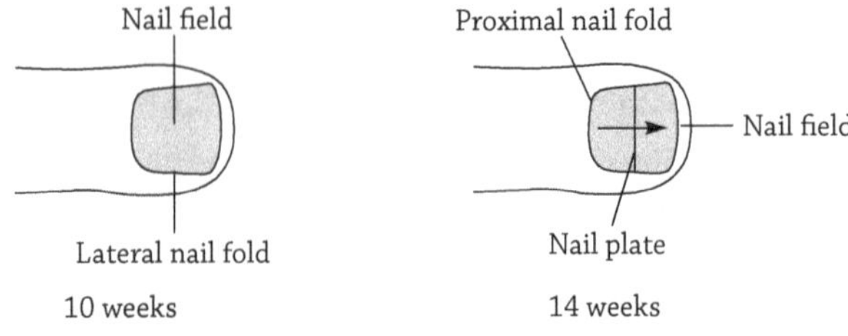

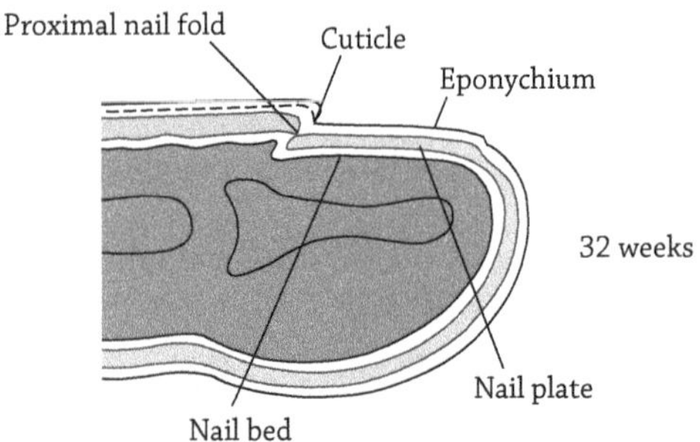

Figure 11.7. Development of nails. From Moore (1982), by permission.

Nail Size, Shape, Quality, and Color

The size of the nail in relation to the nail bed, the shape (e.g., round, oval, long, clubbed, broad [Fig. 11.8]), the quality (e.g., thick, thin, brittle, splitting, ridged, pitted), and any discoloration should be recorded. As with other body structures, photographs are often useful.

Specific changes can be seen in certain syndromes:

Longitudinal ridging occurs in cranio-fronto-nasal syndrome.

Longitudinal ridging and nail dystrophy with the thumbnails most severely affected, including absence of the lateral half of the thumbnail, may be seen in nail-patella syndrome.

Thickened, friable, and darkened fingernails and toenails are seen in pachyonychia congenita.

Subungual fibromas are seen in tuberous sclerosis.

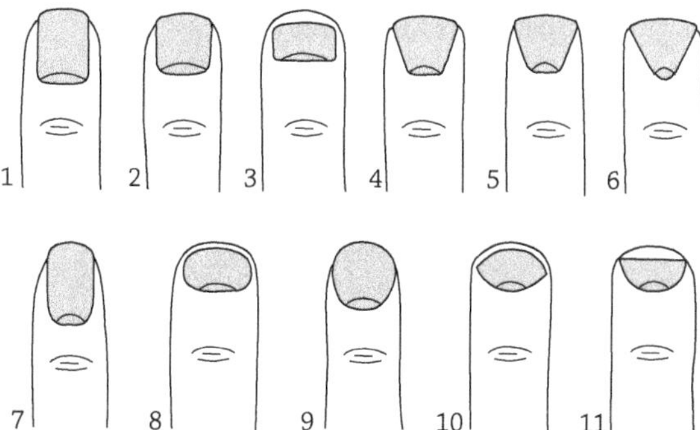

Figure 11.8. Normal variation of fingernail configuration. From Martin and Saller (1962), by permission.

Finger Clubbing

Clubbing of the finger and fingernail is an abnormal axial convex curved shape with enlargement of the distal finger and nail and loss of the angle at the nail fold. Clubbing of the fingers may be associated with an underlying pulmonary disease, as in cyanotic congenital heart disease, cystic fibrosis, and bronchial carcinoma. However, it can also be seen in Crohn's disease, cirrhosis, and thyrotoxicosis. Finger clubbing can be an important clinical sign in the progress of a disease. Inherited differences in finger shape can also resemble pathological clubbing, but the angle at the proximal nail fold is intact. The degree of clubbing can be recorded in photographs taken from the side of the finger. A lateral photograph of the index finger will document the proximal nail fold, cuticle, and nail, as well as the curve of the nail itself (Fig. 11.9).

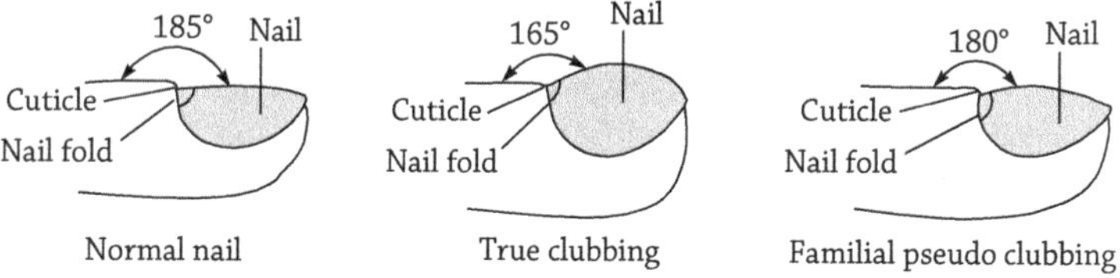

Figure 11.9. Schematic diagram of finger clubbing.

Method to Estimate Nail Growth

The growth of a nail can be followed by marking an area of the nail with silver nitrate or by punching or cutting a hole or mark into the nail (nail plate) itself and measuring the distance from the cuticle over a period of time (see Bibliography).

The average thumbnail takes 150 days to grow from its cuticle to the free edge of the nail. The average rate of nail growth is between 0.10 and 0.123 mm/day. The nails of children grow faster than those of adults.

BIBLIOGRAPHY

Bean, W. B. (1974). Nail growth: 30 years of observation. *Archives of Internal Medicine*, 134, 497–502.

Bentley, D., Moore, A., and Shwachman, H. (1976). Finger clubbing: A quantitative survey by analysis of the shadowgraph. *Lancet*, 2, 164–167.

Fiedler, H. P. (1969). *Der Schweiss*. Aulendorf, Germany: Editio Cantor.

Frias, J. L., and Smith, D. W. (1968). Diminished sweat pores in hypohidrotic ectodermal dysplasia: A new method for assessment. *Journal of Pediatrics*, 72, 606–610.

Gertler, W. (1970). *Systematische Dermatologie und Grenzgebiete* (Bd. I). Leipzig, Germany: Thieme Verlag.

Hamilton, J. B., Terada, H., and Mestler, G. E. (1955). Studies of growth throughout the lifespan in Japanese: Growth and size of nails and their relationship to age, sex, heredity and other factors. *Journal of Geronotology*, 10, 400.

Happle, R. (1985). Lyonization and the lines of Blaschko. *Human Genetics*, 70, 200–206.

Hudson, V. K. (1988). Newborn nail size. *Dysmorphology and Clinical Genetics*, 1, 145.

Jacobs, A. H., and Walton, R. G. (1976). The incidence of birthmarks in the neonate. *Pediatrics*, 58, 218–222.

Jacobs, A. H. (1979). Birthmarks: I. Vascular nevi. *Pediatrics in Review*, 1, 21–24.

Juhlin, L., and Shelley, W. B. (1967). A stain for sweat pores. *Nature*, 213, 408.

Lau, J. T. K., and Ching, R. M. L. (1982). Mongolian spots in Chinese children. *American Journal of Diseases in Children*, 136, 863–864.

Martin, R., and Saller, K. (1962). *Lehrbuch der Anthropologie*. Stuttgart, Germany: Gustav Fischer Verlag.

Moore, K. L. (1982). *The developing human*, pp. 432–446. Philadelphia: W.B. Saunders.

Smith, D. W. (1982). *Recognizable patterns of human malformation* (3rd ed.), p. 576. Philadelphia: W.B. Saunders.

Tan, K. L. (1972). Nevus flammeus of the nape, glabella and eyelids. *Clinical Pediatrics*, 11, 112–118.

Chapter 12

Dermatoglyphics and Trichoglyphics

DERMATOGLYPHICS: INTRODUCTION

In the sixth and seventh weeks of gestation, pads begin to develop on the palmar aspect of the fingertips, on the palm, in the interdigital spaces, as well as on the thenar and hypothenar areas of the proximal palm (Fig. 12.1). The pads show great variation in size and symmetry and influence the pattern of the developing dermal ridges. On the tips of the fingers, large fetal pads develop a whorl pattern, intermediate-sized pads a loop pattern, while a smaller flat pad will usually give rise to an arch pattern (Fig. 12.2). The permanent dermatoglyphic pattern is set by the 19th week of gestation.

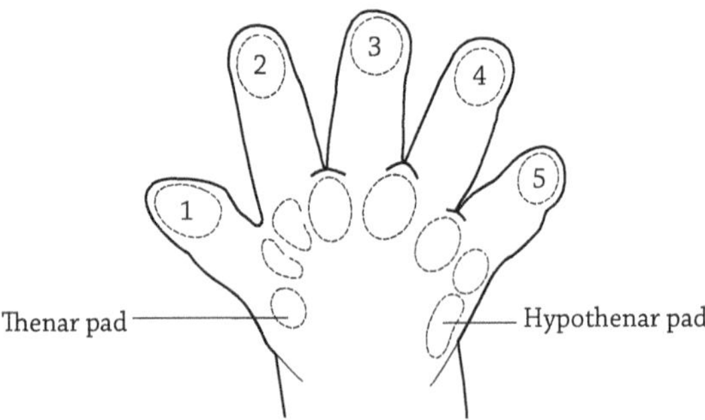

Figure 12.1. Distribution of pads at 10 weeks gestation. From Martin and Saller (1962), by permission.

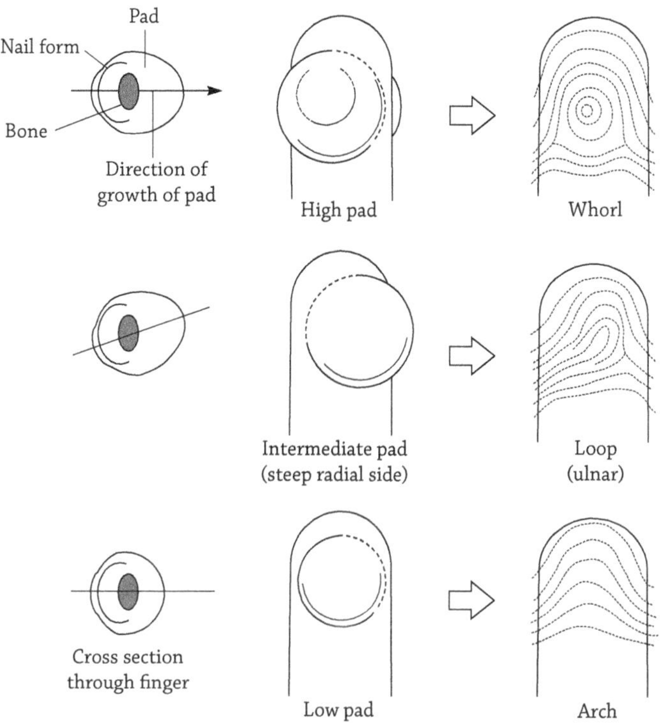

Figure 12.2. Relation of pad height and dermatoglyphic pattern. From Mulvihill and Smith (1969), by permission.

The flexion creases in the skin of the body begin to develop in the second to third gestational month. Those of the limbs are usually present by the sixth month of gestation. In the palms, the pattern of flexion creases appears to be influenced by the size of the pads in the thenar and hypothenar areas, the length of the bones, and intrauterine movement. The flexion creases of the palm do not all develop at the same time but from between the 8th and 13th weeks and are well defined by 13 weeks. They may consist of separate segments that later join (Fig. 12.3).

Strictly speaking, dermatoglyphics is the study of the epidermal ridge pattern of the skin, but, in general use, both the epidermal ridge

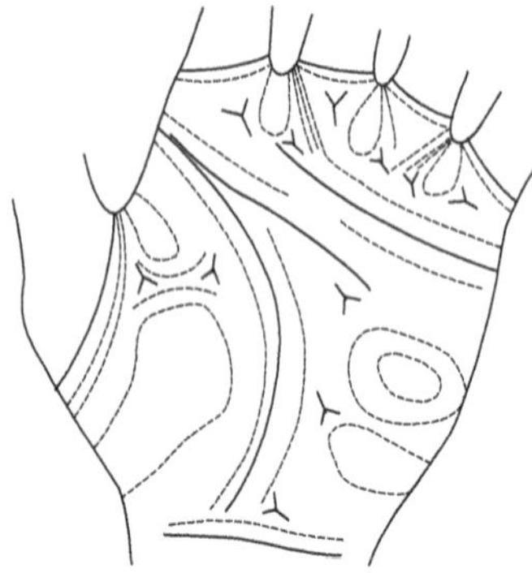

Figure 12.3. Flexion creases in the hand of a 10-week old embryo. From Martin and Saller (1962), by permission.

patterns and flexion creases are discussed together. They reflect structures and relationships that were present at the time they were forming. The epidermal ridge dermatoglyphic pattern consists of ridges (cristae superficiales) and grooves (sulci cutanei). A wide range of normal variation can be seen among dermal ridge patterns. The main patterns on the fingertips are described as arch, loop, and whorl (Fig. 12.2). Pattern variation is also seen in the thenar and hypothenar areas.

METHODS TO RECORD AND ANALYZE DERMATOGLYPHICS

There are several ways to record the dermal ridge patterns of the hands and feet. The first way is to evaluate the patterns with a magnifying glass, preferably one that has an integrated lamp, like an otoscope, or a device used by stamp collectors. For recording the dermal ridge patterns, prints can be made in several ways.

Ink Staining

Ink can be used to stain the patient's hands and feet, applied with a roller on a preinked pad, and distributed as evenly as possible (Fig. 12.4). The

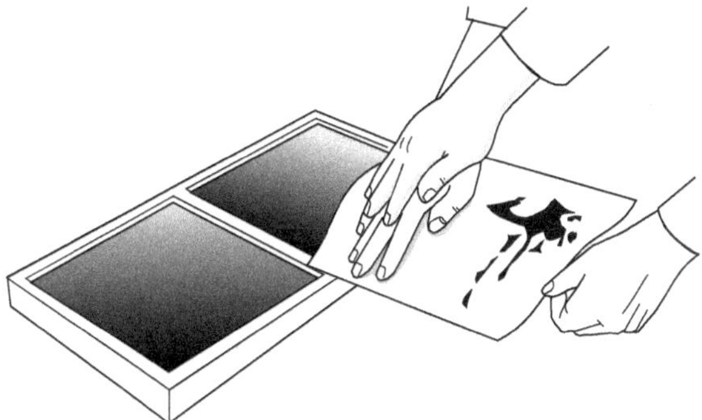

Figure 12.4. Recording dermatoglyphics by the ink-staining method.

print is made by pressing a piece of paper against the palm or letting the patient stand on a piece of paper (it might be easier to have the patient roll the hand over a roller covered with a piece of paper large enough to obtain a print of the whole hand). Backing the paper with a soft material allows the fingers to "sink into" the paper and results in better prints. Usually each fingertip pattern is also recorded by rolling it separately from side to side.

Photographic Emulsion

Instead of ink, a clear resensitizing fluid and photographic paper can be used. The technique for recording is the same. This method does not work as well for infants or on smooth lower ridges.

Graphite

Another alternative is to rub the patient's hands and feet with a soft graphite pencil. A print is taken by placing a broad piece of clear adhesive tape with the sticky side against the palm or sole. The adhesive tape is removed and can then be glued onto a white paper for better contrast and analysis. This method is particularly applicable for infants.

Photocopying

The hands and feet of an individual may be placed on a photocopying machine. The paper photocopies allow analysis of dermatoglyphics, but this is not a very precise method of obtaining dermatoglyphic data.

Scanning

Prints may be photographed by a scanner, similar to the photocopying approach. The images will then be stored, and at times analyzed, using specific computer programs.

ANALYSIS OF RIDGE PATTERNS

Dermal Ridge Count

To count the dermal ridges of a particular pattern, a line is drawn from the middle or center of the pattern to a triradius (a point at which three converging patterns meet) (Fig. 12.5). The number of ridges that are crossed by this line or touch the line is counted. The total dermal ridge count for the individual is the sum of the ridge count of the 10 digits. If there are 2 triradii, as in a whorl, the line is drawn to the most distal triradius. Arch patterns have no ridge counts.

The average dermal ridge count in males is 144; in females, 127.

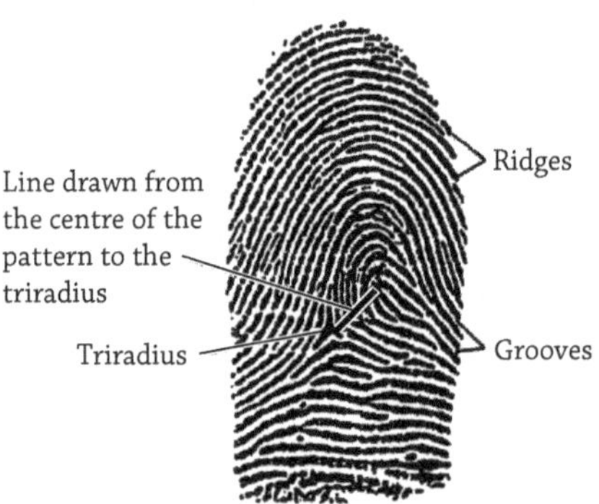

Figure 12.5. Measuring dermal ridge count.

Triradii

Triradii (or deltas) are the points at which three sets of converging ridge patterns meet. They are seen between the bases of the fingers, on the fingertips in loop and whorl patterns, and on the palm. Usually there is a triradius in the proximal part of the palm to the ulnar side of the center, just above the wrist flexion-crease: the proximal axial triradius (*t*). An angle can be established between the triradius at the base of the index finger (*a*), the proximal axial triradius (*t*), and the triradius at the base of the fifth finger (*d*). This is called the *atd* angle. A distal palmar triradius (*t′* or *t″*) may also be present. When the *at″d* angle is calculated, it is usually much larger than the *atd* angle. About 4% of Caucasians have a distal palmar triradius. Distal palmar triradii can be found in a number of syndromes, and their presence should alert the clinician to examine the dermatoglyphics more carefully.

Thenar, Hypothenar, and Hallucal Patterns

Patterns may be present in the thenar and hypothenar areas of the palm. Atypical patterns may be helpful in making a specific diagnosis. A lack of ridges in the hypothenar region of the palm can be seen in Cornelia de Lange syndrome. On the soles of the feet, in the hallucal area, a pattern (loop or whorl) is usually seen. If no pattern is present (i.e., there is an arch), the hallucal area is said to have an "open field." Open hallucal fields are very rarely found in normal individuals, but they are present in about 50% of patients with Down syndrome.

Normal Distribution of Fingerprint Patterns

Evaluation of the fingertips generally reveals a variety of patterns on different fingertips (Fig. 12.6). The patterns tend to be familial. The most frequent patterns are whorls on the thumb and the fourth finger, and ulnar loops on fingers three and five. Among normal

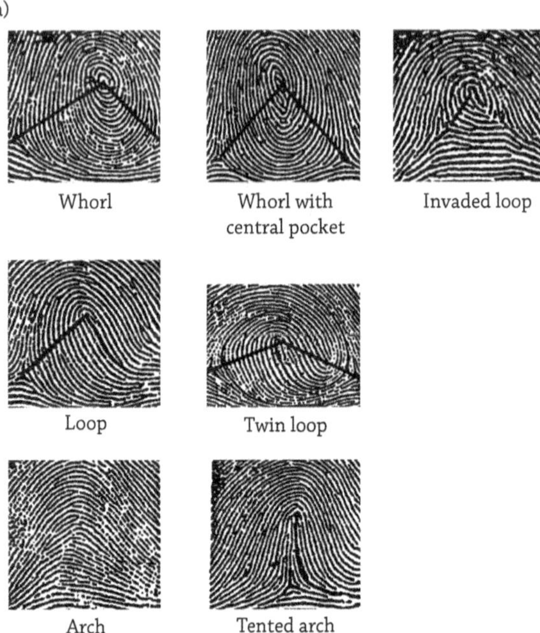

Figure 12.6(a). Normal fingerprint patterns. From Martin and Saller (1962), by permission.

	I(%)	II(%)	III(%)	IV(%)	V(%)	I–V(%)
Figures						
Arches	2.5	11.2	5.0	0.5	1.7	4.2 ± 2.1
Loops	60.7	48.5	73.0	50.7	83.2	63.2 ± 1.3
Whorls	36.7	40.2	22.0	48.7	15.0	32.5 ± 1.8
Toes						
Arches	7.0	9.0	4.2	16.5	58.2	19.0 ± 2.0
Loops	80.7	68.2	36.2	70.2	41.0	59.3 ± 1.4
Whorls	12.2	22.7	59.5	13.2	0.7	21.7 ± 1.9

Figure 12.6(b). Normal distribution of fingerprint pattern. From Martin and Saller (1962), by permission.

individuals, 0.9% have a predominance of arches on the fingertips, (i.e., 6 of 10 fingers show arches). However, this pattern is very frequently seen in patients with trisomy 18.

Three percent of normal individuals show 9–10 fingertips with a whorl pattern. Excessive whorl patterns derive from high fetal pads. They are seen frequently in patients with Turner syndrome or Noonan syndrome.

Radial loops on the fourth and fifth finger are unusual in normal individuals (1.5%) but are common in individuals with Down syndrome (12.4%).

Racial differences exist: Asians and Native Americans have an increased number of whorls.

Remarks

Alterations in the dermal ridge patterns or in the patterns of creases can be recognizable in various syndromes (Fig. 12.7 and Bibliography). They are rarely pathognomonic but may provide an additional clue to diagnosis. Any analysis of dermal ridges should include comparison with parental and/or family patterns.

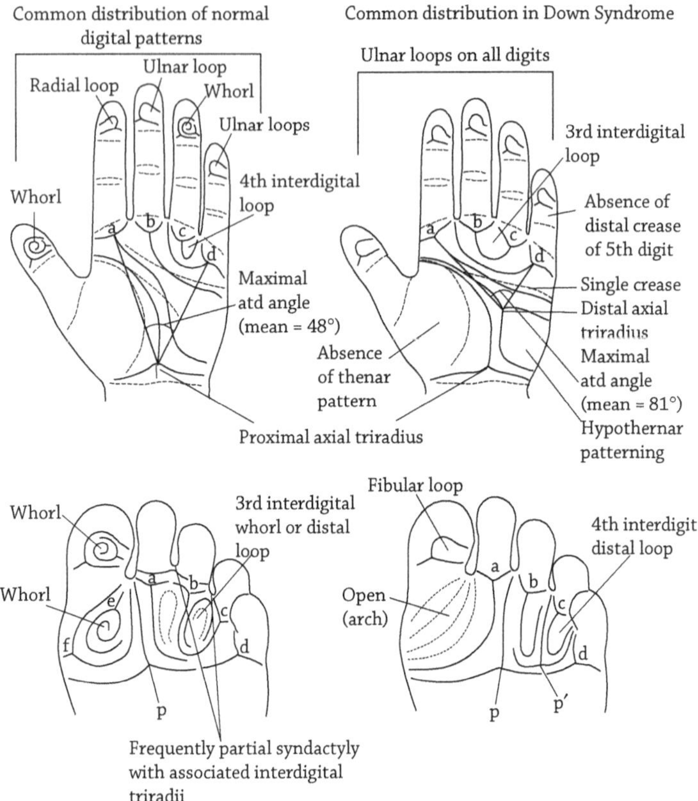

Figure 12.7. Comparison of normal and Down syndrome patterns on hand and foot. From Smith (1982), by permission.

ANALYSIS OF FLEXION CREASES

The flexion creases of fingers reflect flexion at the interphalangeal joint; those of the palm reflect movement of the hand and the digits against the palm early in fetal development.

The flexion creases usually evaluated include those of the fingers and the major flexion creases of the palm. Each finger usually has three transverse creases of similar depth. If a crease is missing, or diminished, in utero movement of the underlying joint may have been absent or abnormal. There are usually three major creases in the palm (Fig. 12.8).

The Five-Finger Crease

The five-finger crease (FFC) starts on the radial side of the hand near the insertion of the index finger and runs across the palm toward the ulnar side. If the FFC is long, it extends below the insertion of fingers 4 and 5. If it is of medium length, it extends below the insertion of the fourth finger, and if short it extends only to the third finger insertion.

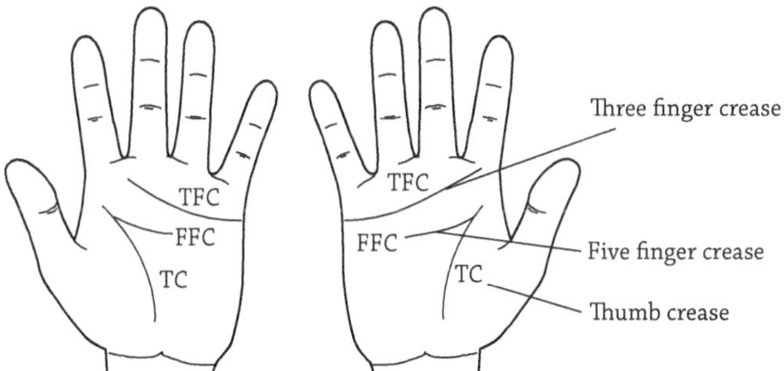

Figure 12.8. Normal flexion crease patterns. From Martin and Saller (1962), by permission.

The Three-Finger Crease

The three-finger crease (TFC) starts on the ulnar side below the insertion of the fifth finger and runs across the palm distally, usually ending below the index and middle finger. The TFC is long if it reaches to the index finger insertion, of medium length if it reaches the interdigital area between the index and middle finger, and short if it only reaches the middle finger.

The Thumb Crease

The thumb crease (TC) starts together with the FFC from the radial side of the palm but runs proximally toward the mid-wrist. It is the consequence of oppositional flexion of the thumb. The TC is long if it reaches down to the wrist crease.

Incomplete development of the FFC and the TFC may give rise to a single palmar crease (which may have different forms, being bridged or split). It may reflect alterations in the slope of the metacarpophalangeal plane of flexion or a short palm.

A single palmar crease (fusion of FFC and TFC) can be found unilaterally in 4% of the normal population and bilaterally in 1% of normal individuals. It is twice as common in males as in females. Single palmar creases are seen with increased frequency in Down syndrome. A Sidney line is said to be present when the FFC extends all the way to the ulnar border.

TRICHOGLYPHICS: INTRODUCTION AND EMBRYOLOGY

The patterning of hair follicles is called *trichoglyphics*. The hair shaft directional slope is secondary to the plane of the stretch exerted on the skin when the hair follicles are forming. During the first 2 months of gestation, the embryo is completely hairless. After the first 2 months of age, primary hair, called *lanugo*, starts to grow (Fig. 12.9).

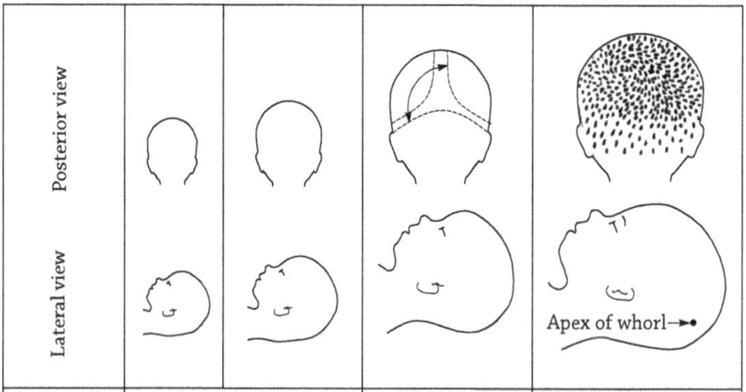

Posterior view				
Lateral view				Apex of whorl→•
Hair	Early hair follicles with sloping downgrowth		Hair being produced	Surface hair patterning evident
Gestational age	11 weeks	12½ weeks	16½ weeks	18 weeks
C–R length	71 mm	83 mm	122 mm	145 mm

Figure 12.9. Time of hair patterning. From Smith and Gong (1974), by permission.

On the scalp, the angle of the hair shaft reflects the prior plane of growth of the skin (e.g., the plane of growth present at the time when the follicle was forming). The plane of growth of the scalp skin is usually determined by the growth of the underlying brain.

The posterior parietal hair whorl is considered to be the focal point from which the growth stretch is exerted by the dome-like outgrowth of the brain during the time of hair follicle development. Central nervous system malformations that antedate hair follicle development, such as encephalocoele or microcephaly, would be expected to produce aberrations in scalp hair patterning. Eighty-five percent of patients with primary microcephaly have altered scalp hair patterning, indicating an early onset of the problem in brain development. Aberrant scalp patterning is also found frequently in association with established syndromes, including Down syndrome. Thus, aberrant scalp hair patterning may be used as an indicator of altered size and/or shape of the brain before 12 weeks gestation.

On the forehead, two normal patterns of hair growth can be distinguished: the forehead stream (growing from the area of inner canthus upwards) and the parietal stream (growing from the parietal whorl to the supraorbital area). As the two streams meet, they give rise to the shape of the eyebrows. Eyebrow shape also reflects the underlying supraorbital ridge shape present in early fetal life. At 18 weeks of gestation, hair grows over the entire scalp and face. Later in gestation, the hair growth in the eyebrow area and over the scalp will predominate, while hair growth over the remainder of the face is suppressed.

Early anomalies in development of the eye and face can secondarily affect hair patterning over the eyebrow and frontal area. Gross anomalies in development of the ear can also secondarily affect hair patterning, especially in the sideburn area.

NORMAL AND ABNORMAL HAIR PATTERNS

The normal location of the parietal hair whorl is several centimeters anterior to the posterior fontanelle, the majority (56%) being located slightly to the left of the midline. Thirty percent of hair whorls in normal individuals are right sided, and 14% have a midline location. Five percent of individuals have bilateral hair whorls posteriorly. Ninety-four percent of hair whorls are clockwise and 5% are counterclockwise.

From the posterior hair whorl, the hair sweeps anteriorly toward the forehead. The growth of the forebrain and the upper face influences the bilateral frontal hairstreams, which emerge from the ocular puncta and arch outward in a lateral direction. Usually the anterior and posterior hairstreams meet on the forehead. If they meet above the forehead, an anterior upsweep of hair will result (cowlick). A mild to moderate anterior upsweep is found in 5% of normal individuals.

Frontal upsweeps to the anterior hairline, as well as unruly hair patterns, have been linked to abnormalities of frontal lobe development. A widow's peak along the frontal scalp line is probably the result of the bilateral periorbital fields of hair growth suppression intersecting lower than usual on the forehead. This can occur when the periorbital fields of hair growth suppression are smaller than usual, or when they are widely spaced. Wide spacing also explains the association between ocular hypertelorism and widow's peak. The only common anomaly of the posterior hairline is low placement with a squared distribution, which may be seen in Turner syndrome, Noonan syndrome, and with abnormalities of cervical spine fusion or segmentation.

LANUGO HAIR PATTERN

Persistence of lanugo hair whorls can be found over the entire back, particularly over the upper spine and in the coccygeal area. A hair whorl over the lower spine can be a sign of a defect of neural tube closure, a congenital tumor, or a neurofibroma. In the coccygeal area there may be a dimple at the point of the whorl (fovea coccygea). The coccygeal whorl may be related to the stretch point of an embryologically existing tail rudiment.

BIBLIOGRAPHY

Aase, J. M., and Lyons, R. B. (1971). Technique for recording dermatoglyphics. *Lancet*, 1, 432–433.

Martin, R., and Saller, K. (1962). *Lehrbuch der Anthropologie*. Stuttgart, Germany: Gustav Fischer Verlag.

Moore, K. L. (1982). *The developing human*, pp. 432–446. Philadelphia: W.B. Saunders.

Mulvihill, J. J., and Smith, D. W. (1969). The genesis of dermatoglyphics. *Journal of Pediatrics*, 75, 579–589.

Rodewald, A., and Zankl, H. (1981). *Hautleistenfibel*. Stuttgart, Germany: Gustav Fischer Verlag.

Smith, D. W. (1982). *Recognizable patterns of human malformation* (3rd ed.), p. 576. Philadelphia: W.B. Saunders.

Smith, D. W., and Cohen, M. M. (1973). Widow's peak scalp-hair anomaly and its relation to ocular hypertelorism. *Lancet*, 2, 1127–1128.

Smith, D. W., and Gong, B. T. (1973). Scalp hair patterning as a clue to early fetal brain development. *Journal of Pediatrics*, 83, 374–400.

Smith, D. W., and Gong, B. T. (1974). Scalp-hair patterning: Its origin and significance relative to early brain and upper facial development. *Teratology*, 9, 17–34.

Smith, D. W., and Greely, M. J. (1978). Unruly scalp hair in infancy: Its nature and relevance to problems of brain morphogenesis. *Pediatrics*, 61, 783–785.

Uchida, I., and Soltan, H. C. (1963). Evaluation of dermatoglyphics in medical genetics. *Pediatric Clinics of North America*, 10, 409.

Chapter 13

Use of Radiographs for Measurement

INTRODUCTION

Two techniques, bone age and pattern profiles, are time honored in describing growth and its variation in children. For other measurements and detailed discussions, the reader is referred to the Bibliography. Limb lengths, specific bone lengths, and asymmetry are often most accurately measured on radiographs. However, correct positioning of the limb or body part is critical to accuracy.

BONE AGE

Bone age is an attempt to quantify bone maturation using radiographs. Bone age can reflect physiological growth and should be compared with height age and chronological age to assess the child's growth status. In normal children, bone age is an accurate reflection of physiological growth; however, in syndromes, growth disturbances, and skeletal dysplasias (either reduced growth or overgrowth), it may be inaccurate. Assessment of bone age is further complicated by differences in the techniques used, and the usefulness of each may vary depending on the circumstances. Despite these problems, an assessment of bone age is an important and useful technique to describe the growth of a child. It can also be used to predict ultimate height with some accuracy.

Assessment of bone age is dependent on the evolving appearance and growth of epiphyseal growth centers, particularly in long bones. In the normal child, there is a predictable pattern of ossification and growth. Two main methods of determining bone age are used:

1. evaluation of the appearance of ossification centers throughout the body;
2. observation of growth and changes in a specific epiphysis or epiphyses and comparison with standards, such as for the hand (Greulich and Pyle) or the knee (Pyle and Hoerr).

In general, appearance of the ossification centers of the feet and knees is thought to be most useful in the young child. After 2 years of age, changes in specific epiphyses (such as in the hands) are most accurate.

Ossification Centers

When taking X-rays to establish bone age, one should estimate approximate age to determine which will be the most useful films. Fig. 13.1 will help to predict which areas should be studied. The observed areas of ossification are identified and compared to the expected age of ossification (Figs. 13.2–13.6). The closest match is determined to be the present bone age.

Comparison with Established Standards

It is necessary to have the standard illustration present in the books by Greulich and Pyle (1959) and by Pyle and Hoerr (1969) to evaluate the shape and growth of phalangeal and knee epiphyses. By comparison with these standards, one arrives at a "best match" and establishes the bone age for the child.

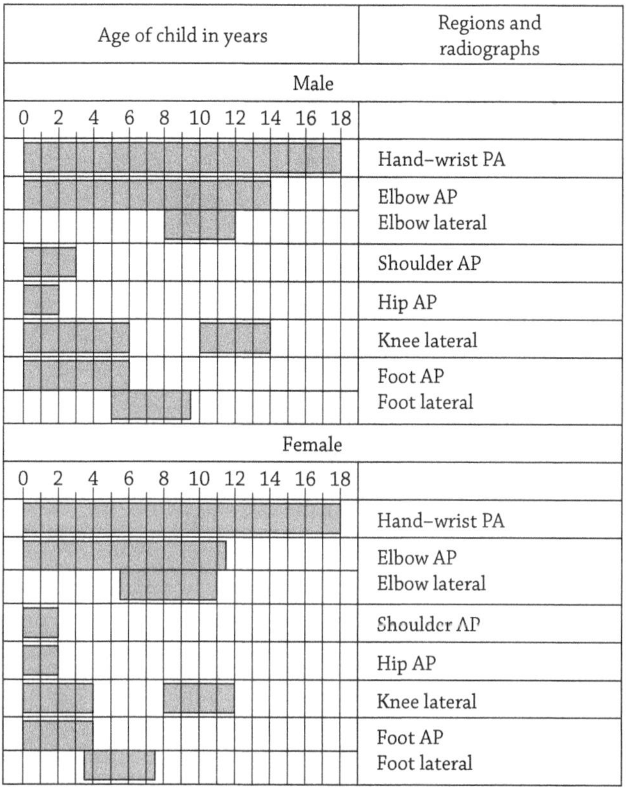

Age of child in years	Regions and radiographs
Male	
0 2 4 6 8 10 12 14 16 18	
	Hand–wrist PA
	Elbow AP Elbow lateral
	Shoulder AP
	Hip AP
	Knee lateral
	Foot AP Foot lateral
Female	
0 2 4 6 8 10 12 14 16 18	
	Hand–wrist PA
	Elbow AP Elbow lateral
	Shoulder AP
	Hip AP
	Knee lateral
	Foot AP Foot lateral

Figure 13.1. Region to sample for bone age for different chronological ages. From Graham (1972), by permission.

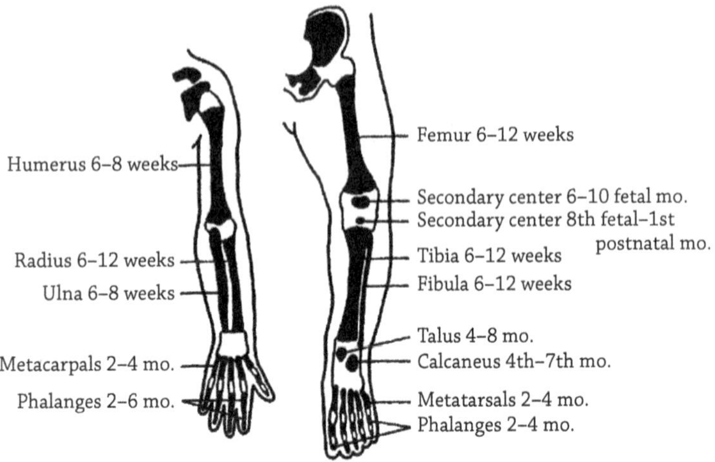

Figure 13.2. Fetal ossification centers. From Lowrey (1986), by permission.

Center	First seen	5%	50%	95%
Humeral head epiphyses	36	37	—	16 postnatal wk
Distal femoral epiphysis	31	31	34	39 wk (male, 40 wk)
	27	—	—	
Proximal tibial epiphysis	34	34	38–39	2 postnatal wk for female and 5 postnatal wk for male
Calcaneus	22	22	—	25 after 26 wk, always present
Talus	25	25	—	31 wk
	26	—	—	Talus may be absent until 34 wk
Cuboid	31	37	—	8 postnatal wk in female and 16 postnatal wk in male
	—	34		

Figure 13.3(a). Appearance time of ossification centers in the newborn (both sexes) in weeks of gestation

Ossification center	Birth weight (g) Under 2000	2000–2499	2500–2999	3000–3499	3500–3999	4000 or more
Calcaneus						
Caucasian Boys	100.0					
girls	100.0					
African American boys	100.0					
girls	100.0					
Talus						
Caucasian boys	72.7	100.0				
girls	83.3	100.0				
African American boys	90.9	100.0				
girls	100.0	100.0				
Distal femoral epiphysis						
Caucasian boys	9.1	75.0	85.3	100.0	100.0	
girls	50.0	91.7	98.0	100.0	100.0	
African American boys	18.2	88.5	90.7	94.0	100.0	
girls	50.2	93.8	99.0	100.0	100.0	
Proximal femoral epiphysis						
Caucasian boys	0.0	18.8	52.9	78.8	84.1	97.1
girls	0.0	54.2	75.5	85.7	90.7	90.5
African American boys	0.0	38.5	62.7	76.0	80.0	92.9
girls	14.3	40.6	76.7	88.1	86.4	100.0
Cuboid						
Caucasian boys	0.0	6.2	14.7	39.8	44.3	60.0
girls	0.0	37.5	57.1	65.2	70.4	76.2
African American boys	0.0	23.1	43.8	58.0	68.2	100.0
girls	21.4	37.5	68.0	78.2	81.8	75.0
Head of humerus						
Caucasian boys	0.0	7.7	13.8	41.9	49.0	59.1
girls	0.0	5.6	25.8	41.9	69.0	86.7
African American boys	0.0	0.0	15.2	27.6	48.4	63.6
girls	0.0	10.7	22.7	52.6	38.9	100.0

Figure 13.3(b). Presence of six ossification centers in roentgenograms of newborns From Kuhns and Poznanski (1980) and Lowrey (1986), by permission.

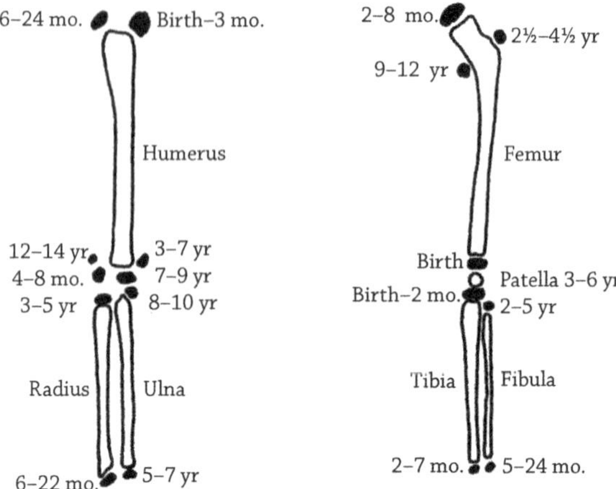

Figure 13.4. Appearance of ossification centers in limbs, both sexes. From Lowrey (1986), by permission.

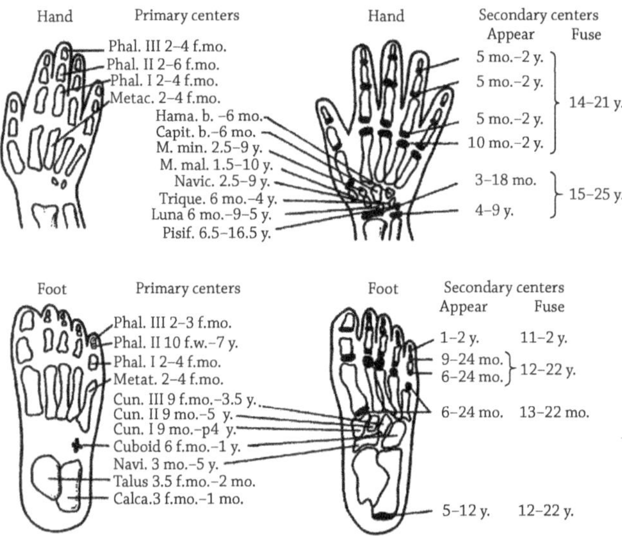

Figure 13.5. Appearance of ossification centers in hands and feet, both sexes. b., birth; Calca., calcaneus; Capit., capitate; Cun., cuneiform; f.mo., fetal months; f.w., fetal weeks; Hama., hamate; Luna., lunate; Metac., metacarpal; Metat., metatarsal; M. maj., multangular major (trapezoid); M. min., multangular minor (trapezium); mo., postnatal months; Navic., navicular; Phal., phalange; Pisif., pisiform; Trique., triquetrum; y., years. From Lowrey (1986), by permission.

	Boys (percentiles)			Girls (percentiles)		
	5th	50th	95th	5th	50th	95th
Wrist						
Capitate	Birth	3m	7m	Birth	2m	7m
Hamate	2w	4m	10m	Birth	2m	7m
Distal radius	6w	1y1m	2y4m	5m	10m	1y8m
Triquetum	6m	2y5m	5y6m	3m	1y8m	3y9m
Lunate	1y6m	4y1m	6y9m	1y1m	2y7m	5y8m
Scaphoid	3y7m	5y8m	7y10m	2y4m	4y1m	6y
Trapezium	3y6m	5y10m	9y	1y11m	4y1m	6y4m
Trapezoid	3y1m	6y3m	8y6m	2y5m	4y2m	6y
Distal ulna	5y3m	7y1m	9y1m	3y3m	5y4m	7y8m
Elbow						
Capitulum	3w	4m	1y1m	3w	3m	9m
Radial head	3y	5y3m	8y	2y3m	3y10m	6y3m
Medical epicondyle	4y3m	6y3m	8y5m	2y1m	3y5m	5y1m
Olecranon of ulna	7y9m	9y8m	11y11m	5y7m	8y	9y11m
Lateral epicondyle	9y3m	11y3m	13y8m	7y2m	9y3m	11y3m
Shoulder						
Head of humerus	37w*		16w	37w*		16w
Coronoid	Birth	2w	4m	Birth	2w	5m
Tubercle of humerus	3m	10m	2y4m	2m	6m	1y2m
Acromion of scapula	12y2n	13y9m	15y6m	10y4m	11y11m	15y4m
Acromion of clavicle	12y	14y	15y11m	10y10m	12y9m	15y4m
Hip						
Head of femur	3w	4m	8m	2w	4m	7m
Greater trochanter	1y11m	3y	4y4m	1y	1y10m	3y
Os acetabulum	11y11m	13y6m	15y4m	9y7m	11y6m	13y5m
Iliac crest	12y	14y	15y11m	10y10m	12y9m	15y4m
Ischial tuberosity	13y7m	15y3m	17y1m	11y9m	13y11m	16y
Knee						
Distal femur	31w*		40w*	31w*		39w*
Proximal tibia	34*		5w	34w*		2w
Proximal fibula	1y10m	3y6m	5y3m	1y4m	2y7m	3y11m
Patella	2y7m	4y	6y	1y6m	2y6m	4y
Tibial tubercle	9y11m	11y10m	13y5m	7y11m	10y3m	11y10m
Foot						
Calcaneus	22w*		25w*	22w*		25w*
Talus	25w*		31w*	25w*		31w*
Cuboid	37w*		16w	37w*		8w
Third cuneiform	3w	6m	1y7m	Birth	3m	1y3m
Os calcis, apophysis	5y2m	7y7m	9y7m	3y6m	5y4m	7y4m

Figure 13.6. Age of appearancJuly 5, 2013 10:30 AMe of perinatal ossification centers, both sexes *Prenatal age. From Poznanski et al. (1976) by permission.

PREDICTION OF ADULT HEIGHT

A number of methods have been developed to predict adult final height (see Chapter 4). Bone age is an important part of accurate predictions.

DENTAL AGE

Teeth can also be used to predict bone age (Fig. 13.7a and b), but this method is not as reliable as radiographic studies. Because tooth development starts in utero, it also may reflect and date prenatal influences on shape, coloration, and enamel formation. Ossification or molars in the jaw seen on a radiograph can also be used to predict gestational age and in utero bone maturation. The first deciduous molar ossification can be seen at 32 weeks gestation. The second deciduous molar ossification occurs at 35 weeks gestation.

	Initiation week in utero	Calcification begins, week in utero	Crown completed, month	Eruption
				Maxillary
Central incisors	7	14 (13–16)	1–3	6–8 mo.
Lateral incisors	7	16 (14½–16½)	2–3	8–11 mo.
Cuspids (canine)	7½	17 (15–18)	9	16–20 mo.
First premolars	—	—	—	—
Second Premolars	—	—	—	—
First molars	8	15½ (14½–17)	6	10–16 mo.
Second molars	10	18½ (16–23½)	10–12	20–30 mo.
Third molars	—	—	—	—

Figure 13.7(a). Dental development: Primary or deciduous teeth.

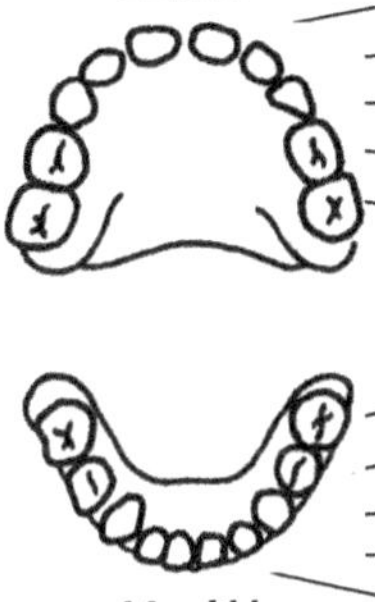

	Age of eruption (mo.): Early	Average	Late	Average age of shedding (yr)
Maxilla	6	9.6	12	7.5
	7	12.4	18	8
	11	18.3	24	11.5
	10	15.7	20	10.5
	13	26.2	31	10.5
	13	26.0	31	11
	10	15.1	30	10
	11	18.2	24	9.5
	7	11.5	15	7
Mandible	5	7.8	11	6

Figure 13.7(b) Sequence of primary tooth eruption and shedding. From Lowrey (1986), by permission.

Eruption	Root completed,	Root resorption	Shedding	
Mandibular	year	begins, year	Maxillary	Mandibular
5–7 mo.	1½–2	5–6	7–8 yr	6–7 yr
7–10 mo.	1½–2	5–6	8–9 yr	7–8 yr
16–20 mo.	2½–3½	6–7	11–12 yr	9–11 yr
—	—	—	—	—
—	—	—	—	—
10–16 mo.	2–2½	4–5	10–11 yr	10–12 yr
20–30 mo.	3	4–5	10–12 yr	11–13 yr
—	—	—	—	—

Figure 13.7(c). Eruption and shedding of primary teeth. From Vaughan et al. (1979), by permission.

	Calcification		Eruption	
	Begins at	Complete at	Maxillary	Mandibular
Central incisors	3–4 mo.	9–10 yr	7–8 yr	6–7 yr
Lateral incisors				
Maxillary	10–12 mo.	10–11 yr	8–9 yr	7–8 yr
Mandibular	3–4 mo.			
Canines	4–5 mo.	12–15 yr	11–12 yr	9–11 yr
First premolars	18–21 mo.	12–13 yr	10–11 yr	10–12 yr
Second premolars	24–30 mo.	12–14 yr	10–12 yr	11–13 yr
First molars	Birth	9–10 yr	6–7 yr	6–7 yr
Second molars	30–36 mo.	14–16 yr	12–13 yr	12–13 yr
Third molars				
Maxillary	7–9 yr	18–25 yr	17–22 yr	17–22 yr
Mandibular	8–10 yr			

Figure 13.7(d). Secondary or permanent teeth. From Harper et al. (1974) by permission.

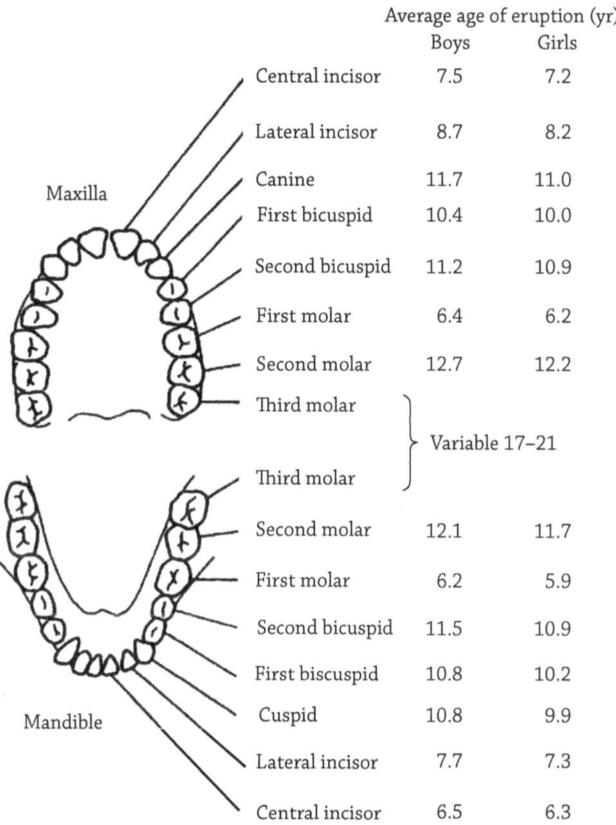

Figure 13.7(e). Average ages of eruption of secondary teeth, males and females. From Lowrey (1986), by permission.

PATTERN PROFILE OF THE HAND

Analysis of the pattern of hand bone lengths is a very useful technique for recognizing specific skeletal dysplasias, syndromes, and familial patterns that affect bone growth. By measuring the length of the 19 tubular bones of the hand from a standardized radiograph of the hand (Fig. 13.8a, b), one can construct a profile of the lengths of each bone in each digit (D1–D5). The lengths are then standardized by age. The measurement for each digit is then plotted by its deviation from the mean for age (Fig. 13.8c–h) giving a profile of the hand.

The normal individual has a flat line with no deviations (Fig. 13.8d), but many syndromes have characteristic patterns. This method is a useful way to characterize and quantify disproportion of the hand in specific conditions. For specific examples, the references at the end of this chapter should be consulted.

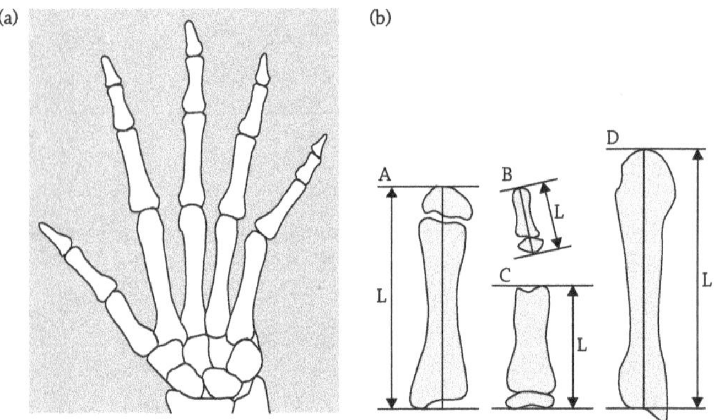

Figure 13.8(a,b). Measuring finger bones. From Poznanski and Gartman (1983), by permission.

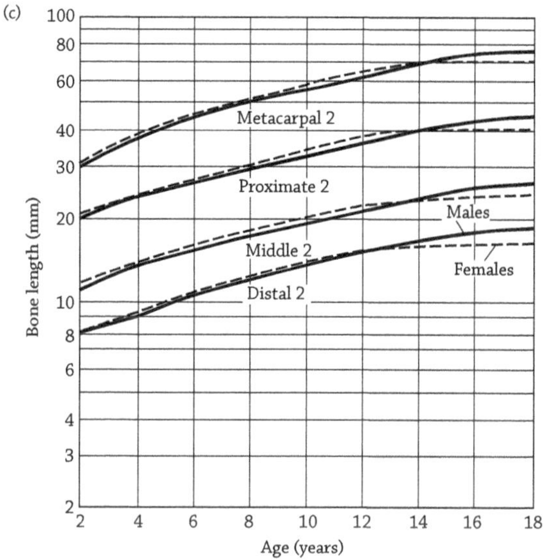

Figure 13.8(c). Normal growth patterns of hand tubular bones.

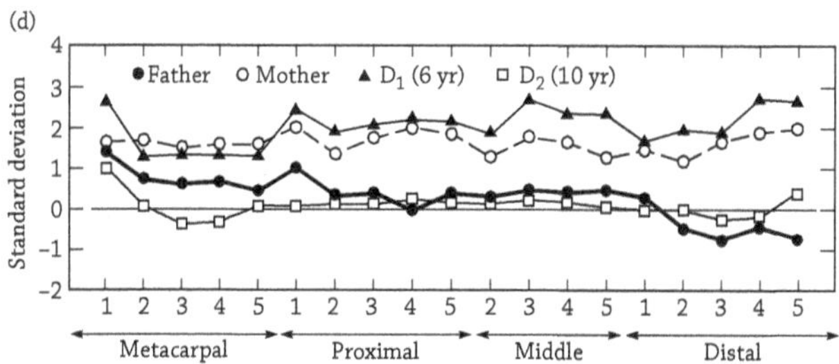

Figure 13.8(d). Normal family pattern profile of finger bones.

Years		2		3		4		5		6		7		8		9		10	
Bones		Mean	SD	Mean	SD	Mean	SD	Mean	SD	Mean	SD	Mean	SD	Mean	SD	Mean	SD	Mean	SD
Males																			
Distal	5	8.8		8.4	0.6	9.0	0.7	9.9	0.6	10.7	0.0	11.4	0.8	12.2	0.9	12.6	1.0	13.5	0.9
	4	9.2	0.7	9.9	0.8	10.5	0.8	11.5	0.9	12.3	0.9	13.1	1.0	13.9	1.0	14.4	1.0	15.3	1.2
	3	8.7	0.9	9.5	0.8	10.2	0.8	11.1	0.8	11.8	0.9	12.7	1.0	13.4	1.0	14.0	1.0	14.8	1.2
	2	8.2	0.5	8.8	—	9.4	0.8	10.1	0.9	10.8	0.9	11.6	1.0	12.4	1.0	13.0	1.0	13.7	1.1
	1	—	—	12.3	—	13.2	1.0	14.4	0.9	15.4	0.9	16.5	1.0	17.4	1.0	17.9	1.2	19.0	1.2
Middle	5	—	—	—	—	10.?	1.0	11.2	1.0	12.0	1.0	12.7	1.1	13.5	1.1	14.3	1.2	15.0	1.2
	4	—	—	—	1.0	15.8	0.0	10.7	0.9	17.7	1.0	18.7	1.1	19.8	1.1	20.9	1.3	21.6	1.4
	3	14.1	0.8	15.1	1.1	16.5	1.0	17.6	1.0	18.7	1.1	19.8	1.2	20.9	1.2	22.0	1.4	22.9	1.4
	2	11.2	0.8	12.3	1.1	13.5	1.0	14.4	0.9	15.3	1.0	16.1	1.1	17.1	1.1	18.1	1.2	18.8	1.2
Proximal	5	16.1	0.7	17.8	0.9	19.2	1.0	20.6	1.0	21.8	1.0	23.0	1.1	24.2	1.3	25.2	1.5	26.4	1.5
	4	20.5	0.9	22.8	1.0	24.7	1.2	26.4	1.2	27.9	1.3	29.5	1.4	31.0	1.6	32.3	1.9	33.9	1.8
	3	21.8	1.0	24.2	1.1	26.3	1.4	28.1	1.4	29.8	1.4	31.5	1.6	33.2	1.8	34.7	2.2	36.1	1.9
	2	19.5	1.0	21.9	1.2	23.7	1.3	25.4	1.4	26.8	1.5	28.3	1.6	29.7	1.8	31.4	1.9	32.5	1.9
	1	15.2		15.9	1.1	17.2	1.1	18.3	1.2	19.6	1.2	20.8	1.3	21.8	1.3	23.1	1.5	24.2	1.4
Metacarpal	5	23.9	1.0	26.3	1.5	28.9	1.9	32.1	2.2	34.6	2.2	36.7	2.1	38.8	2.5	40.6	2.5	42.7	2.9
	4	25.5	1.1	28.9	1.5	31.7	2.1	35.0	2.5	37.9	2.7	40.1	2.5	42.2	3.1	44.1	2.8	46.5	3.5
	3	28.6	1.3	32.3	1.8	35.6	2.3	39.3	2.8	42.6	2.9	45.3	2.8	47.6	3.5	49.8	3.0	52.3	3.7
	2	30.6	1.5	34.5	1.7	37.9	2.3	41.6	2.7	44.9	2.9	47.7	2.8	50.2	3.4	52.6	3.0	55.0	3.9
	1	19.6	1.3	22.0	1.2	24.1	1.6	26.7	1.6	29.0	1.7	30.9	1.8	32.7	2.1	34.4	2.1	36.3	2.3

Figure 13.8e. Norms for finger bone lengths, age 2–10 years, males

Years		2		3		4		5		6		7		8		9		10	
Bones		Mean	SD	Mean	SD	Mean	SD	Mean	SD	Mean	SD	Mean	SD	Mean	SD	Mean	SD	Mean	SD
Females																			
Distal	5	7.8	0.6	8.4	0.6	9.1	0.7	9.9	0.7	10.6	0.8	11.4	0.9	12.1	1.0	12.7	1.1	13.5	1.2
	4	9.1	0.7	9.9	0.7	10.6	0.8	11.5	0.9	12.4	1.0	13.2	1.1	14.0	1.0	14.4	1.2	15.5	1.4
	3	8.8	0.7	9.9	0.8	10.2	0.7	11.1	0.9	12.2	1.3	12.7	1.1	13.0	1.1	14.1	1.1	15.0	1.4
	2	8.0	0.8	8.6	0.7	9.4	0.7	10.1	0.8	10.9	0.9	11.7	1.0	12.3	1.1	13.1	1.1	13.8	1.4
	1	11.3	0.8	12.5	0.8	13.2	0.8	14.4	1.0	15.4	1.1	16.3	1.2	17.3	1.1	17.8	1.3	19.0	1.6
Middle	5	9.0	1.2	9.8	1.1	10.5	1.1	11.2	1.1	12.2	1.2	12.9	1.3	13.6	1.3	14.2	1.4	15.2	1.6
	4	13.5	0.9	14.9	1.0	15.8	1.1	16.9	1.2	18.1	1.3	19.1	1.4	20.1	1.4	20.9	1.5	22.2	1.7
	3	14.2	0.9	15.6	1.1	16.6	1.2	17.9	1.2	19.2	1.3	20.3	1.4	21.4	1.4	22.1	1.6	23.6	1.8
	2	11.6	0.9	12.8	1.0	13.6	1.1	14.8	1.1	16.0	1.2	16.8	1.3	17.8	1.4	18.1	1.5	19.6	1.7
Proximal	5	16.3	1.0	17.9	1.1	19.1	1.1	20.6	1.3	22.0	1.4	23.1	1.6	24.4	1.4	25.2	1.6	27.1	2.0
	4	20.7	1.1	22.9	1.3	24.6	1.3	26.3	1.5	28.2	1.7	29.7	1.9	31.2	1.6	32.4	2.0	34.5	2.4
	3	22.2	1.2	24.5	1.3	26.4	1.4	28.3	1.8	30.4	1.8	32.1	2.0	33.7	2.0	35.0	2.2	37.3	2.6
	2	20.1	1.2	22.3	1.3	24.0	1.8	25.8	1.7	27.7	1.7	29.2	1.9	30.7	2.2	31.5	2.4	34.0	2.4
	1	14.9	1.0	16.3	1.1	17.2	1.3	18.8	1.3	20.2	1.3	2.14	1.5	22.7	2.0	23.5	2.0	25.5	2.1
Metacarpal	5	23.7	1.5	26.9	2.1	29.4	1.8	32.6	2.0	35.1	2.1	37.2	2.4	39.4	1.6	40.8	2.5	43.8	2.8
	4	26.0	1.9	29.6	2.7	32.2	2.0	35.6	2.5	38.4	2.7	40.5	2.8	43.1	3.0	44.3	2.8	47.5	3.5
	3	29.4	2.1	33.4	2.9	36.3	2.2	40.3	2.7	43.3	3.1	45.8	3.1	48.7	3.2	49.9	3.2	53.6	3.8
	2	31.3	1.9	35.2	2.7	38.2	2.3	42.3	2.7	45.6	3.2	48.1	3.3	51.2	3.3	52.6	3.4	56.6	4.1
	1	19.9	1.6	22.7	1.6	24.8	1.7	27.3	1.8	29.6	1.9	31.5	2.0	33.5	2.1	34.8	2.4	37.4	2.6

Figure 13.8f. Norms for finger bone lengths, age 2–10 years, females. * For each sex, N = 150 at age 4, 124 at age 9, 78 in adulthood, and 30–85 at intermediate ages. All values are in millimeters.

Years		11		12		13		14		15		16		17		18		Adults	
Bones		Mean	SD	Mean	SD	Mean	SD	Mean	SD	Mean	SD	Mean	SD	Mean	SD	Mean	SD	Mean	SD
Males																			
Distal	5	14.2	0.9	15.0	0.9	15.8	0.9	16.8	1.0	17.6	1.1	17.9	1.0	18.1	1.0	18.1	1.2	18.7	1.3
	4	16.1	1.2	17.0	1.3	17.8	1.4	18.8	1.3	19.6	1.4	20.0	1.3	20.3	1.3	20.0	1.3	20.5	1.2
	3	15.6	1.2	16.4	1.2	17.1	1.3	18.2	1.3	19.0	1.4	19.3	1.4	19.5	1.3	19.4	1.3	20.1	1.2
	2	14.3	1.1	15.0	1.0	15.7	1.4	16.7	1.2	17.5	1.2	17.8	1.3	18.2	1.3	18.1	1.3	18.8	1.4
	1	19.7	1.2	20.6	1.3	21.7	1.4	22.8	1.3	24.1	1.4	24.5	1.4	24.9	1.4	24.8	1.5	25.2	1.4
Middle	5	15.7	1.4	16.5	1.5	17.5	1.5	18.9	1.6	19.9	1.4	20.5	1.4	20.6	1.4	21.0	1.4	21.6	1.6
	4	22.6	1.5	23.6	1.5	24.8	1.7	26.5	1.6	27.7	1.5	28.4	1.5	28.7	1.4	29.1	1.5	29.6	1.6
	3	24.0	1.8	24.9	1.4	26.3	1.6	28.0	1.5	29.2	1.6	30.5	1.6	30.2	1.6	30.6	1.8	31.1	1.8
	2	19.8	1.7	20.4	1.3	21.6	1.6	23.2	1.5	24.3	1.5	25.0	1.5	25.3	1.4	25.6	1.7	26.1	1.6
Proximal	5	27.6	2.0	28.9	2.0	30.5	2.4	32.9	2.4	34.9	2.0	35.6	1.8	36.1	1.8	35.9	2.0	36.3	2.0
	4	35.3	2.3	37.0	2.4	38.8	2.8	41.6	2.8	43.7	2.6	44.9	2.3	45.4	2.2	45.2	2.5	45.5	2.3
	3	37.8	2.1	39.5	2.6	41.5	2.9	44.4	2.8	46.6	2.5	47.8	2.4	48.3	2.3	48.2	2.7	48.5	2.6
	2	33.9	1.6	35.5	2.4	37.2	2.6	39.8	2.6	41.8	2.2	42.8	2.0	43.3	2.1	43.4	2.4	43.7	2.2
	1	25.4	2.8	26.7	2.0	28.5	2.2	30.9	2.2	32.9	1.8	33.8	1.5	34.6	2.6	34.7	1.8	35.0	1.9
Metacarpal	5	44.6	3.1	47.1	3.2	49.1	4.0	52.2	3.9	55.4	3.6	57.1	2.8	57.9	2.5	57.5	2.9	58.0	3.0
	4	48.4	3.4	5.10	3.7	53.1	4.6	56.4	4.5	59.5	4.1	61.5	3.7	62.6	3.1	61.7	3.4	62.1	3.5
	3	54.6	3.5	57.3	4.0	59.5	5.1	63.1	4.9	66.7	4.4	68.7	4.1	69.7	3.3	69.0	3.7	69.0	3.8
	2	57.3	2.4	60.6	3.9	63.5	5.1	67.1	4.8	70.6	4.3	73.2	3.8	74.2	2.9	73.9	3.5	73.7	3.8
	1	38.2		40.2	2.7	42.5	3.0	45.1	2.8	47.6	2.6	48.8	2.3	49.5	2.1	49.4	2.7	49.6	2.9

Figure 13.8g. Norms for finger bone lengths, ages 11 years to adult, males.

Years		11		12		13		14		15		16		17		18		Adults	
Bones		Mean	SD	Mean	SD	Mean	SD	Mean	SD	Mean	SD	Mean	SD	Mean	SD	Mean	SD	Mean	SD
Females																			
Distal	5	14.2	1.3	15.0	1.3	15.4	1.3	15.6	1.3	15.9	1.4	15.9	1.4	16.2	1.3	16.0	1.2	16.2	1.2
	4	16.2	1.4	17.1	1.4	17.6	1.2	17.9	1.3	18.0	1.4	18.0	1.3	18.1	1.4	17.9	1.3	18.0	1.3
	3	15.8	1.3	16.6	1.4	17.1	1.4	17.3	1.3	17.6	1.5	17.5	1.4	17.6	1.4	17.4	1.3	17.7	1.3
	2	14.4	1.3	15.2	1.5	15.7	1.5	15.8	1.5	16.1	1.6	16.0	1.6	16.3	1.5	16.2	1.3	16.6	1.3
	1	20.0	1.7	20.9	1.7	21.4	1.6	21.7	1.6	22.0	1.7	22.0	1.7	22.1	1.8	22.0	1.6	22.1	1.6
Middle	5	16.2	1.8	17.2	1.7	17.9	1.8	18.1	1.6	18.4	1.7	18.5	1.7	18.5	1.9	18.6	1.7	18.7	1.7
	4	23.4	1.9	24.7	1.8	25.7	1.9	25.9	1.6	26.3	1.8	26.4	1.8	26.5	1.9	26.3	1.8	26.4	1.7
	3	24.9	1.8	26.2	1.9	27.2	2.0	27.5	1.7	28.1	1.8	28.0	1.9	28.0	1.8	27.8	1.8	27.9	1.7
	2	20.9	2.1	21.8	1.9	22.7	1.8	23.0	1.8	23.5	2.2	23.3	1.9	23.4	1.9	23.1	1.6	23.2	1.6
Proximal	5	28.7	2.5	30.5	2.2	31.9	2.2	32.3	2.1	32.9	2.5	32.8	2.3	32.8	2.3	32.5	2.0	32.5	1.9
	4	36.5	2.7	38.8	2.6	40.3	2.5	40.9	2.3	41.5	2.6	41.6	2.6	41.7	2.6	41.1	2.2	40.8	2.4
	3	39.5	2.6	41.7	2.8	43.5	2.8	44.1	2.4	44.8	2.6	44.8	2.7	44.8	2.2	44.2	2.4	44.0	2.3
	2	36.5	2.3	38.0	2.6	39.5	2.6	39.9	2.4	40.6	2.0	40.6	2.6	40.7	2.7	39.9	2.3	40.0	2.3
	1	35.9	2.9	29.2	2.4	30.6	2.2	31.1	1.9	31.8	2.0	31.7	2.1	31.9	3.5	31.3	1.9	31.4	2.0
Metacarpal	5	27.2	3.8	48.7	2.9	50.8	2.8	52.1	2.8	52.6	3.0	52.8	3.0	53.0	4.0	52.0	2.7	51.9	3.6
	4	46.3	4.0	52.8	3.7	55.1	3.6	56.2	3.6	56.9	3.6	57.2	3.9	57.2	4.1	56.1	2.9	56.0	3.5
	3	50.2	4.3	59.5	4.2	62.1	4.0	63.4	3.9	63.9	3.9	64.3	4.0	64.5	2.6	63.2	3.4	62.6	4.0
	2	56.5	3.0	63.2	4.4	66.2	4.2	67.4	3.9	68.1	4.2	68.6	4.3	68.9		67.5	3.4	66.9	4.3
	1	59.9		42.0	3.0	43.8	2.7	44.4	2.5	45.3	2.4	45.0	2.8	45.0		44.6	2.2	44.2	2.6
		39.7																	

Figure 13.8h. Norms for finger bone lengths, age 11 years to adult, females. *For each sex, N= 150 at age 4, 124 at age 9, 78 in adulthood, and 30–85 at intermediate ages. All values are in millimeters. From Garn et al. (1972) by permission.

CARPAL ANGLE

The angle that the carpal bones make at the wrist is useful in alerting the clinician to disproportionate growth elsewhere. Norms have been established for age, sex, and racial group.

The carpal angle is defined as the angle resulting from the intersection of two lines, one tangent to the proximal edge of the lunate and scaphoid and one tangent to the proximal edge of the lunate and triquetrum.

Imaginary lines are drawn on the X-ray, and the angles are measured (Fig. 13.9a). The angle should be compared with normal standards (Fig. 13.9b).

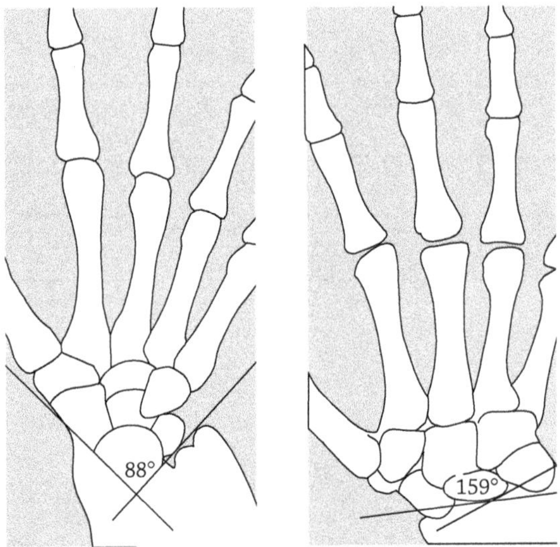

Figure 13.9(a). Measurement of carpal angle using X-rays.

	Carpal angle in degrees							
Age		Percentiles				Percentiles		
groups	Sample				Sample			
(years)	size	5th	50th	95th	size	5th	50th	95th
		White males				White females		
4–6	10	116.0	122.0	132.5	120.0	126.5	143.0	
6–8	36	111.0	124.0	153.5	115.0	130.5	147.5	
8–10	25	122.0	133.5	147.0	115.5	129.5	139.5	
10–12	24	155.5	133.0	143.0	123.0	134.0	152.5	
12–14	24	117.0	132.0	142.5	116.0	130.0	143.0	
14–24	49	119.0	134.0	149.0	115.0	129.0	139.5	
24–40	30	114.0	136.0	145.5	112.0	130.5	142.5	
40–83	33	113.5	134.0	146.5	113.0	130.5	149.0	
		African American males				African American females		
4–6	9	124.0	131.0	143.0	16	116.5	130.5	140.5
6–8	32	119.0	128.5	147.5	22	121.0	133.0	146.5
8–10	31	128.0	139.0	142.0	16	125.0	139.0	155.0
10–12	28	121.0	138.0	152.5	23	125.5	138.5	151.0
12–14	32	125.5	141.0	143.0	28	123.0	141.0	153.5
14–24	52	128.0	146.0	139.5	67	123.0	139.0	150.0
24–40	14	128.0	136.0	142.5	18	127.0	136.5	151.0
40–83	32	125.5	140.0	149.0	46	126.5	140.5	153.5

Figure 13.9b. Carpal angle—norms From Vaughan et al. (1979), by permission.

BIBLIOGRAPHY

Garn, S. M., Hertzog, K. P., Poznanski, A. K., and Nagy, J. M. (1972). Metacarpophalangeal length in the evaluation of skeletal malformation. *Radiology*, 105, 375–381.

Graham, C. B. (1972). Assessment of bone maturation—methods and pitfalls. *Radiologic Clinics of North America*, 10, 185–202.

Greulich, W. W., and Pyle, S. I. (1959). *Radiographic atlas of skeletal development of the hand and wrist* (2nd ed.). Stanford, CA: Stanford University Press.

Harper, H. A. S., Poznanski, A. K., and Garn, S. M. (1974). The carpal angle in American populations. *Investigative Radiology*, 9, 217–221.

Kuhns, L. R., and Poznanski, A. K. (1980). Radiological assessment of maturity and size of the newborn infant. *CRC Critical Reviews in Diagnostic Imaging, Vol.* 0, 245–308.

Lowrey, G. H. (1986). *Growth and development of children* (8th ed.). Chicago: Year Book Medical Publishers.

Lunt, R. C., and Law, D. B. (1974). A review of the chronology of calcification of the deciduous teeth. *Journal of the American Dental Association*, 89, 599–606.

Poznanski, A. K., Kuhns, L. R., and Garn, S. M. (1976). *Radiology evaluation of maturation. Practical approaches to pediatric radiology,* pp. 293–310. Chicago: Year Book Medical Publishers.

Poznanski, A. K., Garn, S. M. Nagy, J. M., and Gal, J. C., Jr. (1972). Metacarpophalangeal pattern profiles in the evaluation of skeletal malformations. *Radiology*, 104, 1–11.

Poznanski, A. K., Garn, S. M., and Shaw, H. A. (1975). The carpal angle in the congenital malformation syndromes. *European Society of Pediatric Radiology*, 19, 141–150.

Poznanski, A. K., and Gartman, S. (1983). Pattern profile comparisons: Differences and similarities. *European Society of Pediatric Radiology*, 89–96.

Pyle, S. I., and Hoerr, N. L. (1969). *Radiographic standard reference for the growing knee*. Springfield, IL: Charles C. Thomas.

Vaughan, V. C., McKay, R. J., and Behrman, R. E. (1979). *Nelson's textbook of pediatrics*, p. 32. Philadelphia: W.B. Saunders.

Chapter 14

Developmental Data

INTRODUCTION

Behavioral development depends on the growth and functional maturation of the central nervous system. In the evaluation of the infant or child, there is considerable overlap between the neurological and the behavioral aspects. The behavioral or developmental assessment is a measure of a person's achievements or accomplishments in functional areas. This involves a steady, largely predictable gain in abilities with increasing age as a result of the interaction between the central nervous system and environmental experiences. The neurological assessment measures the integrity of neural mechanisms appropriate to the age of the subject. Although these two different assessments will usually parallel or complement each other, exceptions can exist.

Evaluation of the individual begins in utero with documentation of appropriate growth and movement (see Chapter 15). The fetus exhibits reflex movements as early as 8 or 9 weeks. These consist of flexion of the trunk, retraction of the head, and retraction or backward movement of the arms. By 14 to 16 weeks, the fetus is quite active, showing elementary movements of short excursion involving the extremities, trunk, and neck. The motor and most of the reflex behavior in later fetal life is mainly under the control of the medulla and spinal cord. Many of the so-called primitive reflexes, especially those involving the limbs, depend on the tonic and myotactic reflexes—that is, recoil from stretch. These reflexes appear at or after 32 weeks of gestation. One of the earliest reflex patterns to develop is that of sucking. By 14 to 16 weeks gestation, the fetus will protrude the lips in preparation for sucking. The tongue and pharynx can adequately adapt to swallowing by this time. Figure 14.1 provides detail of the evolution of neonatal reflexes.

After birth, the first neurodevelopmental assessment is the assignment of an Apgar score based on heart rate, respiratory effort, muscle tone, color, and reflex (Fig. 14.2). At birth, tonicity and activity are equal bilaterally and the resting position assumed is one in which there is a tendency for all extremities to be flexed in an attitude of the fetal position (Fig. 14.3). There is usually good tone throughout the body, and this is particularly exemplified by the resistance to exten-

Reflex	Appears (fetal week)	Disappears (postnatal mo.)
Tonic-neck	20	7–8
Moro	28	2–3
Palmar grasp	28	3–4
Trunk in-curve	28	4–5
Doll's eyes*	32	10 days
Babinski	38	12–16

Figure 14.1. Evolution of neonatal reflexes. *Eyes open, head is rotated from side to side. Positive response is contraversive conjugate deviation of eyes. From Lowrey (1986), by permission.

Score	Heart rate	Respiratory effort	Muscle tone	Color	Reflex
2	Over 100	Strong cry	Good, active movement	Completely pink	Irritability (response to stimulation of foot) Normal cry
1	Below 100	Slow, irregular respirations	Fair, some flexion of limbs	Baby pink limbs blue	Moderately depressed grimace
0	No beat obtained	No respirations	Flaccid	Blue, pale	Absent

Figure 14.2. Apgar test.

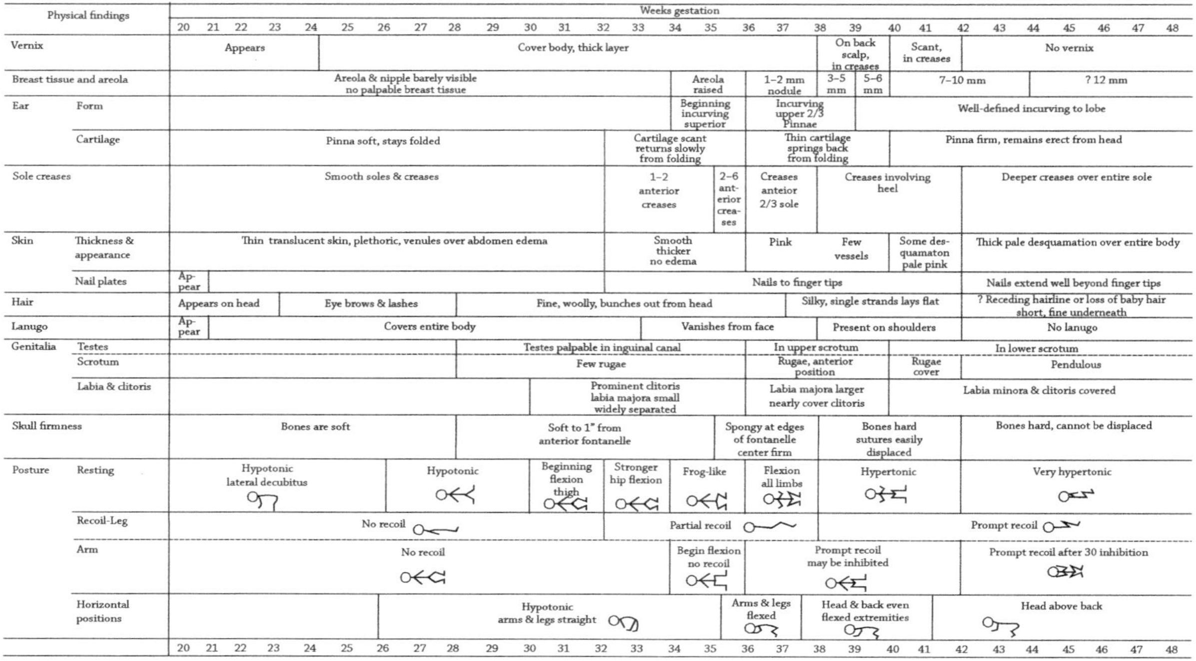

Physical findings		Weeks gestation (20 21 22 23 24 25 26 27 28 29 30 31 32 33 34 35 36 37 38 39 40 41 42 43 44 45 46 47 48)							
Vernix		Appears	Cover body, thick layer	On back scalp, in creases	Scant, in creases	No vernix			
Breast tissue and areola		Areola & nipple barely visible no palpable breast tissue	Areola raised	1–2 mm nodule	3–5 mm	5–6 mm	7–10 mm	? 12 mm	
Ear	Form		Beginning incurving superior	Incurving upper 2/3 Pinnae	Well-defined incurving to lobe				
	Cartilage	Pinna soft, stays folded	Cartilage scant returns slowly from folding	Thin cartilage springs back from folding	Pinna firm, remains erect from head				
Sole creases		Smooth soles & creases	1–2 anterior creases	2–6 anterior creases	Creases anteior 2/3 sole	Creases involving heel	Deeper creases over entire sole		
Skin	Thickness & appearance	Thin translucent skin, plethoric, venules over abdomen edema	Smooth thicker no edema	Pink	Few vessels	Some desquamaton pale pink	Thick pale desquamation over entire body		
	Nail plates	Ap-pear		Nails to finger tips	Nails extend well beyond finger tips				
Hair		Appears on head	Eye brows & lashes	Fine, woolly, bunches out from head	Silky, single strands lays flat	? Receding hairline or loss of baby hair short, fine underneath			
Lanugo		Ap-pear	Covers entire body	Vanishes from face	Present on shoulders	No lanugo			
Genitalia	Testes		Testes palpable in inguinal canal	In upper scrotum	In lower scrotum				
	Scrotum		Few rugae	Rugae, anterior position	Rugae cover	Pendulous			
	Labia & clitoris		Prominent clitoris labia majora small widely separated	Labia majora larger nearly cover clitoris	Labia minora & clitoris covered				
Skull firmness		Bones are soft	Soft to 1" from anterior fontanelle	Spongy at edges of fontanelle center firm	Bones hard sutures easily displaced	Bones hard, cannot be displaced			
Posture	Resting	Hypotonic lateral decubitus	Hypotonic	Beginning flexion thigh	Stronger hip flexion	Frog-like	Flexion all limbs	Hypertonic	Very hypertonic
	Recoil-Leg	No recoil	Partial recoil	Prompt recoil					
	Arm	No recoil	Begin flexion no recoil	Prompt recoil may be inhibited	Prompt recoil after 30 inhibition				
	Horizontal positions		Hypotonic arms & legs straight	Arms & legs flexed	Head & back even flexed extremities	Head above back			

Figure 14.3. Clinical estimation of gestational age. From Lubchenko (1986), by permission.

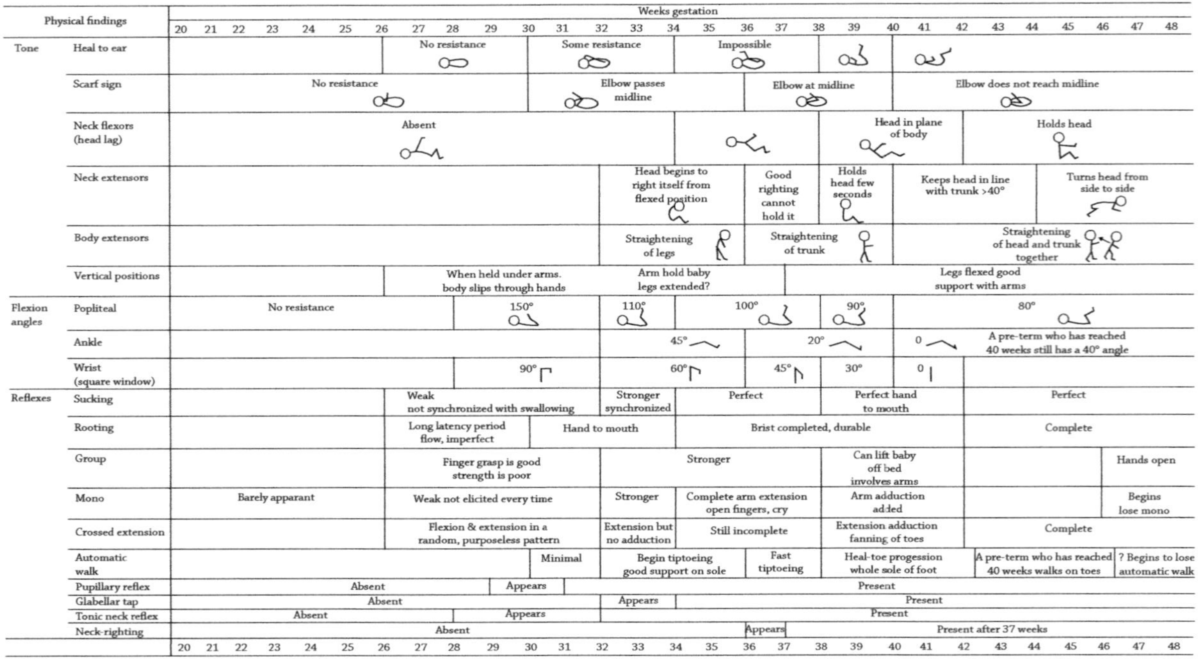

Physical findings		Weeks gestation																												
		20	21	22	23	24	25	26	27	28	29	30	31	32	33	34	35	36	37	38	39	40	41	42	43	44	45	46	47	48
Tone	Heal to ear							No resistance				Some resistance				Impossible														
	Scarf sign	No resistance										Elbow passes midline						Elbow at midline				Elbow does not reach midline								
	Neck flexors (head lag)	Absent																		Head in plane of body				Holds head						
	Neck extensors													Head begins to right itself from flexed position				Good righting cannot hold it		Holds head few seconds		Keeps head in line with trunk >40°				Turns head from side to side				
	Body extensors													Straightening of legs				Straightening of trunk				Straightening of head and trunk together								
	Vertical positions							When held under arms. body slips through hands						Arm hold baby legs extended?					Legs flexed good support with arms											
Flexion angles	Popliteal	No resistance								150°				110°		100°				90°		80°								
	Ankle													45°				20°				0		A pre-term who has reached 40 weeks still has a 40° angle						
	Wrist (square window)									90°				60°				45°		30°		0								
Reflexes	Sucking							Weak not synchronized with swallowing						Stronger synchronized		Perfect				Perfect hand to mouth				Perfect						
	Rooting							Long latency period flow, imperfect				Hand to mouth				Brist completed, durable								Complete						
	Group							Finger grasp is good strength is poor						Stronger						Can lift baby off bed involves arms								Hands open		
	Mono	Barely apparant						Weak not elicited every time						Stronger		Complete arm extension open fingers, cry				Arm adduction added								Begins lose mono		
	Crossed extension							Flexion & extension in a random, purposeless pattern						Extension but no adduction		Still incomplete				Extension adduction fanning of toes				Complete						
	Automatic walk											Minimal		Begin tiptoeing good support on sole				Fast tiptoeing		Heal-toe progession whole sole of foot				A pre-term who has reached 40 weeks walks on toes				? Begins to lose automatic walk		
	Pupillary reflex	Absent									Appears		Present																	
	Glabellar tap	Absent												Appears		Present														
	Tonic neck reflex	Absent								Appears				Present																
	Neck-righting	Absent																Appears	Present after 37 weeks											
		20	21	22	23	24	25	26	27	28	29	30	31	32	33	34	35	36	37	38	39	40	41	42	43	44	45	46	47	48

Figure 14.3 (*Continued*)

sion of all extremities. Full details of the various neonatal reflexes will not be provided here.

INTELLIGENCE

Most people would probably agree that individuals vary in their capacity for adaptive thinking and action. There is considerable controversy about the extent to which these variations in intelligence are genetically determined, the extent to which they remain constant throughout the life cycle, and the point in development at which such variations become measurable and predictable entities. The reliability and validity of infant intelligence tests are questionable. During the first 2 years of life, there is little consistency between an infant's performance on the same test at different times, or between an individual's performance on different tests given at the same time. At any given point in development, it is not possible to predict from a child's score on one test what his or her score might be on another test. Infants' test scores are poor indices of performance on intelligence tests for older children such as the Stanford Binet and the Wechsler Intelligence Scale for Children (WISC). This may be explained by the fact that infant tests measure primarily sensorimotor functions, while tests at later age levels are based on verbal and reasoning skills.

A general rule of thumb in interpreting infant intelligence test scores is that their predictive value increases directly as the age of the child increases and inversely with the amount of time between successive testing. Infant tests can also reveal children who are exceedingly advanced or who are exceedingly slow. Infant tests are less useful in the middle range of intellectual ability, where finer discriminations are necessary. Unfortunately, it is in just this middle range where tests are most needed, since an experienced clinician does not usually need a mental test to recognize the exceptional child at either end of the ability scale.

General intellectual functioning is defined as an intelligence quotient (IQ) obtained by assessment with one or more of the individually administered general intelligence tests. Figure 14.4 outlines the suggested age at which many of these available tests are applicable. Each test measures specific areas and has particular strengths and weaknesses. The interested reader is referred to literature cited at the end of this chapter for more detailed information.

Significantly decreased intellectual functioning is defined as an IQ of 70 or less on an individually administered IQ test. Since any measurement is fallible, an IQ score is generally thought to have an error of measurement of approximately 5 points. Hence, an IQ of 70 is considered to represent a band or zone of 65 to 75. An IQ level of 70 was chosen because most people with an IQ below 70 require special services and care, particularly during the school age years. The arbitrary IQ ceiling values outlined in Figure 14.5 are based on data indicating a positive association between intelligence and adaptive behavior at lower IQ levels. This association declines at the mild and moderate levels of intellectual disability.

Adaptive functioning refers to a person's effectiveness in areas such as social skills, communication and daily living skills, and how

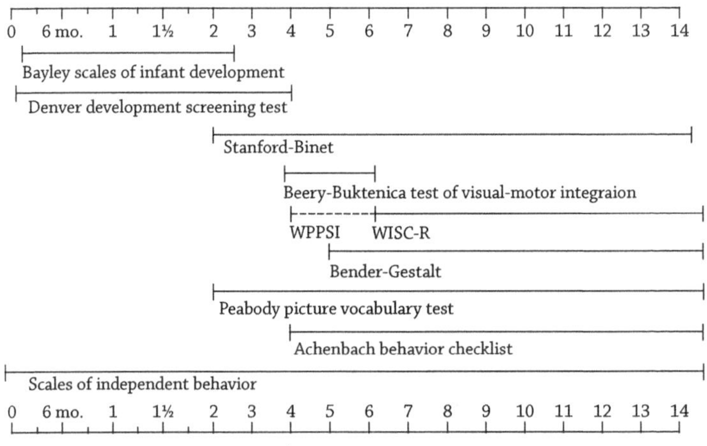

Figure 14.4. Age-appropriate psychometric testing.

Degree of intellectual disability	IQ
Mild	50–55~70
Moderate	35–40 to 50–55
Severe	20–25 to 35–40
Profound	Below 20 or 25
Intelligence	
Borderline	70–79
Dull average/normal	80–89
Average	90–109
Upper average/bright	110–119
Superior	120 or above

Figure 14.5. Classification of intelligence and intellectual disability From American Psychiatric Association (1987) by permission.

well he or she meets the standards of personal independence and social responsibility expected of certain age level or cultural group. Adaptive functioning in people with intellectual disability is influenced by personality, motivation, education, and social and vocational opportunities. Adaptive behavior is more likely to improve with support services than is IQ, which tends to remain more stable.

The Expanded Interview of the Vineland Adaptive Behavior Scales II assesses the personal and social skills of disabled and nondisabled individuals, ranging in age from birth to 90 years (Sparrow et al., 2005).

DEVELOPMENTAL SCREENING

Developmental screening is viewed as a necessary strategy for the primary detection of developmental disabilities. Early detection can be adequately achieved only by the use of standardized, valid, reliable instruments to assess the developmental status of young children. If one relies on a developmental history and a child's performance in a clinical situation, mild developmental delay is frequently overlooked.

This situation may be compounded by denial by the physicians or parents.

The Denver Developmental Screening Test (DDST) was devised in 1967 because of the need for standardized screening for early detection of developmental delays so that a child suspected to have difficulties could have further detailed investigations and opportunities for effective treatment. It was revised in 1981, and the most recent version was published in 1990 as Denver II. The test is simple to administer, easy to score and interpret, and useful for repeated evaluations. A graphic format was designed so that the user could easily compare the individual with the standard for age. Each item was represented by a horizontal bar marked to indicate the 25th, 50th, 75th, and 90th percentiles. Four categories were designated: gross motor, fine motor–adaptive, language, and personal–social. The results were validated by good correlation with the Yale Developmental Schedule.

Failure to pass a particular item may represent inability to pass or unwillingness to pass secondary to illness, fatigue, or fear of separation from the parent. The separation of items into developmental domains has important prescriptive, diagnostic, and predictive value. The typically developing infant may demonstrate uniformity across all domains of assessment, but a delayed infant can exhibit unique patterns and inconsistencies. A single global score will not provide enough information to indicate the direction of further assessment and intervention.

The (Denver II) is easy to use and is a reliable developmental screening instrument (Fig. 14.6). Through its agreement with diagnostic tests such as the Stanford Binet or the revised Bayley, the Denver II attains predictive validity. More than 78% of the children who initially fail a Denver II have educational disability and low intelligence or learning problems in school. It requires that the clinician be trained to proficiency in the administration and interpretation of the Denver II. Improper administration or interpretation of test items invalidates the norms. The Denver II and its abbreviated modifications assess only a limited number of developmental aspects. For example, it does not evaluate the home environment, which is a

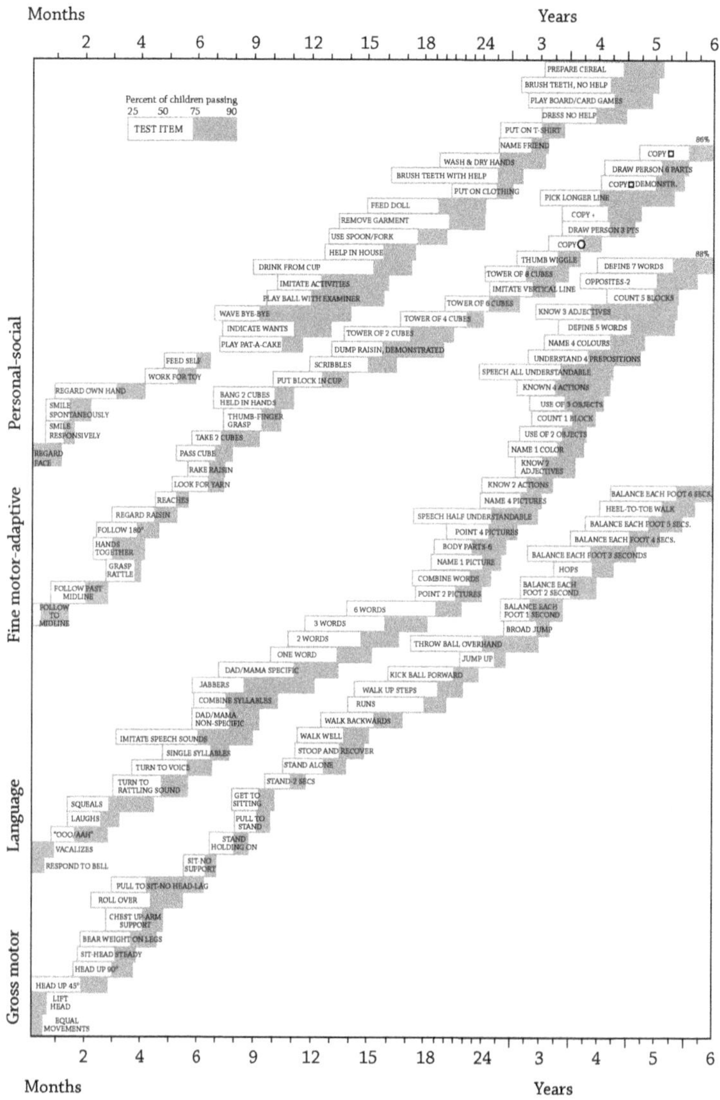

Figure 14.6(a). Denver Developmental Screening Test; Denver II. From Frankenburg and Dodds (1990), by permission.

DIRECTION FOR ADMINISTRATION

1. Try to get child to smile by smiling, talking or waving. Do not touch him/her.
2. Child must stare at hand several seconds.
3. Parent may help guide toothbrush and put toothpaste on brush.
4. Child does not have to be able to tie shoes or button/zip in the back.
5. Move yarn slowly in an arc from one side to the other, about 8" above child's face.
6. Pass if child grasps rattle when it is touched to the backs or tips of fingers.
7. Pass if child tries to see where yarn went. Yarn should be dropped quickly from sight from tester's had without arm movement.
8. Child must transfer cube from hand to hand without helf of body, mouth, or table.
9. Pass if child picks up raisin with any part of thumb and finger.
10. Line can vary only 30 degrees or less from tester's line.
11. Make a fist with thumb pointing upward and wiggle only the thumb. Pass if child imitates and does not move any fingers other than the thumb.

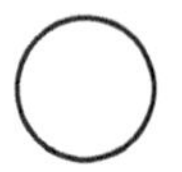

12. Pass any enclosed form. Fail continuous round motions.

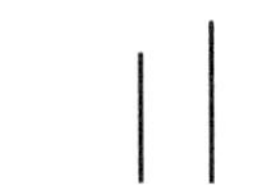

13. Which line is longer? (Not bigger.) Turn paper upside down and repeat (pass 3 of 3 or 5 of 6)

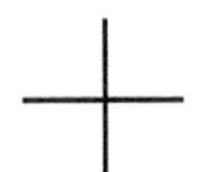

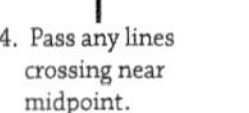

14. Pass any lines crossing near midpoint.

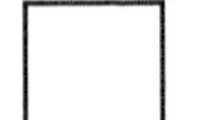

15. Have child copy first. If failed, demonstrate.

When giving items 12, 14 and 15, do not name the forms. Do not demonstrate 12 and 14.

16. When scoring, each pair (2 arms, 2 legs, etc.) counts as one part.
17. Place one cube in cup and shake gently near child's ear, but out of sight. Repeat for other ear.
18. Point to picture and have child name it. (No credit is given for sounds only.) If less than 4 pictures are named correctly, have child point to picture as each is named by tester.

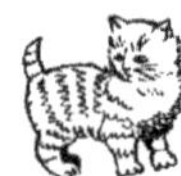

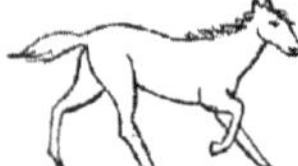

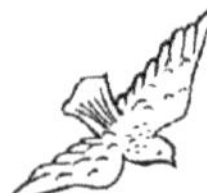

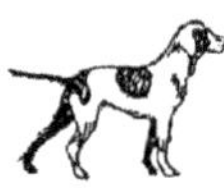

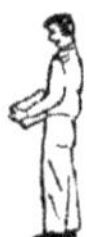

19. Using doll, tell child: Show me the nose, eyes, ears, mouth, hands, feet, tummy, hair. Pass 6 of 8.
20. Using pictures, ask child: Which one files?... says meow?...talks?... barks?...gallops? Pass 2 of 5, 4 of 5.
21. Ask child: What do you do when you are cold?... tired?... hungry? Pass 2 of 3, 3 of 3.
22. Ask child: What do you do with a cup? What is a chair used for? What is a pencil used for? Action words must be included in answers.
23. Pass if child correctly places <u>and</u> say how many blocks are on paper. (1, 5).
24. Tell child: Put block **on** table; **under** table; **in front of** me, **behind** me. Pass 4 of 4. (Do not help child by pointing, moving head or eyes.)
25. Ask child:What is ball?... Lake?... desk?... house...? banana?... curtain?... fence?... ceiling?... Pass if defined in terms of use, shape, what it is made of, or general category (such as banana is fruit, not just yellow). Pass 5 of 8, 7 of 8.
26. Ask child: if a horse is big, a mouse is____? If fire is hot, ice is ___? If the sun shines during the day, the moon shines during the ____? Pass 2 of 3/
27. Child may use wall or rail only, not person. May not crawl.
28. Child must throw ball overhand 3 feet to within arm's reach of tester.
29. Child must perform standing broad jump over width of test sheet (8 1/2 inches).
30. Tell child to walk forward, ∞∞∞∞→ heel within 1 inch of toe. Tester may demonstrate. Child must walk 4 consecutive steps.
31. In the second year, half or normal children are non-compliant.

OBSERVATIONS:

Figure 14.6(b). Denver Developmental Screening Test; Denver II. From Frankenburg and Dodds (1990), by permission.

major determinant of later development. Thus, reassuring Denver II scores for a particular child who may be having developmental problems should not lull the clinician into a false sense of security, since the test does not examine all aspects of development. Furthermore, even if a child's development seems to be progressing appropriately, it is important to realize that development is an ongoing, dynamic process which requires periodic rescreening.

BIBLIOGRAPHY

American Psychiatric Association. (1987). *Diagnostic and statistical manual of mental disorders* (3rd ed.), pp. 28–33. Washington, DC: American Psychiatric Association.

Elkind, D. (1973). Infant intelligence. *American Journal of Diseases in Children*, 126, 143–144.

Frankenburg, W. K., and Dodds, J. B. (1967). The Denver Developmental Screening Test. *Journal of Pediatrics*, 71, 181–191.

Frankenburg, W. K., Dick, N. P., and Carland, J. (1975). Development of preschool-aged children of different social and ethnic groups: Implications for developmental screening. *Journal of Pediatrics*, 87, 125–132.

Frankenburg, W. K., and Dodds, J. B. (1990). *The Denver Development Assessment [Denver II]*. Denver, Colorado: University of Colorado Medical School.

Frankenburg, W. K., Dodds, J., Archer, P., Shapiro, H., and Bresnick, B. (1992). The DENVER II: A major revision and restandardization of the Denver Developmental Screening Test. Pediatrics, 89, 91–97.

Katoff, L., and Reuter, J. (1980). Review of developmental screening tests for infants. *Journal of Clinical Child Psychology*, 9, 30–34.

Lowrey, G. H. (1986). Behaviour and personality. In *Growth and development of children* (8th ed.), pp. 143–219. Chicago: Year Book Medical Publishers.

Lubchenko, L. (1986). In G. H. Lowery, *Growth and development of children* (8th ed.). Chicago: Year Book Medical Publishers.

Sattler, J. M. (1982). *Assessment of children's intellect and special abilities* (2nd ed.). Boston: Allyn and Bacon.

Sparrow, S. S., Cicchetti, D. V., and Ball, D. A. (2005). *Vineland Adaptive Behavior Scales* (2nd ed.). Circle Pines, MN: American Guidance Service.

Chapter 15

Prenatal Ultrasound Measurements

INTRODUCTION

With the advent of prenatal diagnosis, standards for intrauterine growth have become important. Ultrasound measurements of the fetus help not only to establish the gestational age but also to determine whether the fetus is growing normally. Comparison of measurements in different areas of the body can establish normal proportions in the fetus, in the same manner as postnatal measurements. Comparisons over time can establish normal or atypical growth patterns, which can allow specific diagnosis and improved pregnancy management.

Accurate norms for various body structures at different stages of gestation are available. However, the quality and accuracy of the measurements in a particular case are very much a function of the experience of the technician and the quality of the equipment used. Most ultrasound departments, with a large volume of prenatal diagnostic studies, establish their own age-related norms.

CHOICE OF MEASUREMENT IN RELATION TO GESTATIONAL AGE

At different gestational ages, different measurements are most accurate. Studies should be adapted to the gestational age and the particular circumstances of the case. Measurements can be made and compared with the appropriate standards, given in Figures 15.1–15.23.

- From 7 to 10 weeks:
  - Crown–rump length (Fig. 15.5)
- From 10 to 14 weeks:
  - Crown–rump length (Fig. 15.5)
  - Biparietal diameter (Fig. 15.6)
  - Femur length (Fig. 15.8)
  - Humerus length (Fig. 15.9)
- From 15 to 28 weeks:
  - Biparietal diameter (Fig. 15.6)
  - Femur length (Fig. 15.8)
  - Humerus length (Fig. 15.9)
  - Binocular distance (Fig. 15.19)
  - Other long bone lengths (Figs. 15.10–15.14)
- After 28 weeks:
  - Biparietal diameter (Fig. 15.6)
  - Femur length (Fig. 15.8)
  - Humerus length (Fig. 15.19)
  - Other long bone lengths (Figs. 15.10–15.14)
  - Binocular distance (Fig. 15.19)

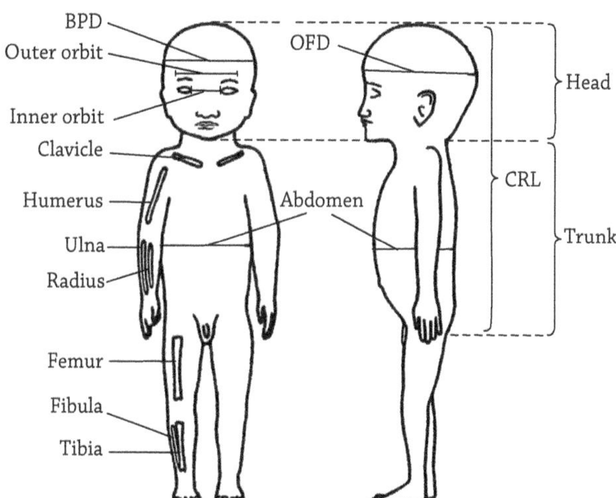

Figure 15.1. Positions of ultrasound measurements.

Week	BPD	OFD	HC	TTD	AC	Femur	CRL	Weight
12	2.0 cm	—	—	1.7	5.3	—	4.7	—
13	2.4	—	—	2.0	6.3	1.0	6.0	14g
14	2.8	3.1	10.6	2.4	7.5	1.2	7.3	25
15	3.2	3.8	11.5	2.7	8.5	1.6	8.6	50
16	3.5	4.1	12.7	3.1	9.7	1.8	9.7	80
17	3.8	4.6	14.0	3.4	10.7	2.2	11.0	100
18	4.2	5.0	15.2	3.7	11.6	2.5	12.0	150
19	4.6	5.4	16.4	4.0	12.6	2.8	13.0	200
20	4.9	5.8	17.6	4.4	13.5	3.1	14.0	250
21	5.2	6.3	19.0	4.7	14.5	3.4	CHL	300
22	5.6	6.7	20.3	5.0	15.5	3.6	▼	350
23	5.9	7.2	21.5	5.3	16.5	3.9	28	450
24	6.2	7.6	22.6	5.6	17.3	4.1		530
25	6.5	8.0	24.0	5.9	18.3	4.4	31	700
26	6.8	8.4	25.1	6.2	19.1	4.7		850
27	7.1	8.8	26.3	6.5	20.2	4.9	34	1000
28	7.4	9.1	27.4	6.9	21.1	5.1		1100
29	7.7	9.5	28.4	7.2	22.2	5.4	37	1250
30	8.0	9.8	29.3	7.4	23.0	5.6		1400
31	8.2	10.0	30.3	7.8	24.0	5.9	40	1600
32	8.5	10.3	31.1	8.1	24.9	6.1		1800
33	8.7	10.5	31.8	8.3	25.8	6.3	43	2000
34	8.9	10.7	32.5	8.6	26.8	6.5		2250
35	9.1	10.9	33.2	8.9	27.7	6.7	45	2550
36	9.3	11.1	33.7	9.2	28.7	6.9		2750
37	9.5	11.2	34.0	9.4	29.6	7.1	47	2950
38	9.6	11.3	34.4	9.7	30.6	7.3		3100
39	9.8	11.4	34.7	9.9	31.5	7.4	50	3250
40	9.9	11.5	34.9	10.1	32.0	7.5		3400

Figure 15.2. Fetal biometric data from ultrasound measurements. AC, abdominal circumference; BPD, biparietal diameter; CHL, crown–heel length; CRL, crown–rump length; HC, head circumference; OFD, occipitofrontal diameter; TTD, transthoracic diameter. From Hansmann (1985), by permission.

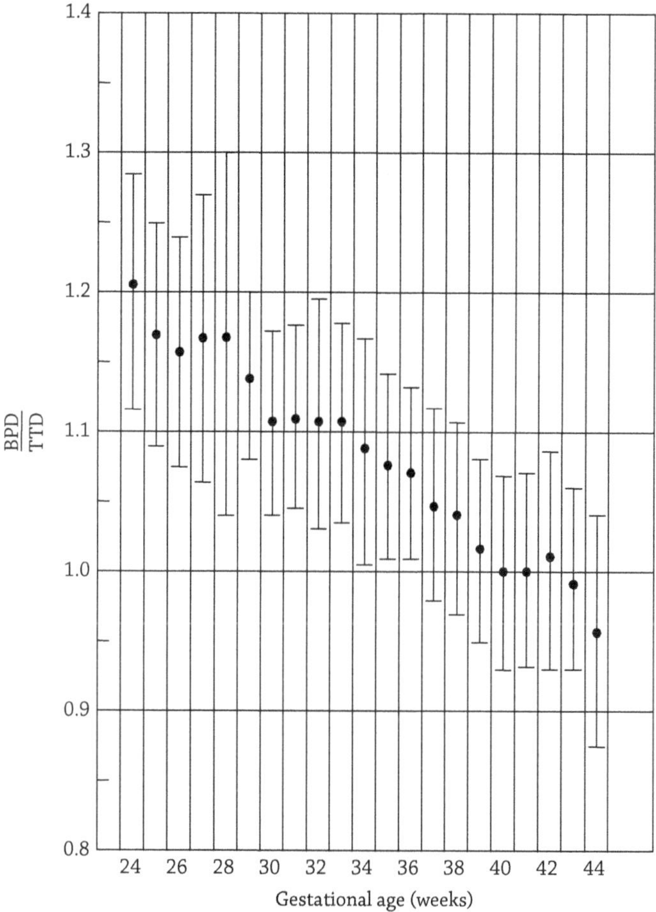

Figure 15.3. Head-to-trunk ratio as a function of gestational age. BPD, biparietal diameter; TTD, transthoracic diameter. From Hansmann (1985), by permission.

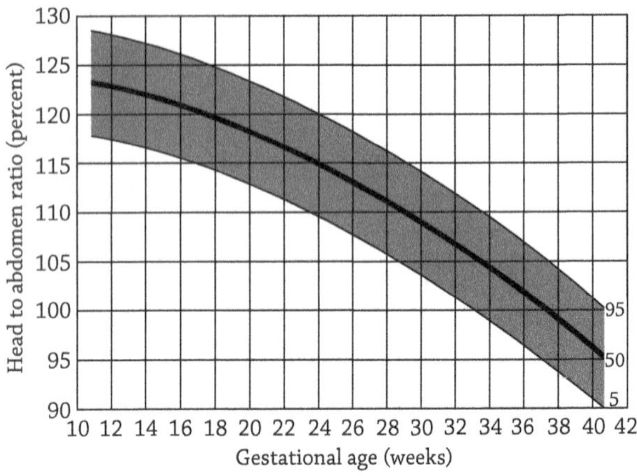

Figure 15.4. Head-to-abdomen circumference ratio. From Hansmann (1985), by permission.

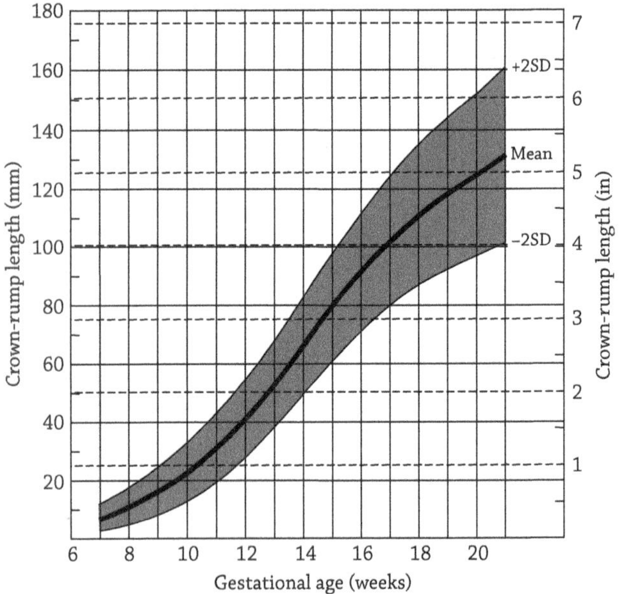

Figure 15.5. Crown–rump length as a function of gestational age. From Hansmann (1985), by permission.

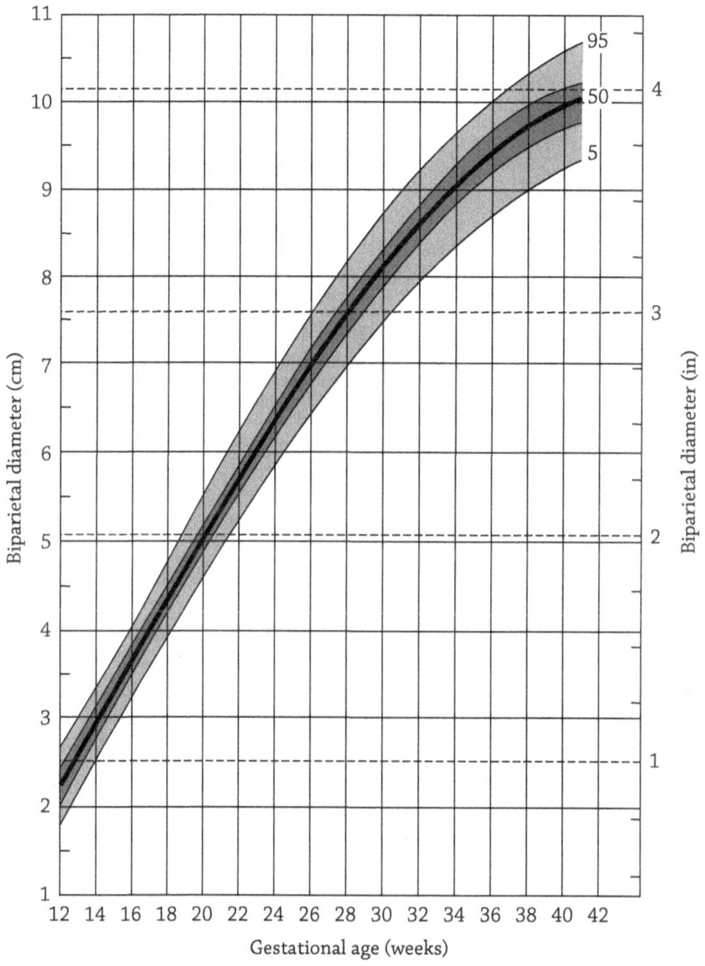

Figure 15.6. Biparietal diameter as a function of gestational age. From Sabbagha et al. (1978), by permission.

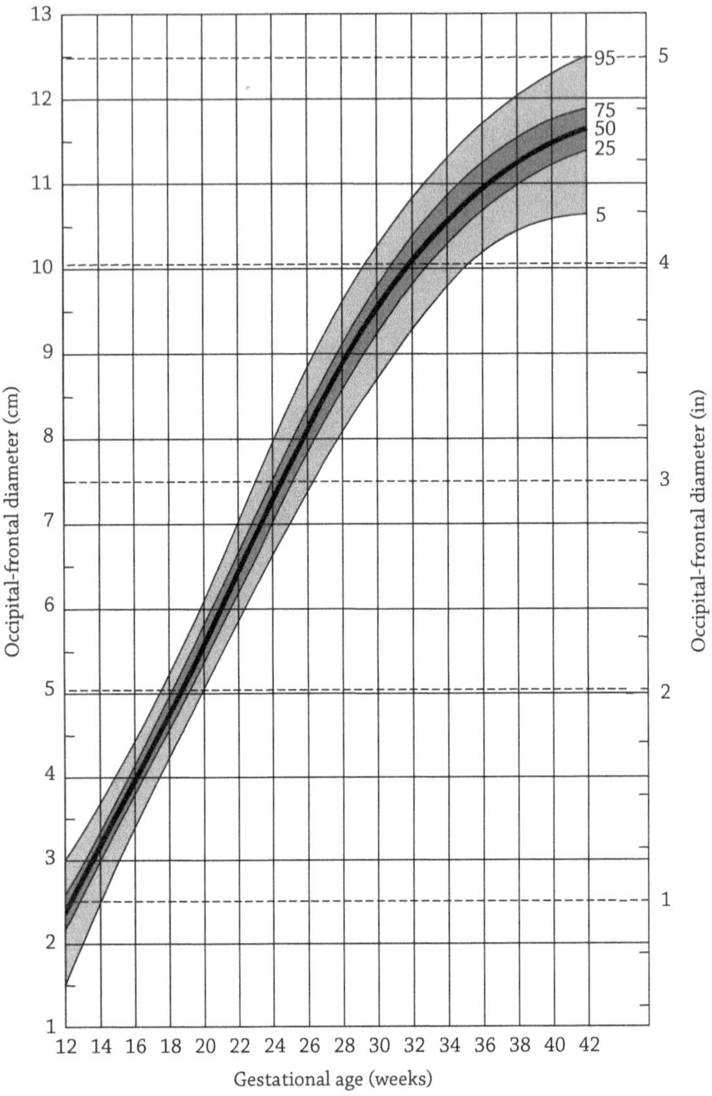

Figure 15.7. Occipital–frontal diameter—percentile growth curves. From Hansmann (1985), by permission.

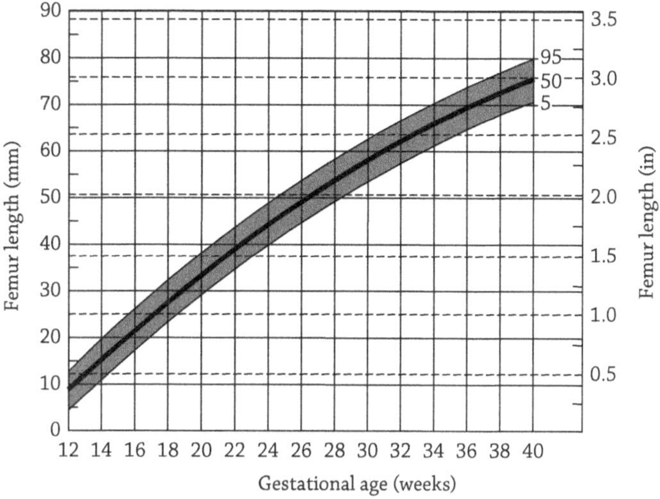

Figure 15.8. Growth of femur as a function of gestational age. From Hansmann (1985), by permission.

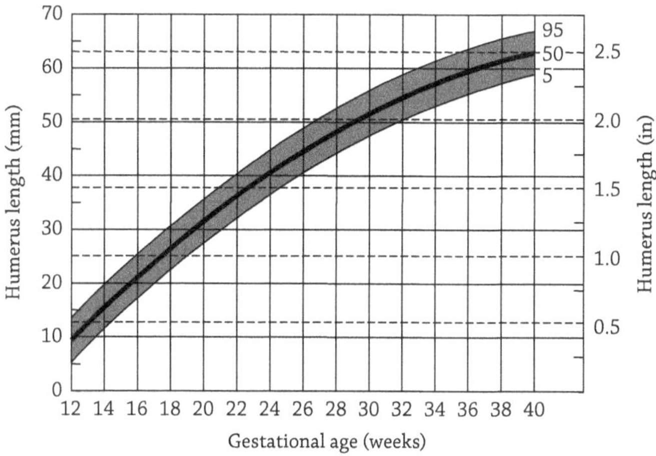

Figure 15.9. Growth of humerus length as a function of gestational age. From Jeanty and Romero (1984), by permission.

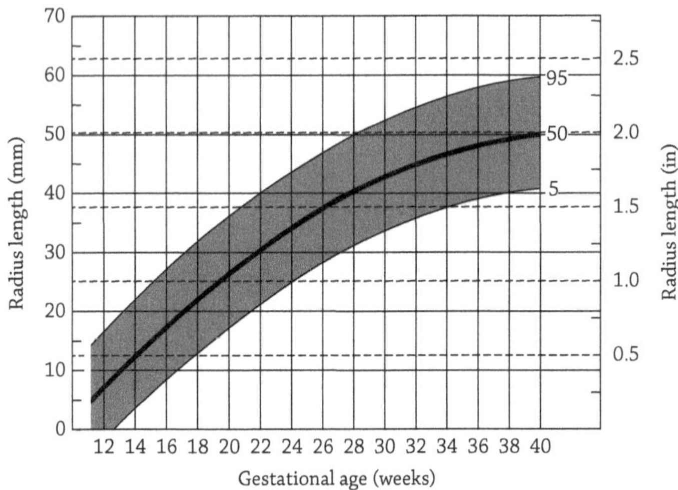

Figure 15.10. Growth of radius length as a function of gestational age. From Jeanty and Romero (1984), by permission.

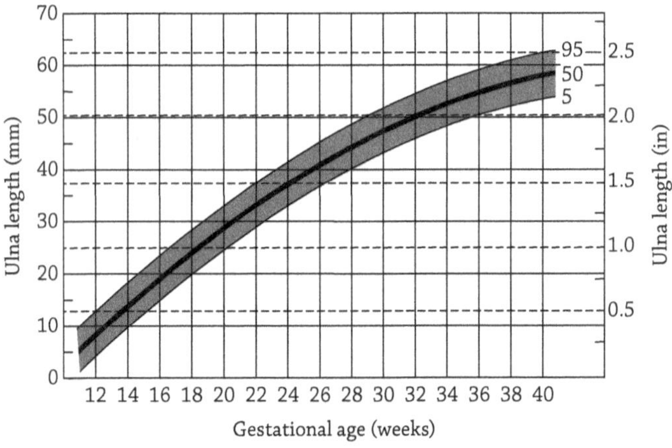

Figure 15.11. Growth of ulna length as a function of gestational age. From Jeanty and Romero (1984), by permission.

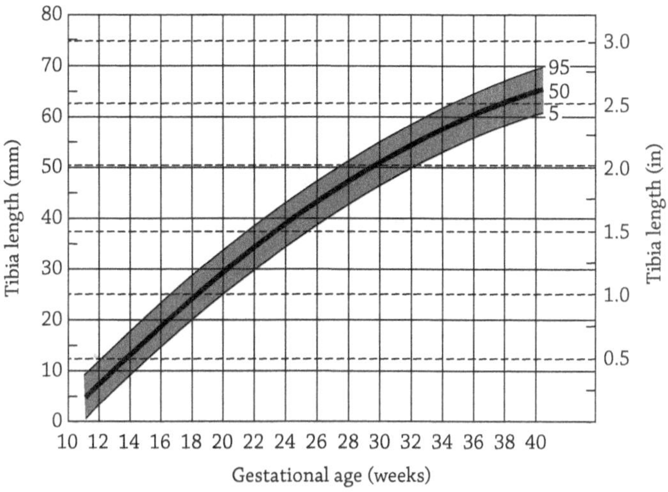

Figure 15.12. Growth of tibia length as a function of gestational age. From Jeanty and Romero (1984), by permission.

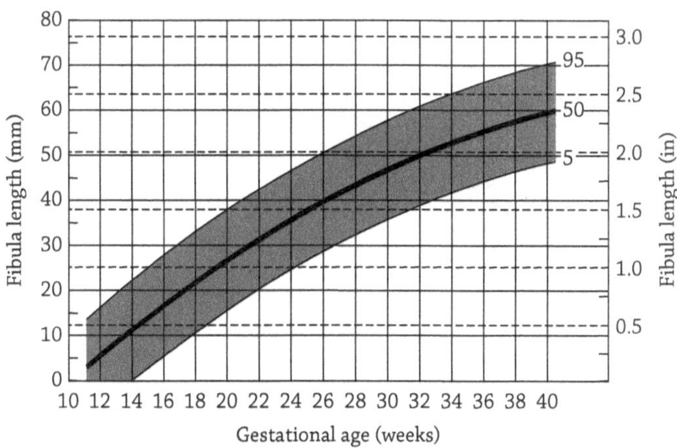

Figure 15.13. Growth of fibula length as a function of gestational age. From Jeanty and Romero (1984), by permission.

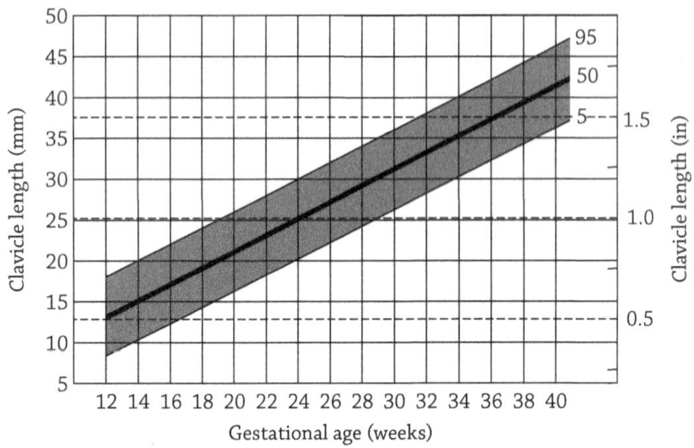

Figure 15.14. Growth of clavicle length as a function of gestational age. From Hansmann (1985), by permission.

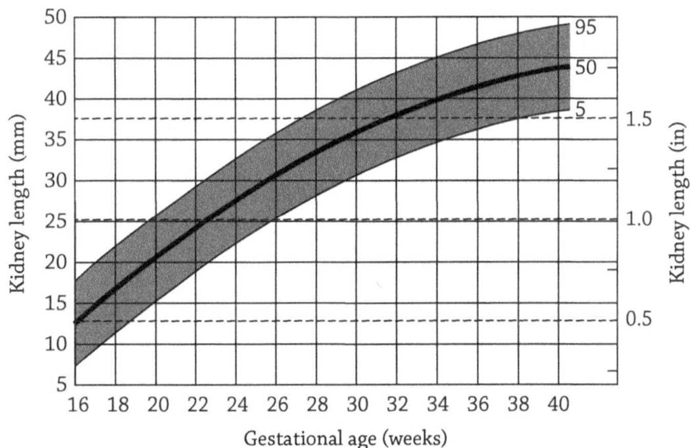

Figure 15.15. Growth of kidney length as a function of gestational age. From Hansmann (1985), by permission.

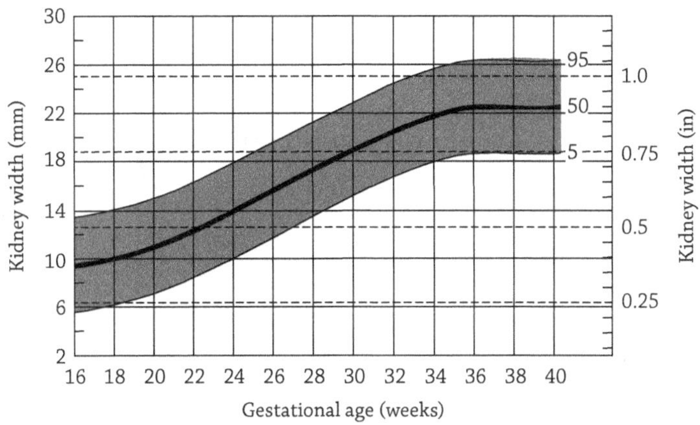

Figure 15.16. Growth of kidney width as a function of gestational age. From Hansmann (1985), by permission.

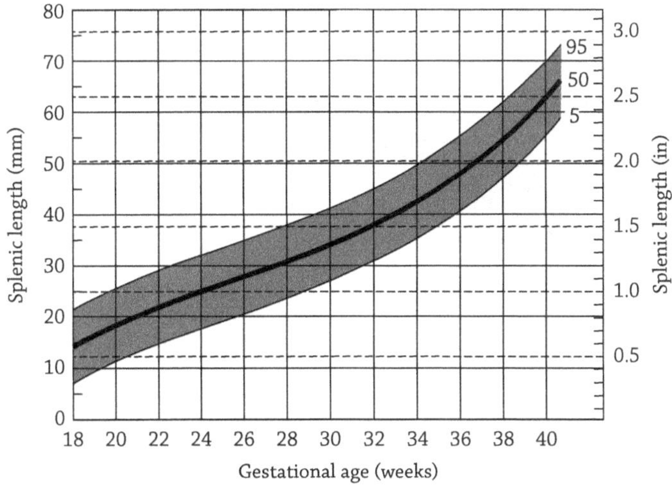

Figure 15.17. Growth of splenic length as a function of gestational age. From Hansmann (1985), by permission.

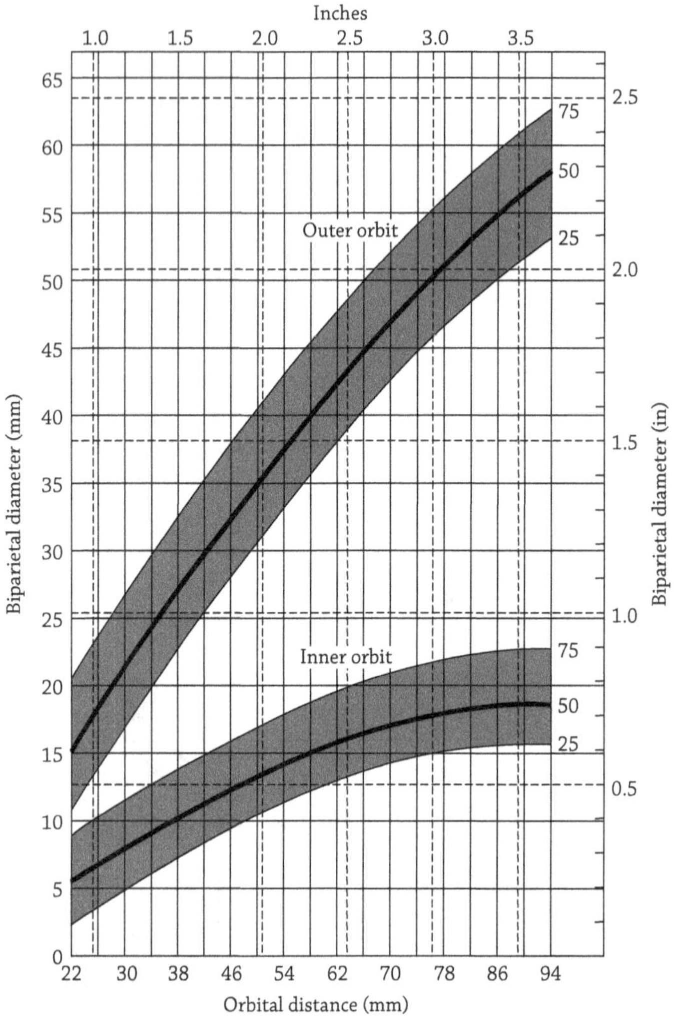

Figure 15.18. Growth of orbit size in relation to biparietal diameter. From Mayden et al. (1982), by permission.

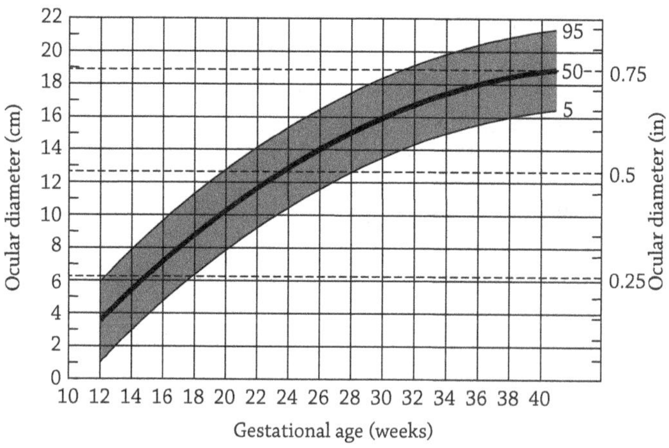

Figure 15.19. Growth of ocular diameter as a function of gestational age. From Mayden et al. (1982), by permission.

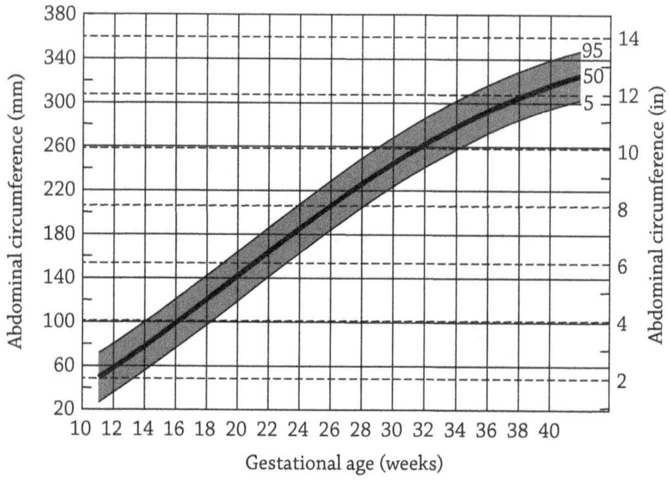

Figure 15.20. Growth of abdominal circumference as a function of gestational age. From Hadlock et al. (1982), by permission.

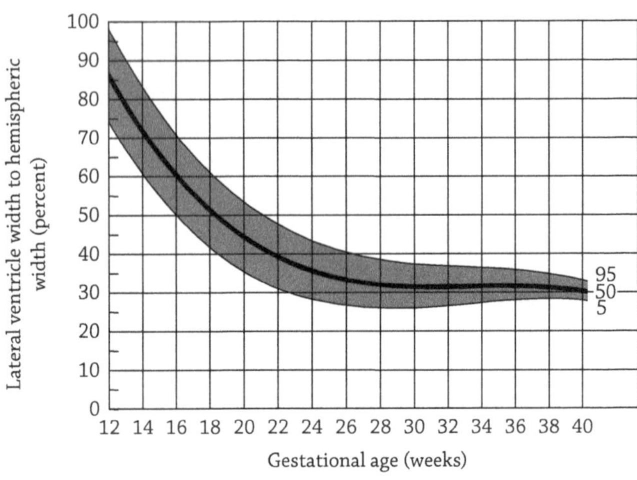

Figure 15.21. Lateral ventricle width as a function of hemispheric width. From Hansmann (1985), by permission.

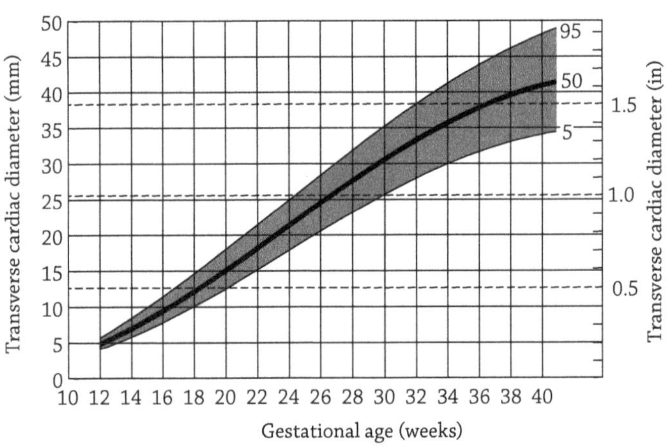

Figure 15.22. Growth of transverse cardiac diameter as a function of gestational age. From Hansmann (1985), by permission.

PRENATAL MEASUREMENTS

In general, ultrasound measurements use the longest dimension of a particular structure, whether it is a bone, such as the femur, or an organ, such as the kidney. Ratios help to determine whether there is disproportionate growth, reduced growth, or overgrowth of a structure. When assessing brain growth, ventricular size must be evaluated (Fig. 15.21) and when assessing renal size and function, the amount of amniotic fluid must be evaluated (Fig. 15.23). Fetal magnetic resonance imaging is increasingly being used as a more sensitive imaging technology, in particular when a fetal brain abnormality is suspected.

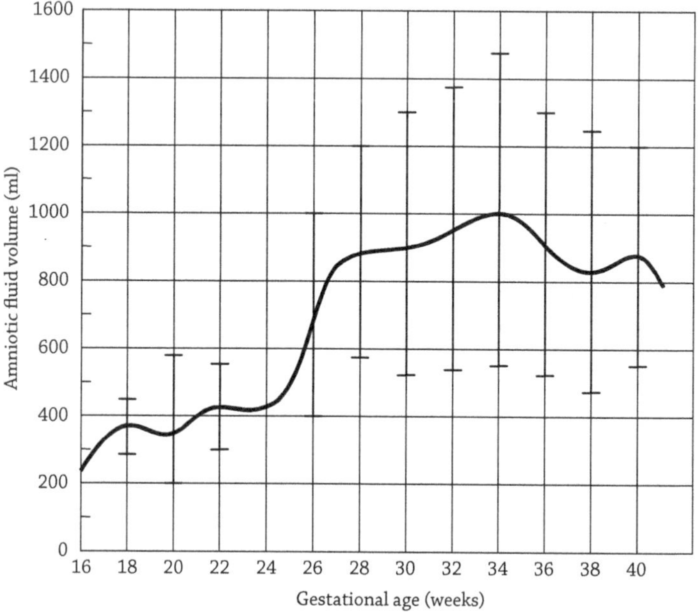

Figure 15.23. Amniotic fluid volume in relation to gestational age. At 20 weeks, the fetus swallows about 12 mL of amniotic fluid every 24 hours and urinates 15–17 mL of urine into the amniotic fluid every 24 hours. From Hansmann (1985), by permission.

NORMAL FETAL ACTIVITY DURING GESTATION

Patterns of fetal activity indicate fetal well-being and help to determine maturation.

Type of movement	Normal activity	Movement observed
Embryo movement	From 7 wk	
Limb movement	From 10 wk, increases up to 20 wk	Mean movement 120/hr
	Decreases from 20–40 wk	Mean movement 60–80/hr
Breathing	12–24 wk	Seen 5%–17% of time
	28–40 wk	Present 30% of time; episodic and irregular; may go up to 2 hr without breathing movements
	30 wk onward	20–60 breaths/min Coordinated and synchronized breathing movements
Hiccoughing	From 12 wk	Abrupt thoracic and abdominal movement
Sucking	From 12 wk	Hands are held around the face; regular thumb sucking in third trimester
Swallowing	From 12 wk	Amniotic fluid increases if no swallowing occurs
Bladder emptying	From 12 wk	Fills over 45 min period, then empties

Figure 15.24. Fetal movement during gestation.

BIBLIOGRAPHY

Abramovich, D. R. (1970). The volume of amniotic fluid in early pregnancy. *British Journal of Obstetrics and Gynaecology*, 77, 865.

Campbell, S., and Newman, G. B. (1973). Growth of the fetal biparietal diameter during normal pregnancy. *British Journal of Obstetrics and Gynaecology*, 78, 513.

Campbell, S., Waldimiroff, J. W., and Dewhyrst, C. J. (1973). The antenatal measurements of fetal urine production. *British Journal of Obstetrics and Gynaecology*, 80, 680.

de Vries, J. I. P., Visser, G. H. A., and van Prechtl, H. F. R. (1982). *Behavioural states in the human fetus during labour*. Proceedings, 1st Conference, The Society for the Study of Fetal Physiology, Oxford, England.

Hadlock, F. P., Deter, R. L., Harrist, R. B., and Park, S. K. (1982). Fetal abdominal circumference as a predictor of menstrual age. *AJR, American Journal of Roentgenology*, 139, 367–370.

Hansmann, M. (1985). *Ultrasonic diagnosis in obstetrics and gynecology*. Berlin: Springer.

Jeanty, P., and Romero, R. (1984). *Obstetrical ultrasound*. New York: McGraw-Hill.

Levi, S. (1973). Intra-uterine fetal growth studied by ultrasonic biparietal measurement. The percentiles of biparietal distribution. *Acta Obstetrica Gynecologica Scandinavica*, 52, 193.

Mayden, K. L., Tortora, M., Berkowitz, R. L., Braken, M., and Hobbins, J. C. (1982). Orbital diameters. *American Journal of Obstetrics and Gynecology*, 144, 289–297.

Meire, H. B. (1981). Ultrasound assessment of fetal growth patterns. *British Medical Bulletin*, 37, 253–258.

Queenan, J. T., and Thompson, P. (1972). Amniotic fluid volumes in normal pregnancies. *American Journal of Obstetrics and Gynecology*, 114, 34–48.

Sabbagha, R. E., and Hughey, M. (1978). Standardization of sonar cephalometry and gestational age. *Obstetrics & Gynecology*, 52(4), 402–406.

Chapter 16

Postmortem Organ Weights

EMBRYO AND FETAL PATHOLOGY

Intrauterine fetal death during the late second or third trimester of pregnancy is reported to occur once in every 100 births. Although the risk is less with improved fetal surveillance and testing, a stillbirth requires thorough investigation for proper patient counseling. After delivery, obvious abnormalities are uncommon on gross inspection of the fetus or placenta. The clinical history is often unremarkable, and any preexisting antepartum medical or obstetric complications may not relate directly to the cause of the stillbirth.

In 25% of stillbirths, there is a fetal abnormality. One-half of these have a single gene or chromosomal cause with a risk for recurrence. In approximately two-thirds, the recurrence risk is greater than 1%. In 25%, the recurrence risk is greater than 10%. Prenatal diagnosis is possible in 50% of the cases where there is a recurrence risk.

Current recommendations for the evaluation of all stillbirths and infants dying within 24 hours after birth (neonatal deaths) include gross and microscopic autopsy of the fetus and the placenta, postmortem photography and radiography, analysis of bacterial cultures, molecular karyotyping through array-based comparative genomic hybridization (aCGH), and saving tissue for further DNA studies when indicated (Fig. 16.1).

Detailed clinical examination of the placenta will reveal abnormalities in more than 80% of cases, autopsy examination of the placenta will reveal abnormalities in 70%, and placental histological evaluation will reveal abnormalities in 98% of cases. The placental abnormalities are the sole findings in 10% of cases. The most frequent placental anomalies are hemorrhagic endovasculitis, severe acute chorioamnionitis, retroplacental hematomas, erythroblastosis/hydrops, and villus changes indicative of uteroplacental vascular insufficiency. A two-vessel cord, which may be associated with underlying congenital anomalies, may go undetected without microscopic examination.

Often the single most useful tool for establishing a specific diagnosis is the gross postmortem examination. Careful and complete histopathological evaluation may further understanding of the mechanisms of embryogenesis, pregnancy loss, and early neonatal mortality in addition to providing a specific diagnosis. Since full details of specific organ weights proportional to total fetal body weight at varying gestational ages are not widely available, the data are provided here (Figs. 16.2–16.9). Additional syndrome specific data may be available in the literature, such as measurements of deceased fetuses with Turner syndrome in Barr and Oman-Ganes (2002).

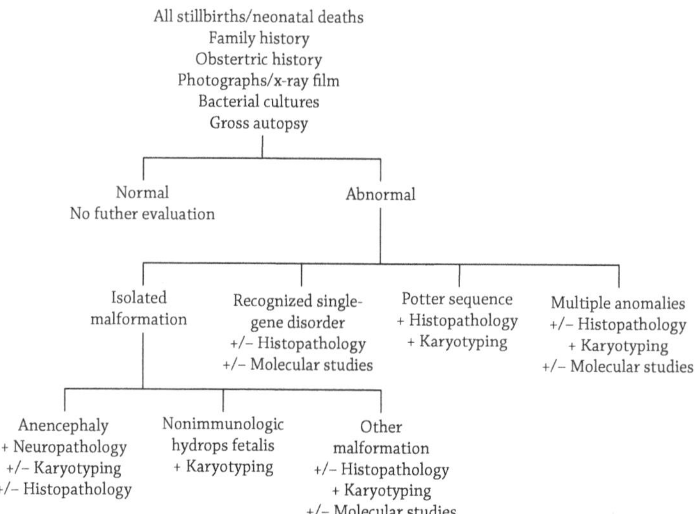

Figure 16.1. Protocol for selective evaluation of stillbirths and early neonatal deaths. From Mueller et al. (1983), by permission. Karyotyping should include array-based comparative genomic hybridization whenever possible (Raca et al., 2009).

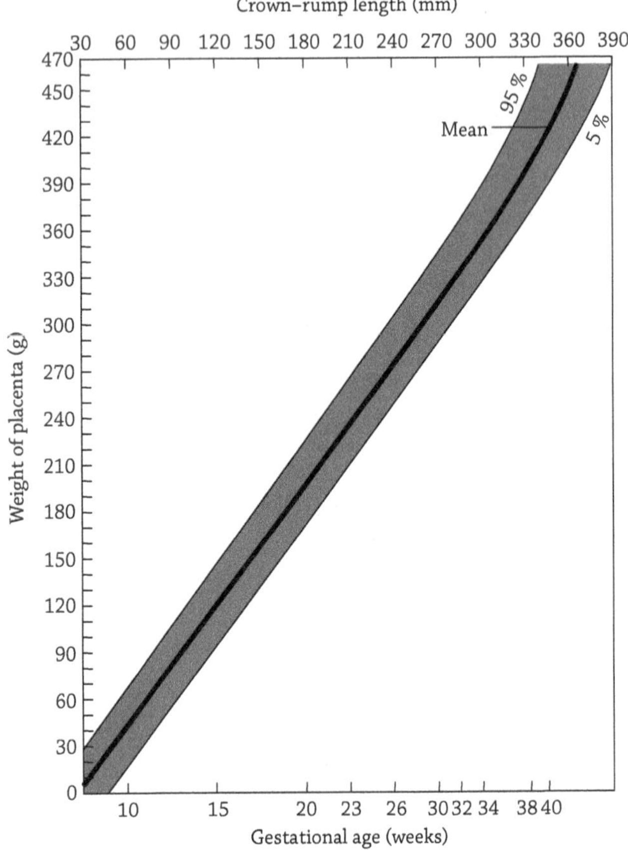

Figure 16.2. Placental weight at term; average weight is 500 g (range: 350–600 g).

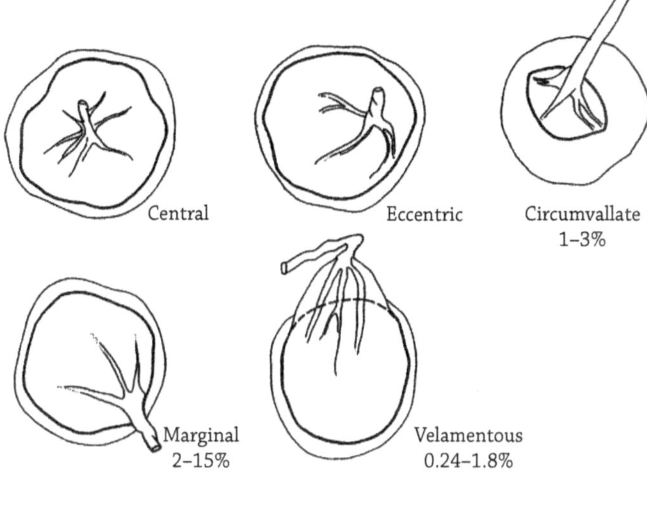

Menstrual age (week)	Umbilical cord length (cm ± 1SD)
20 to 21	32.4 ± 8.6
22 to 23	36.4 ± 9.0
24 to 25	40.1 ± 10.1
26 to 27	42.5 ± 11.3
28 to 29	45.0 ± 9.7
30 to 31	47.6 ± 11.3
32 to 33	50.2 ± 12.1
34 to 35	52.5 ± 11.2
36 to 37	55.6 ± 12.6
38 to 39	57.4 ± 12.6
40 to 41	59.6 ± 12.6
42 to 43	60.3 ± 12.7
44 to 45	60.4 ± 12.7
46 to 47	60.5 ± 13.0

Figure 16.3. Placenta cord insertion and umbilical cord length. From Naeye (1985), by permission.

(a)

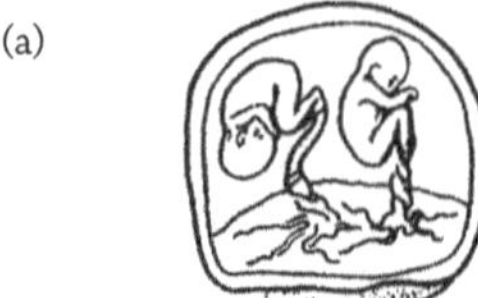

Monochorionic monoamniotic placenta indicative of fertilization of one ovum by one sperm and separation into two embryonic discs 8 days or more after ovulation. About 1% of all twin pregnancies. About 7% of monozygous twin pregancies.

(b)

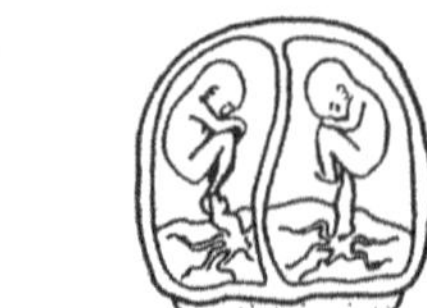

Monochorionic diamniotic placenta indicative of fertilization of one ovum by one sperm and separation into two embryonic discs between 3 and 8 days after ovulation. 20–30% of all twin pregnancies. 70–75% of all monozygous twin pregnancies.

(c)

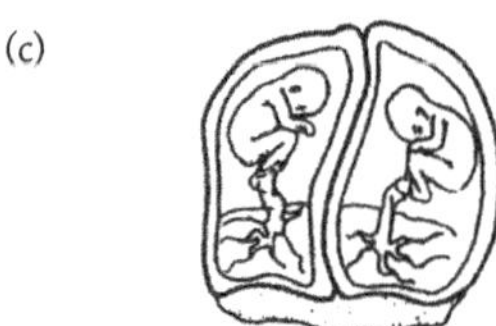

Fused dichorionic diamniotic placenta (35–40% of all twin pregnancies) indicative of: (i) fertilization of the one ovum by one sperm and early separation of the blastomere (0–3 days post-ovulation) 10% of all monozygous twin pregnancies; (ii) fertilization of two ova by two sperm and implantation in juxtaposition. 35–40% of all dizygous twin pregnancies.

(d)

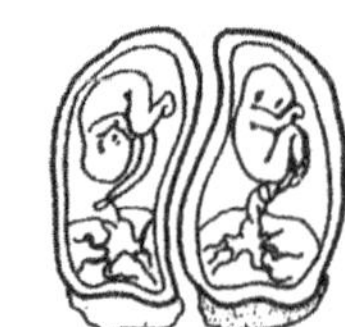

Separate dichorionic diamniotic placentas (35–50% of all twin pregnancies) indicative of: (i) fertiliztion of one ovum by one sperm, early separation of blastomeres and separate implanation sites (0–3 days post-ovulation) 15% of all monozygous twin pregnancies; (ii) fertilization of two ovam by two sperm which implant at separate sites 60–65% of all dizygous twin pregnancies.

(e)

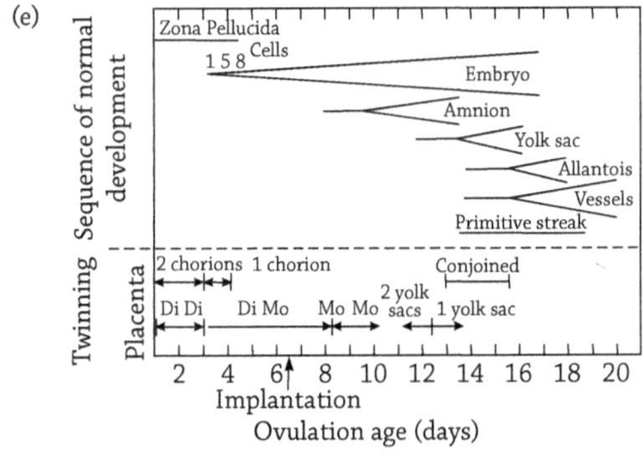

Figure 16.4. Twinning, timing, and membranes. From MacGillivray et al. (1975), by permission.

Ovulation	Weight	CR length	Brain	Heart	Lungs	Liver	Kidneys	Adrenals	Thymus	Spleen	Pancreas
age (days)	(g)	(mm)	(g)	(g)	(g)	(g)	(g)	(g)	(g)	(g)	(g)
49	0–4	3	0.8	0.1	0.1	0.2	0.1	0.1	—	—	—
66	5–9	5	1.2	0.1	0.1	0.2	0.1	—	—	—	—
67	10	6	1.5	0.2	0.3	0.7	0.1	0.1	—	—	—
71	15	6	2.6	0.2	0.4	0.8	0.1	0.1	—	—	—
73	20	7	4.3	0.3	0.4	1.1	0.2	0.1	—	—	—
76	25	7	4.8	0.4	0.7	1.1	0.2	—	—	—	—
79	30	8	5.4	0.4	1.0	1.3	0.2	0.2	—	—	—
84	35	9	6.2	0.5	1.4	2.0	0.3	0.2	—	—	—
88	40	9	—	—	—	—	—	—	—	—	—
89	45	9	7.4	0.5	1.9	2.5	0.4	0.4	—	—	—
90	50	10	8.5	0.5	1.9	3.0	0.5	0.5	0.1	0.1	—
91	60	10	10	0.5	2.5	3.4	0.6	0.6	0.2	0.1	—
92	70	11	11	0.6	3.0	3.6	0.8	0.6	0.2	0.1	0.1
96	80	11	12	0.7	3.0	4.3	0.8	0.6	0.2	0.2	0.1
100	90	12	14	0.9	3.0	4.7	0.9	0.7	0.2	0.2	0.2
105	100	12	17	1.1	3.9	5.6	1.4	0.7	0.3	0.2	0.2
109	125	13	23	1.3	4.1	7.4	1.4	0.7	0.3	0.2	0.2
115	150	14	23	1.4	5.3	9.2	1.4	0.8	0.3	0.3	0.2
117	175	14	23	1.4	5.6	11	1.8	0.8	0.3	0.4	0.4
118	200	15	33	1.7	7.2	12	2.2	1.1	0.4	0.4	0.4
124	250	16	39	2.2	9.1	15	2.7	1.2	0.4	0.5	0.4
130	300	17	46	2.4	10	17	3.1	1.5	0.7	0.6	0.5
133	350	18	54	2.9	11	21	3.8	2.0	0.8	0.7	0.5
143	400	18	61	3.4	11	23	4.2	2.2	1.0	0.8	0.6
149	450 +	19	70	3.4	12	23	4.7	2.3	1.0	0.8	0.6

Figure 16.5a. Fetal organ weights by ovulation age After Potter and Craig (1975), by permission.

Body weight (g)	Organ weights (g)									
	Brain	Heart	Lungs	Liver	Kidneys	Adrenals	Thymus	Spleen	Pancreas	Thyroid
500–999	109 ± 45	6 ± 2	18 ± 6	39 ± 11	7 ± 3	3 ± 1	2 ± 1	2 ± 3	1.0 ± 1.3	0.8 ± 0.7
1000–1499	180 ± 53	9 ± 5	27 ± 7	60 ± 16	12 ± 4	4 ± 1	4 ± 2	3 ± 3	1.4 ± 1.0	0.8 ± 0.8
1500–1999	250 ± 55	13 ± 5	38 ± 10	76 ± 17	16 ± 4	5 ± 2	7 ± 3	5 ± 3	2.0 ± 1.3	0.9 ± 0.6
2000–2499	308 ± 76	15 ± 5	44 ± 10	98 ± 25	20 ± 4	6 ± 2	8 ± 4	7 ± 5	2.3 ± 1.1	1.0 ± 0.7
2500–2999	359 ± 67	19 ± 5	49 ± 11	127 ± 31	23 ± 5	8 ± 3	9 ± 4	9 ± 4	3.0 ± 1.2	1.3 ± 0.9
3000–3499	403 ± 60	21 ± 4	55 ± 13	155 ± 33	25 ± 5	10 ± 3	11 ± 4	10 ± 4	3.5 ± 1.2	1.6 ± 0.9
3500–3999	421 ± 72	23 ± 5	58 ± 12	178 ± 38	28 ± 7	11 ± 3	13 ± 5	12 ± 5	4.0 ± 1.5	1.7 ± 0.8
4000–4499	424 ± 55	28 ± 5	66 ± 15	215 ± 36	31 ± 7	12 ± 4	14 ± 5	14 ± 5	4.6 ± 2.1	1.9 ± 0.9
4500 +	406 ± 56	36 ± 10	74 ± 16	275 ± 54	33 ± 8	15 ± 4	17 ± 6	17 ± 7	6.0 ± 6.2	2.3 ± 1.1

Figure 16.5b. Fetal organ weights, by body weight After Potter and Craig (1975), by permission.

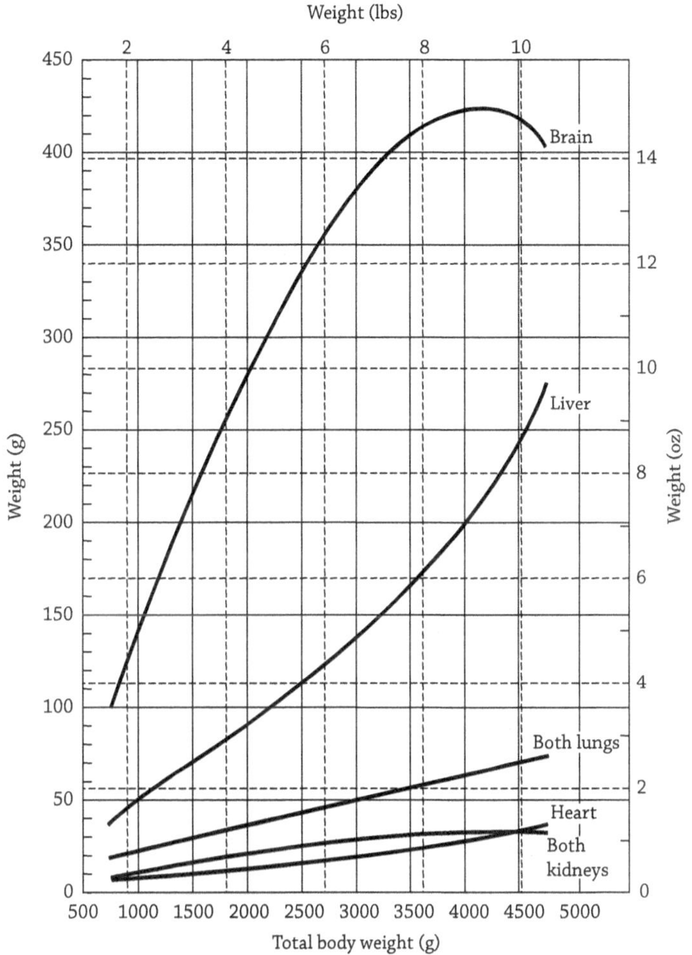

Figure 16.6. Fetal tissue weights, part 1.

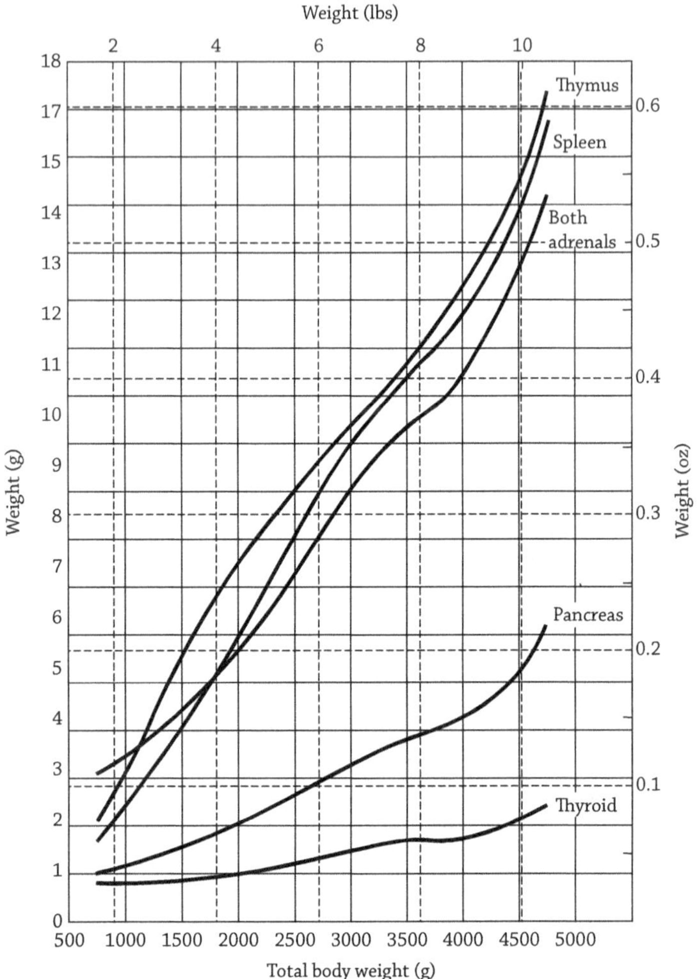

Figure 16.7. Fetal tissue weights, part 2.

Age	Sex	Weight (kg)	Length (cm)	Brain (g)	Heart (g)	Lungs Right (g)	Lungs Left (g)	Liver (g)	Kidneys Right (g)	Kidneys Left (g)	Adrenals (g)	Thymus (g)	Spleen (g)	Pancreas (g)
Birth-3 days	Both Sexes	3.4	49	335	17	21	18	78	13	14			8	
3–7 days			49	355	18	24	22	96	14	14			9	
1–3 weeks			52	382	19	29	26	123	15	15	5.0	7.2	10	6.1
3–5 weeks			52	413	20	31	27	127	16	16			12	
5–7 weeks			53	422	21	32	28	133	19	18			13	
7–9 weeks			55	489	23	32	29	136	19	18	4.9	8.0	13	7.2
3 months		6.5	56	516	23	35	30	140	20	19	4.9		14	8.0
4 months			59	540	27	37	33	160	22	21		9.8	16	10.0
5 months			61	614	29	38	35	188	25	25		13.0	16	11.0
6 months		8.5	62	660	31	42	39	200	26	25	4.9	10.0	17	11.0
7 months			63	691	34	49	41	227	30	30	5.3		99	
8 months			65	714	37	52	45	254	31	30	5.3		20	
9 months		9.8	67	750	37	53	47	260	31	30	5.4		20	11.0
10 months			69	809	39	54	51	274	32	31	5.7		22	14
11 months		10.8	70	852	40	59	53	277	34	33	6.1		25	15
12 months			73	925	44	64	57	288	36	35	6.2		26	14
14 months			74	944	45	66	60	304	36	35			26	
16 months			77	1010	48	72	64	331	39	39			28	
18 months			78	1042	52	72	65	345	40	43		26.6	30	
20 months			79	1050	56	80	74	370	43	44			30	

(continued)

						Lungs			Kidneys					
Age	Sex	Weight (kg)	Length (cm)	Brain (g)	Heart (g)	Right (g)	Left (g)	Liver (g)	Right (g)	Left (g)	Adrenals (g)	Thymus (g)	Spleen (g)	Pancreas (g)
3 years		15.2	88	1141	59	89	77	418	48	49			39	
4 years		17.3	99	1191	73	90	85	516	55	56			47	
5 years		19.4	108	1237	85	107	104	596	65	64			58	
6 years		21.9	109	1243	94	121	122	642	68	67			66	
7 years		24.6	113	1263	100	130	123	680	69	70			69	
8 years		27.7	119	1273	110	150	140	736	74	75			73	
9 years		31.0	125	1275	115	174	152	756	82	83			85	
10 years		34.8	130	1290	116	177	166	852	92	95			87	
11 years		38.8	135	1320	122	201	190	909	94	95			93	
12 years		43.2	139	1351	124	—	—	936	95	96			—	
17–19	M			1340	219							190		
	F			1242	210						25	120		
20–29	M			1396				1820						
	F			1234				1440						
30–39	M			1365				1830					155	
	F			1233				1460				20	120	
40–49	M			1366				1840					145	
	F			1240				1440					120	

50–59	M	1375				1840		16	145	
	F	1200				1430			110	
60–69	M	1323				1740				
	F	1178				1380				
All adult ages	Both sexes			450	375					
	M		300 (270–360)			1840 (900–3000)	313 (230–440)	9.7 (7–20)	145 (75–245)	110 (60–135)
	F		250 (200–280)			1700 (910–2130)	288 (240–350)	8.3 (7–18)	115 (55–190)	

Figure 16.8. Normal mean organ weight by age. From Sunderman and Boerner (1949), by permission.

Organ	Age	Weight (g)	Length (cm)
Thyroid	Adult	40 (30–70)	
Parathyroids	Adult	0.12–0.18	
Pituitary	10–20 yr	0.56	
	20–70 yr	0.61	
	Pregnancy	0.95 (0.84–1.06)	
Combined ovaries	Birth–5 yr	0.4–2.1	
	6–10 yr	2.2–3.1	
	11–16 yr	3.3–4.0	
	Adult	14	
Combined testes	Birth–5 yr	0.4–1.8	
	6–10 yr	1.6–3.0	
	11–16 yr	3.0–13.0	
	Adult	25 (20–27)	
Uterus	Birth–	4.6	
	1 mo–5 yr	1.9–2.9	
	6–10 yr	2.9–3.4	
	11–16 yr	5.3–25	
	Adult	35 (33–41)	
	After pregnancy	110 (102–117)	
Prostate	Birth–5 yr	0.9–1.2	
	6–10 yr	1.2–1.4	
	11–16 yr	2.3–6.1	
	20–30 yr	15	
	31–50 yr	20	
	51–80 yr	40	
Gastrointestinal tract (adults)			
Esophagus		25	
Duodenum		30	
Small intestine		550–650	
Colon		150–170	
Spinal cord		Average weight 27 g	Average length 45 cm
		Frontal	Sagittal
	Cervical	1.3–1.4 cm	Average 0.9
	Thoracic	Average 1.0 cm	Average 0.8
	Lumbar	Average 1.2 cm	Average 0.9

Figure 16.9. Miscellaneous organ sizes. From Minckler and Boyd (1968) and Sunderman and Boerner (1949), by permission.

BIBLIOGRAPHY

Barr, M., and Oman-Ganes, L. (2002). Turner syndrome morphology and morphometrics: Cardiac hypoplasia as a cause of midgestation death. *Teratology*, 66, 65–72.

Kissane, J. M. (1975). *Pathology of infancy and childhood* (2nd ed.). St. Louis: C.V. Mosby.

Kronick, J. B., Scriver, C. R., Goodyer, P. R., and Kaplan, P. B. (1983). A perimortem protocol for suspected genetic disease. *Pediatrics*, 71, 960–963.

MacGillivray, I., Nylander, P. P. S., and Corney, G. (1975). *Human multiple reproduction*. Philadelphia: W.B. Saunders.

MacLeod, P. M., Dill, F., and Hardwick, D. F. (1979). Chromosomes, syndromes, and perinatal deaths: The genetic counseling value of making a diagnosis in a malformed abortus, stillborn and deceased newborn. *Birth Defects*, 15(5A), 105–111.

Minckler, T. M., and Boyd, E. (1968). Physical growth of the nervous system and its coverings. In *Pathology of the nervous system* (ed. J. Minckler), Vol. 1, pp. 120–137. New York; McGraw-Hill.

Moore, K. L. (1982). *The developing human* (3rd ed.). Philadelphia: W.B. Saunders.

Mueller, R. F., Sybert, V. P., Johnson, J., Brown, Z. A., and Chen, W. -J. (1983). Evaluation of a protocol for post-mortem examination of stillbirths. *New England Journal of Medicine*, 309, 586–590.

Naeye, R. L. (1985). Umbilical cord length: Clinical significance. *Journal of Pediatrics*, 107(2), 278–281.

Raca, G., Artzer, A., Thorson, L., Huber, S., Modaff, P., Laffin, J., and Pauli, R. M. (2009). Array-based comparative genomic hybridization (aCGH) in the genetic evaluation of stillbirth. *American Journal of Medical Genetics Part A*, 149A, 2437–2443.

Poland, B. J., and Lowry, R. B. (1974). The use of spontaneous abortuses and stillbirths in genetic counseling. *American Journal of Obstetrics and Gynecology*, 118, 322–331.

Potter, E. L., and Craig, J. M. (1975). *Pathology of the fetus and the infant* (3rd ed.). Chicago, IL: Year Book Medical Publishers.

Rayburn, W., Sander, C., Barr, M. Jr., and Rygiel, R. (1985). The stillborn fetus: Placental histologic examination in determining a cause. *Obstetrics and Gynecology*, 65, 637–641.

Sunderman, F. W., and Boerner, F. (1949). *Normal values in clinical medicine*. Philadelphia: W.B. Saunders.

Chapter 17

Measurements for Specific Syndromes

INTRODUCTION

As the natural history of various specific conditions is defined, it is possible to generate growth curves for those conditions. Although inevitably there are many problems with such growth curves (e.g., heterogeneity, lack of longitudinal data, complicating factors as part of the natural history, use of growth hormone), they are still very useful because they allow comparison between the individual and what is considered "typical" for the specific condition.

We are including growth curves for specific syndromes in the hope that they will be useful and will also encourage the collection of additional measurement data to enlarge the number of cases and the number of disorders for which such information is available.

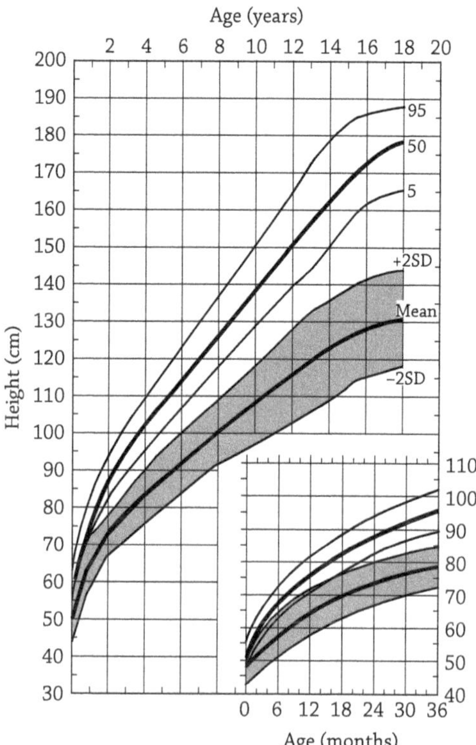

Figure 17.1 Achondroplasia, height, males, birth to 18 years. Mean and two standard deviations are depicted as indicated. For comparison, range of measurements in typical persons is included. Adapted from Horton et al. (1978).

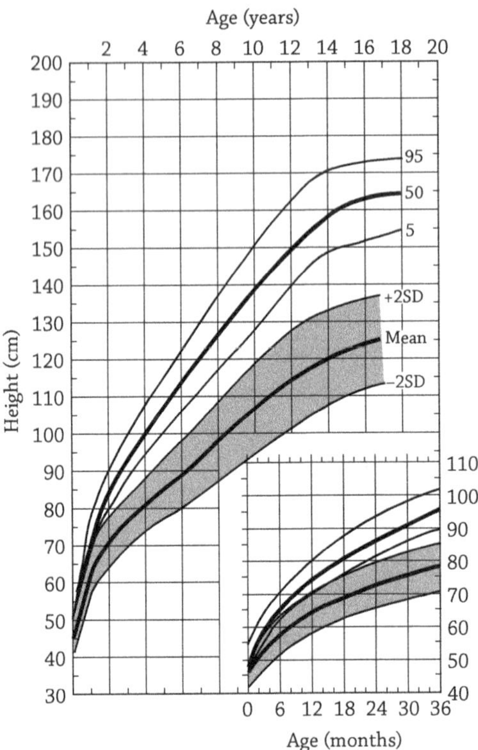

Figure 17.2 Achondroplasia, height, females, birth to 18 years. Mean and two standard deviations are depicted as indicated. For comparison, range of measurements in typical persons is included. Adapted from Horton et al. (1978).

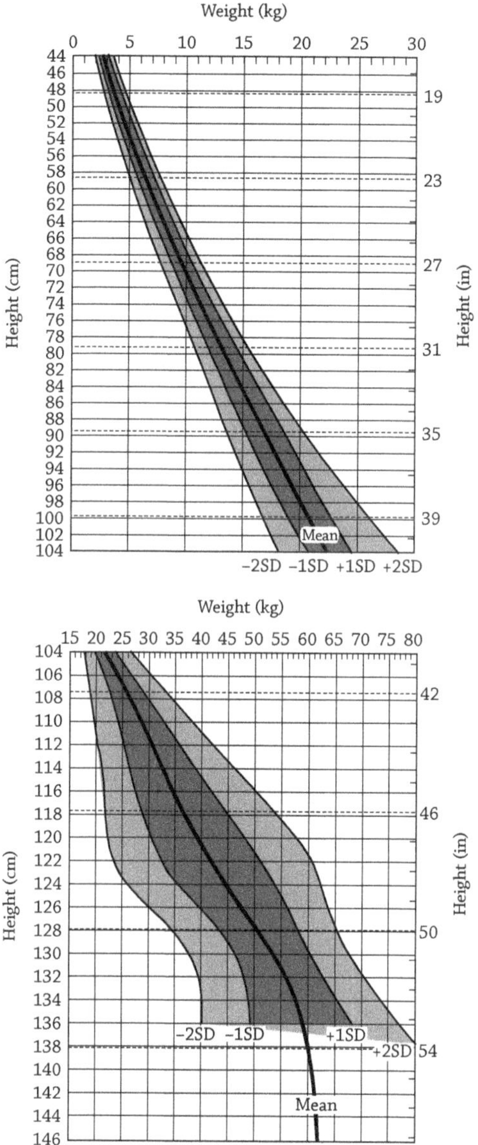

Figure 17.3 Achondroplasia, weight for height, males. Mean, one standard deviation, and two standard deviations are shown. Data for height to 104 cm is shown in the upper figure, with data for height above 104 cm shown in the lower figure. Adapted from Hunter et al. (1996a).

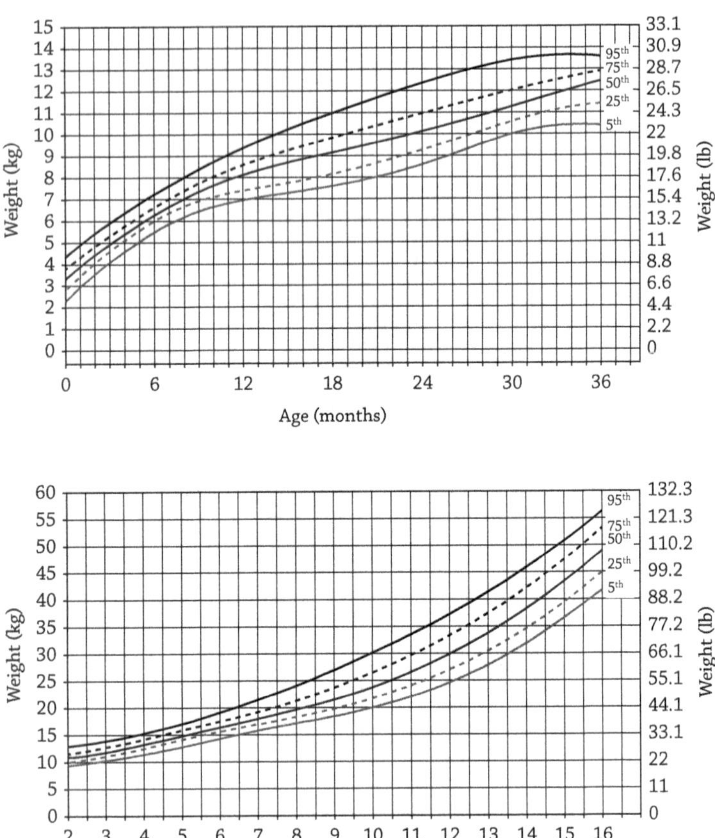

Figure 17.4 Achondroplasia, weight for age, males. Adapted from Hoover-Fong et al. (2007).

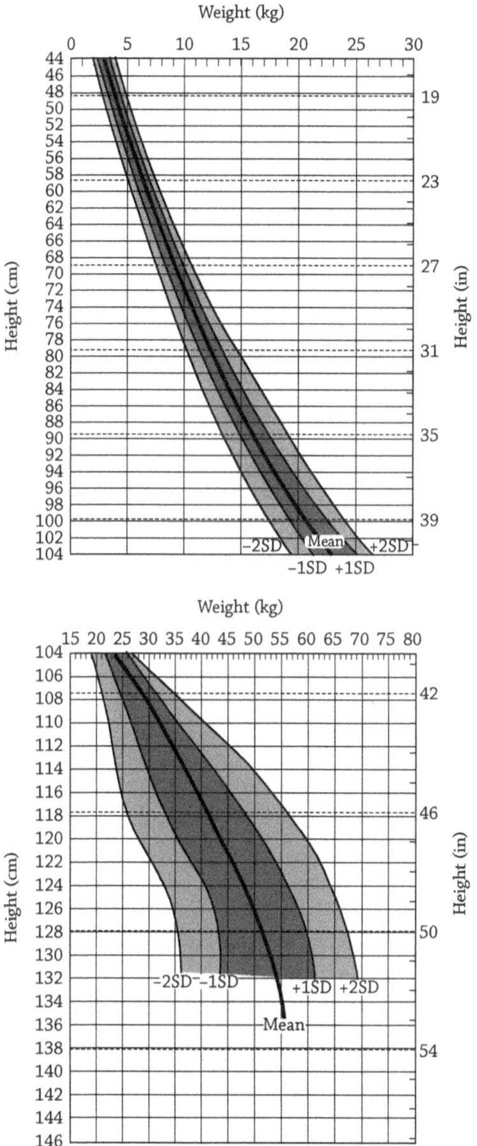

Figure 17.5 Achondroplasia, weight for height, females. Mean, one standard deviation, and two standard deviations are shown. Data for height to 104 cm is shown in the upper figure, with data for height above 104 cm shown in the lower figure. Adapted from Hunter et al. (1996a).

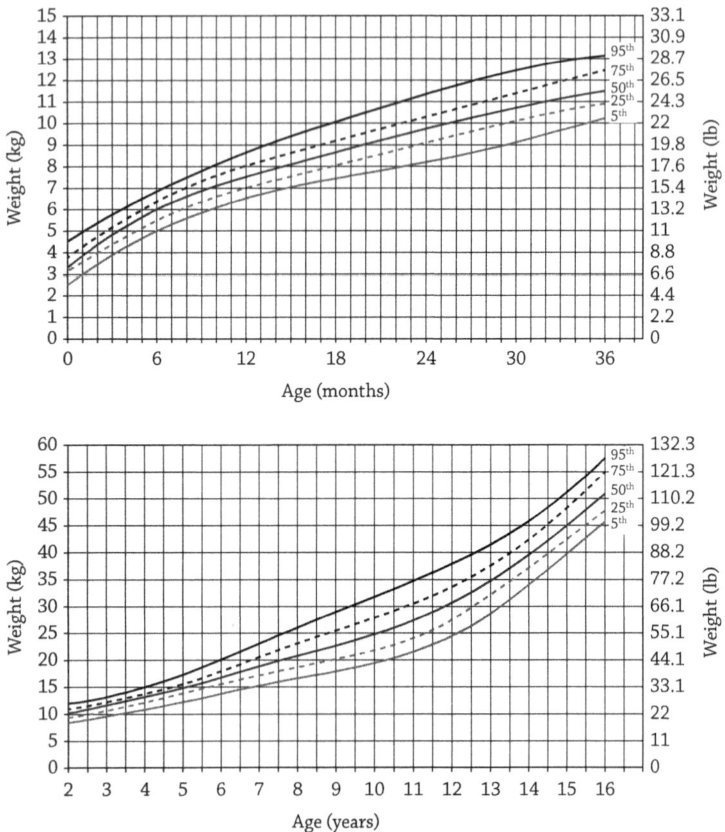

Figure 17.6 Achondroplasia, weight for age, females. Adapted from Hoover-Fong et al. (2007).

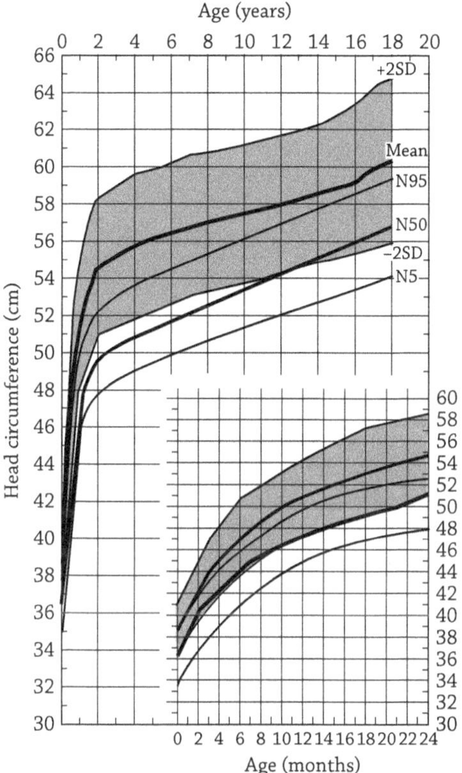

Figure 17.7 Achondroplasia, head circumference, males, birth to 18 years. Mean and two standard deviations are depicted as indicated. For comparison, range of measurements in typical persons is included. Adapted from Horton et al. (1978).

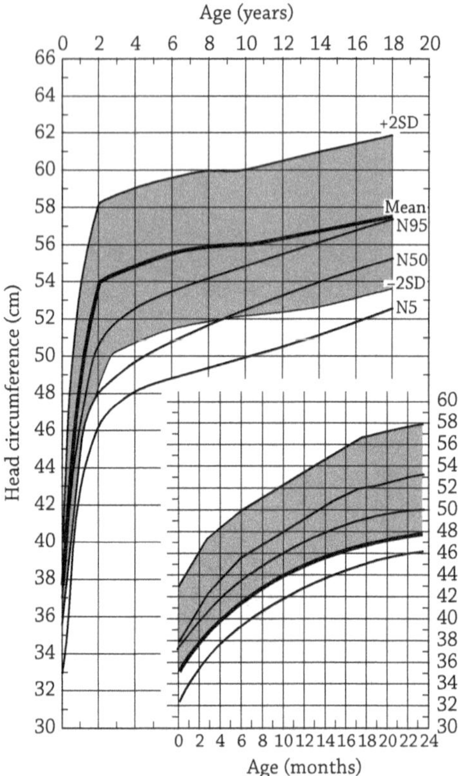

Figure 17.8 Achondroplasia, head circumference, females, birth to 18 years. Mean and two standard deviations are depicted as indicated. For comparison, range of measurements in typical persons is included. Adapted from Horton et al. (1978).

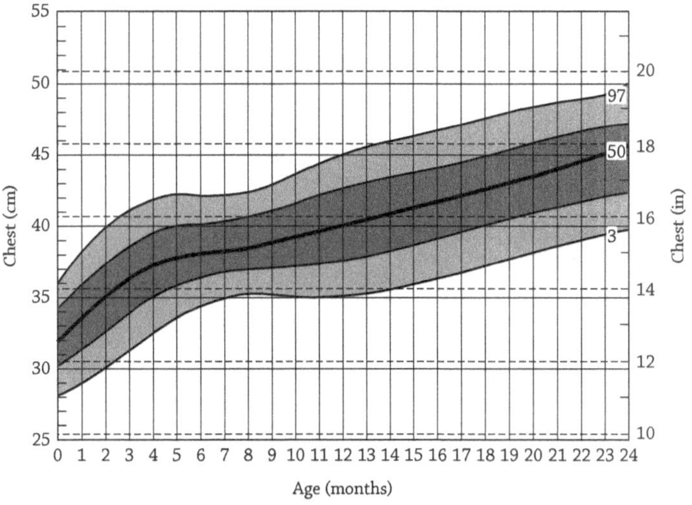

Figure 17.9 Achondroplasia, smoothed curve of mean chest circumference, males, birth to 24 months. Adapted from Horton et al. (1978).

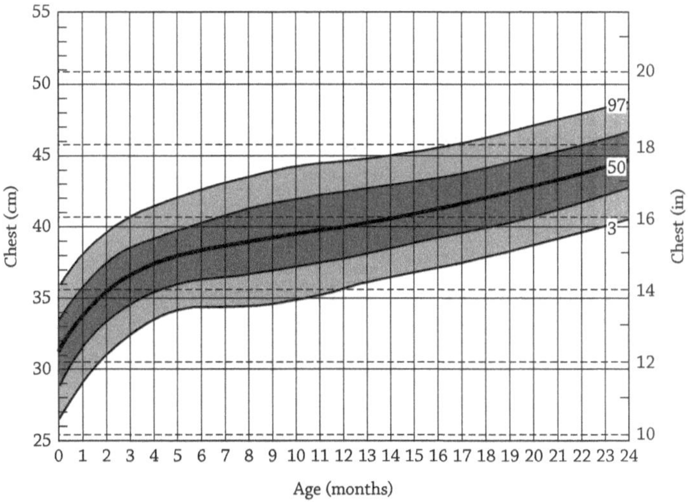

Figure 17.10 Achondroplasia, smoothed curve of mean chest circumference, females, birth to 24 months. Adapted from Horton et al. (1978).

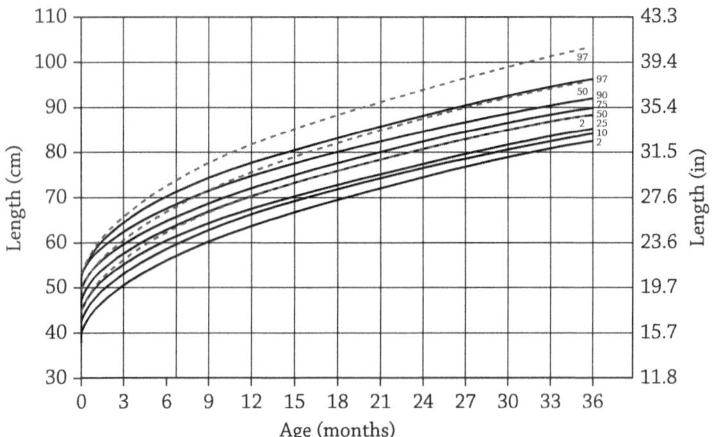

Figure 17.11 Barth syndrome, height from birth to 36 months. Dashed lines show 3rd, 50th, and 97th centiles for typical males. Data derived from 73 individuals. Adapted from Roberts et al. (2012).

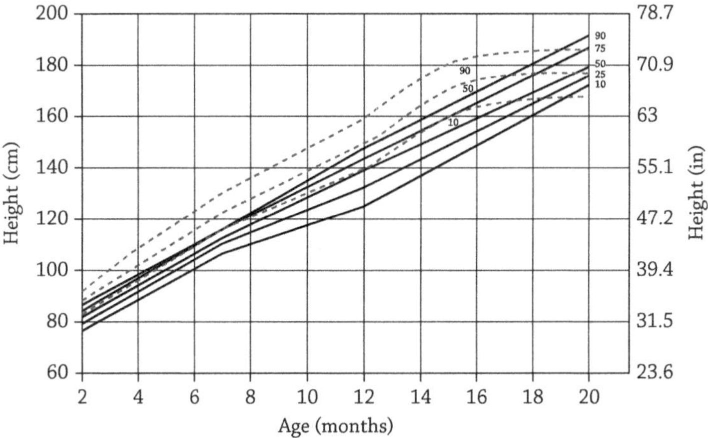

Figure 17.12 Barth syndrome, height from 2 to 20 years. Dashed lines show 10th, 50th, and 90th centiles for typical males. Data derived from 73 individuals. Adapted from Roberts et al. (2012).

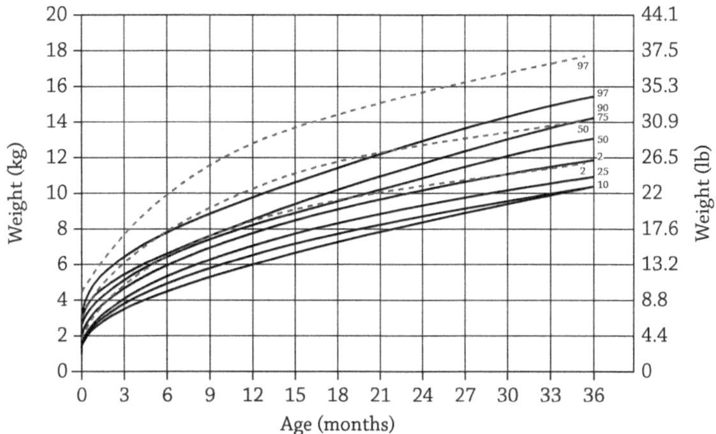

Figure 17.13 Barth syndrome, weight from birth to 36 months. Dashed lines show 3rd, 50th, and 97th centiles for typical males. Data derived from 73 individuals. Adapted from Roberts et al. (2012).

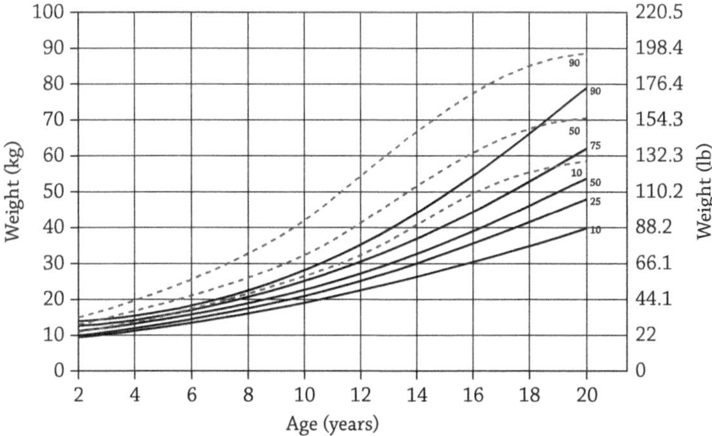

Figure 17.14 Barth syndrome, weight from 2 to 20 years. Dashed lines show 10th, 50th, and 90th centiles for typical males. Data derived from 73 individuals. Adapted from Roberts et al. (2012).

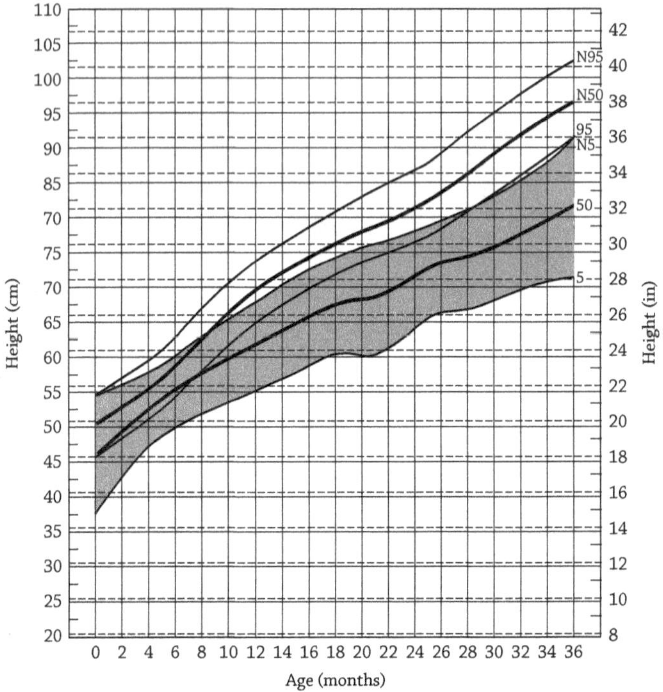

Figure 17.15 Cornelia de Lange syndrome, height, males, birth to 36 months. For comparison, range of measurements in typical persons (N) is included. Adapted from Kline et al. (1993); all Cornelia de Lange syndrome graphs were derived from a total of 180 patients.

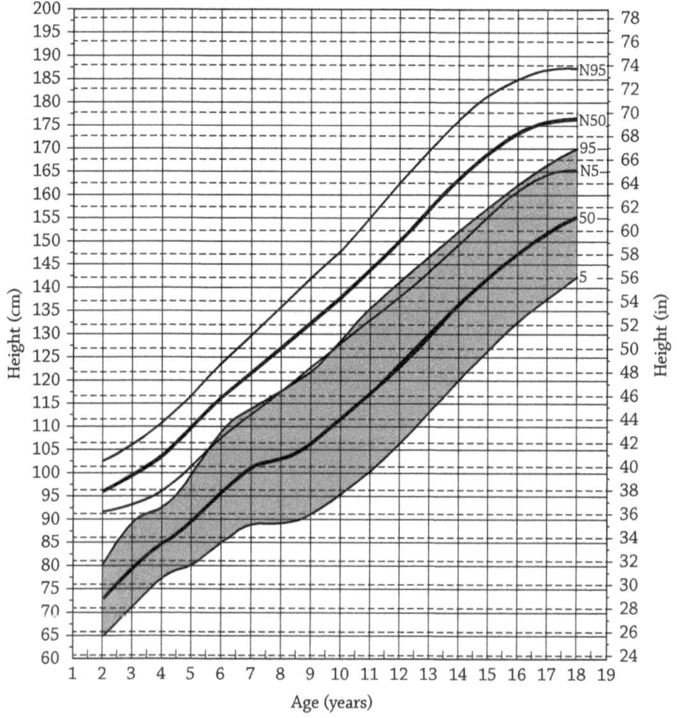

Figure 17.16 Cornelia de Lange syndrome, height, males, 2 to 18 years. For comparison, range of measurements in typical persons (N) is included. Adapted from Kline et al. (1993); all Cornelia de Lange syndrome graphs were derived from a total of 180 patients.

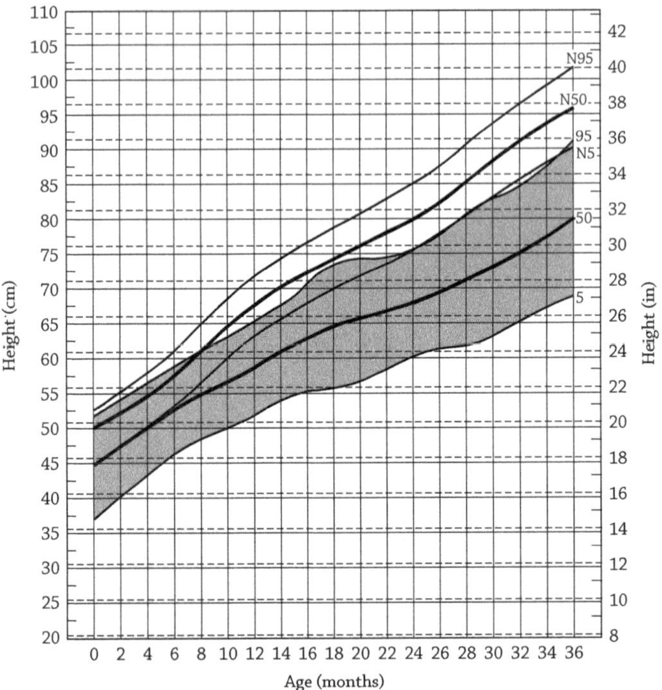

Figure 17.17 Cornelia de Lange syndrome, height, females, birth to 36 months. For comparison, range of measurements in typical persons (N) is included. Adapted from Kline et al. (1993); all Cornelia de Lange syndrome graphs were derived from a total of 180 patients.

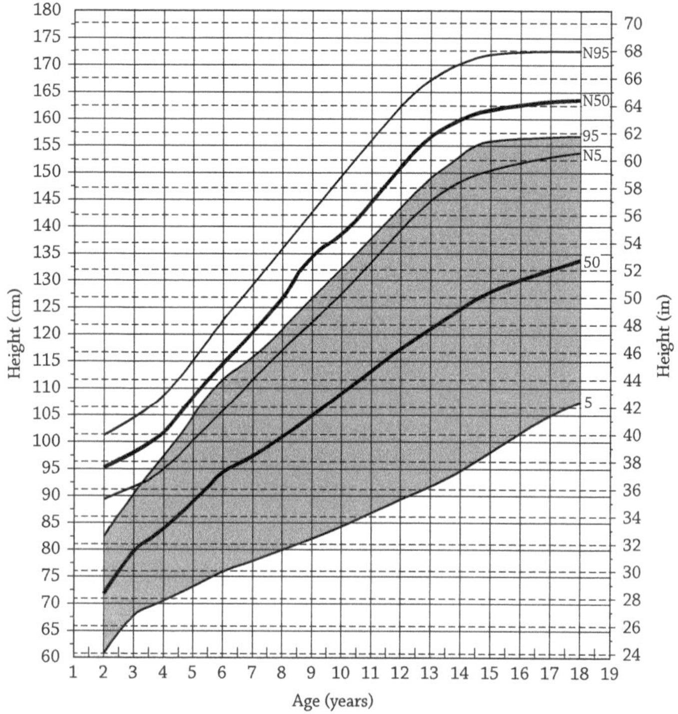

Figure 17.18 Cornelia de Lange syndrome, height, females, 2 to 18 years. For comparison, range of measurements in typical persons (N) is included. Adapted from Kline et al. (1993); all Cornelia de Lange syndrome graphs were derived from a total of 180 patients.

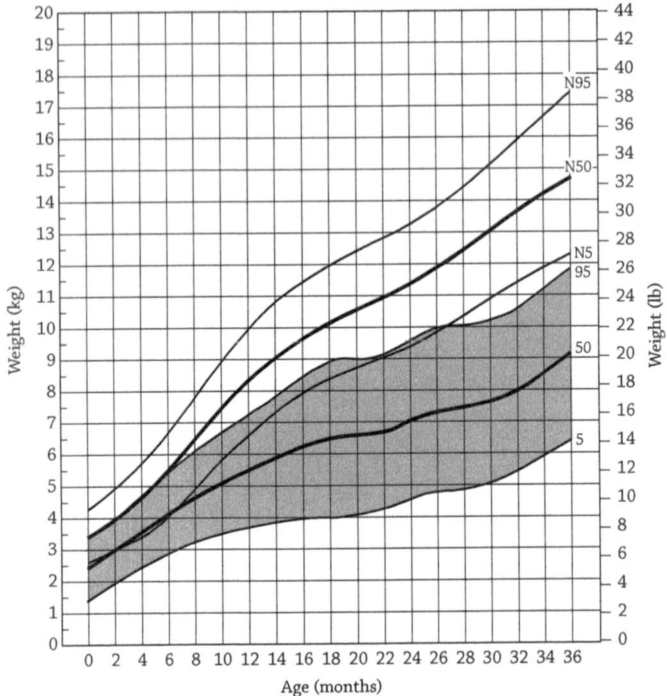

Figure 17.19 Cornelia de Lange syndrome, weight, males, birth to 36 months. For comparison, range of measurements in typical persons (N) is included. Adapted from Kline et al. (1993); all Cornelia de Lange syndrome graphs were derived from a total of 180 patients.

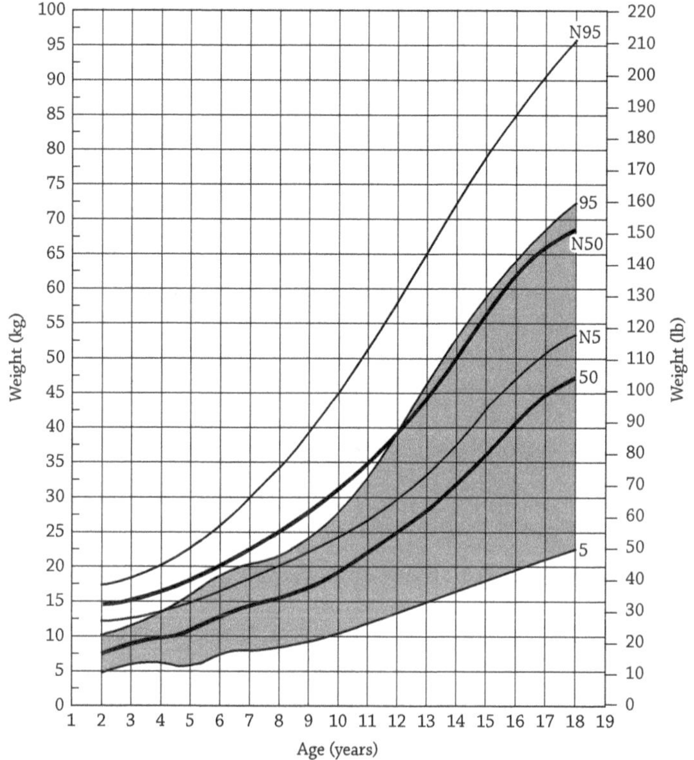

Figure 17.20 Cornelia de Lange syndrome, weight, males, 2 to 18 years. For comparison, range of measurements in typical persons (N) is included. Adapted from Kline et al. (1993); all Cornelia de Lange syndrome graphs were derived from a total of 180 patients.

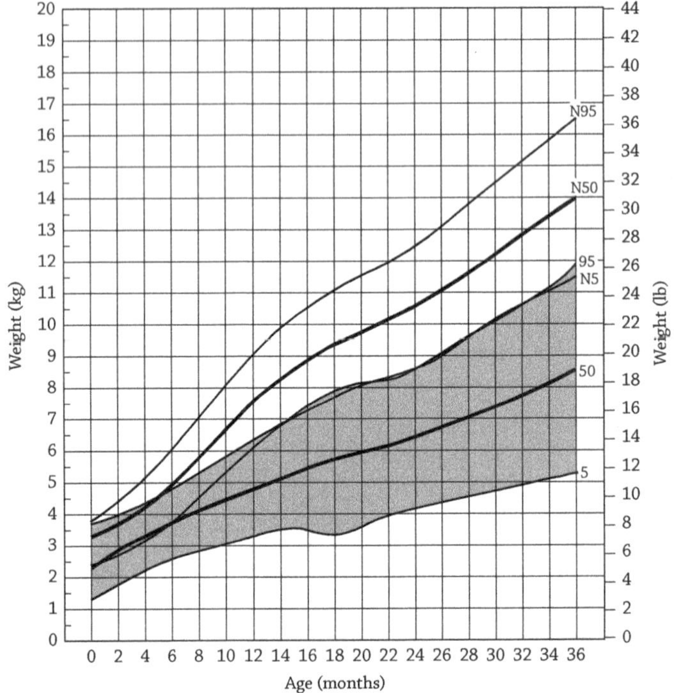

Figure 17.21 Cornelia de Lange syndrome, weight, females, birth to 36 months. For comparison, range of measurements in typical persons (N) is included. Adapted from Kline et al. (1993); all Cornelia de Lange syndrome graphs were derived from a total of 180 patients.

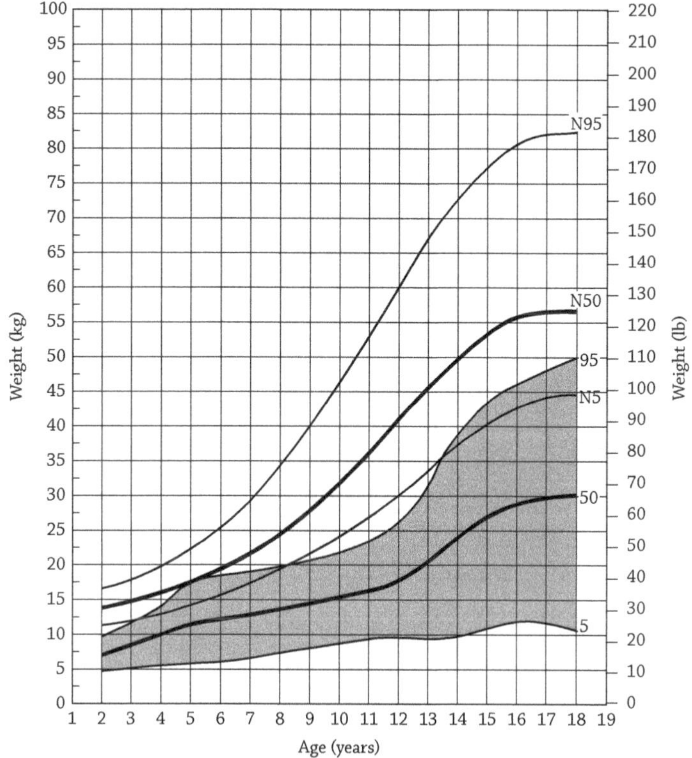

Figure 17.22 Cornelia de Lange syndrome, weight, females, 2 to 18 years. For comparison, range of measurements in typical persons (N) is included. Adapted from Kline et al. (1993); all Cornelia de Lange syndrome graphs were derived from a total of 180 patients.

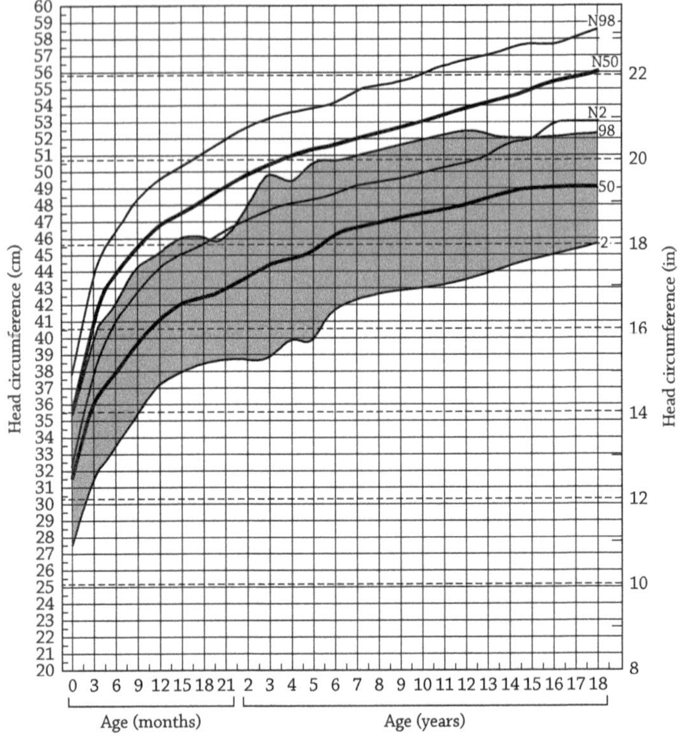

Figure 17.23 Cornelia de Lange syndrome, head circumference, males, birth to 18 years, compared with normal males (N). Adapted from Kline et al. (1993); all Cornelia de Lange syndrome graphs were derived from a total of 180 patients.

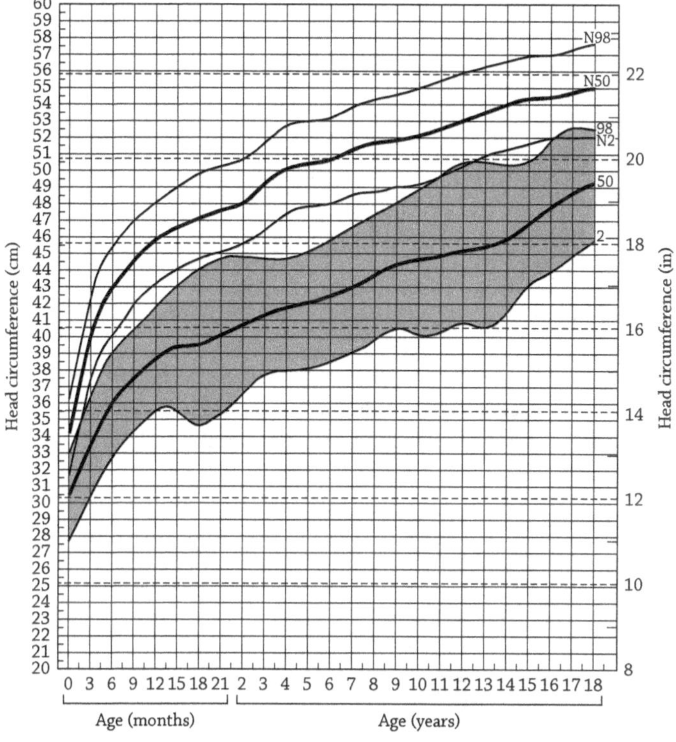

Figure 17.24 Cornelia de Lange syndrome, head circumference, females, birth to 18 years, compared with normal females (N). Adapted from Kline et al. (1993); all Cornelia de Lange syndrome graphs were derived from a total of 180 patients.

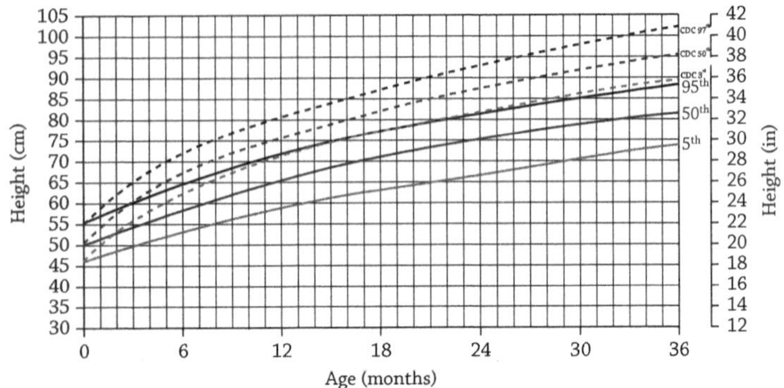

Figure 17.25 Costello syndrome (mutation in *HRAS*), height in males and females combined from birth to 36 months (solid lines), compared to typical male CDC 3rd, 50th, and 97th centiles (dashed lines). Adapted from Sammon et al. (2012).

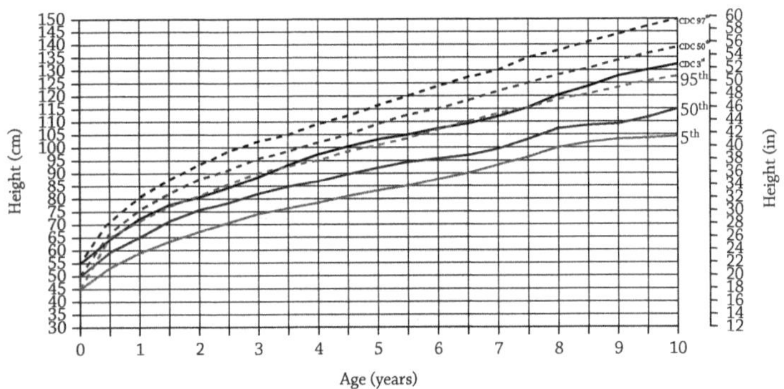

Figure 17.26 Costello syndrome (mutation in *HRAS*), height in males and females (solid lines) combined from birth to 10 years, compared to typical male CDC 3rd, 50th, and 97th centiles (dashed lines). Adapted from Sammon et al. (2012).

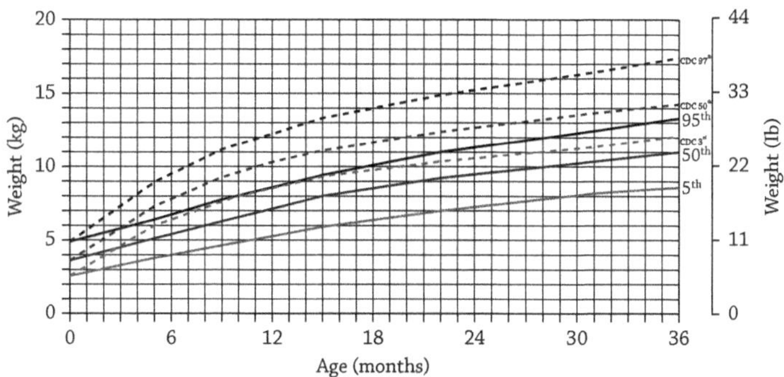

Figure 17.27 Costello syndrome (mutation in *HRAS*), weight in males and females combined from birth to 36 months (solid lines), compared to typical male CDC 3rd, 50th, and 97th centiles (dashed lines). Adapted from Sammon et al. (2012).

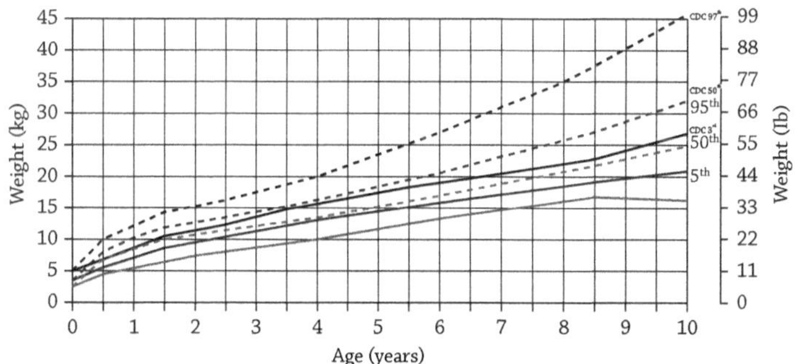

Figure 17.28 Costello syndrome (mutation in *HRAS*), weight in males and females combined from birth to 10 years (solid lines), compared to typical male CDC 3rd, 50th, and 97th centiles (dashed lines) Adapted from Sammon et al. (2012).

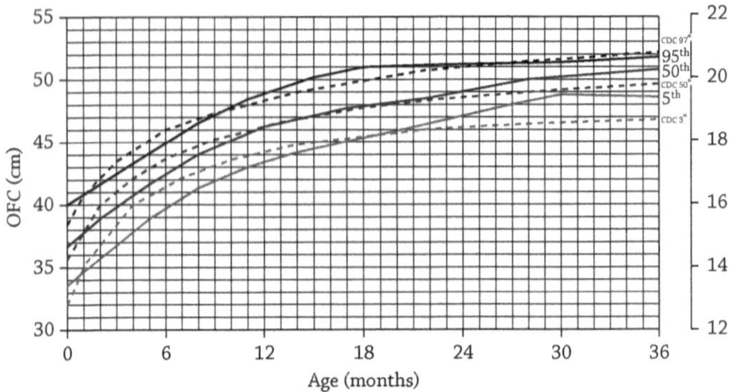

Figure 17.29 Costello syndrome (mutation in *HRAS*), head circumference in males and females combined from birth to 36 months (solid lines), compared to typical male CDC 3rd, 50th, and 97th centiles (dashed lines). Adapted from Sammon et al. (2012).

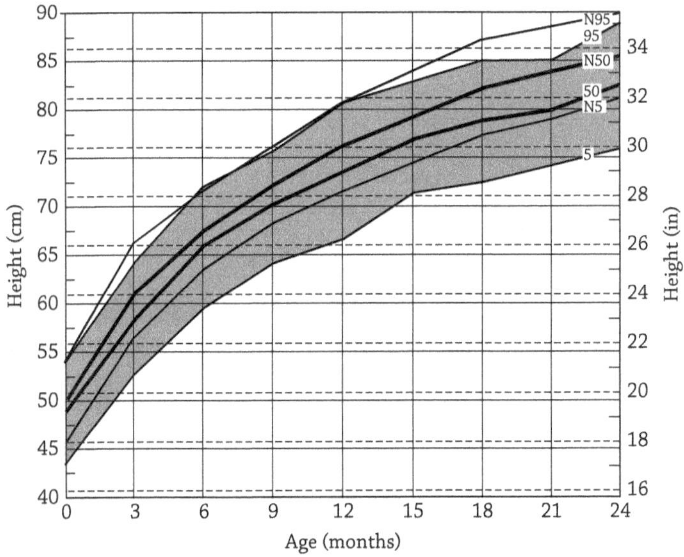

Figure 17.30 Cri-du-chat syndrome, height, males, birth to 2 years. Normal growth curves (N) are included. Adapted from Marinescu et al. (2000); all Cri-du-chat syndrome graphs were derived from a total of 374 patients.

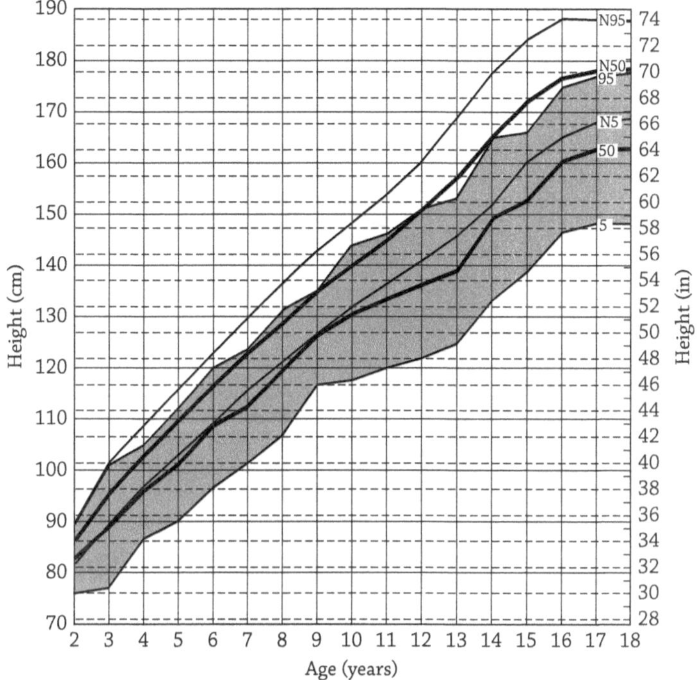

Figure 17.31 Cri-du-chat syndrome, height, males, 2 to 18 years. Normal growth curves (N) are included. Adapted from Marinescu et al. (2000); all Cri-du-chat syndrome graphs were derived from a total of 374 patients.

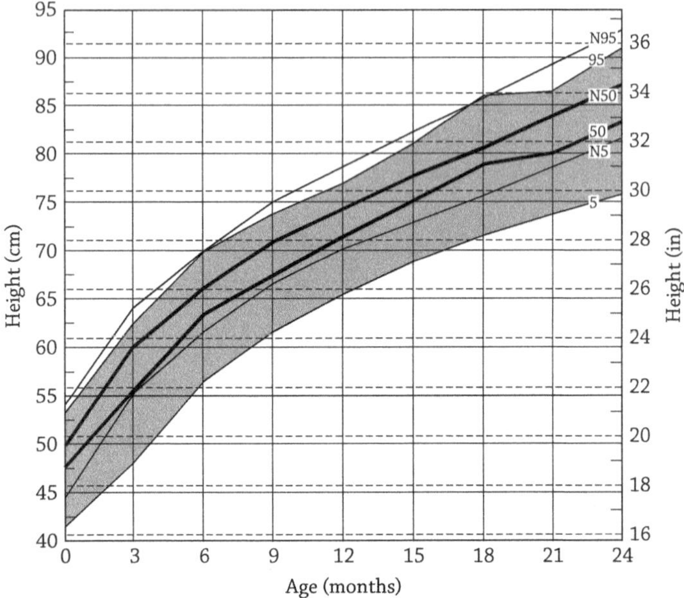

Figure 17.32 Cri-du-chat syndrome, height, females, birth to 2 years. Normal growth curves (N) are included. Adapted from Marinescu et al. (2000); all Cri-du-chat syndrome graphs were derived from a total of 374 patients.

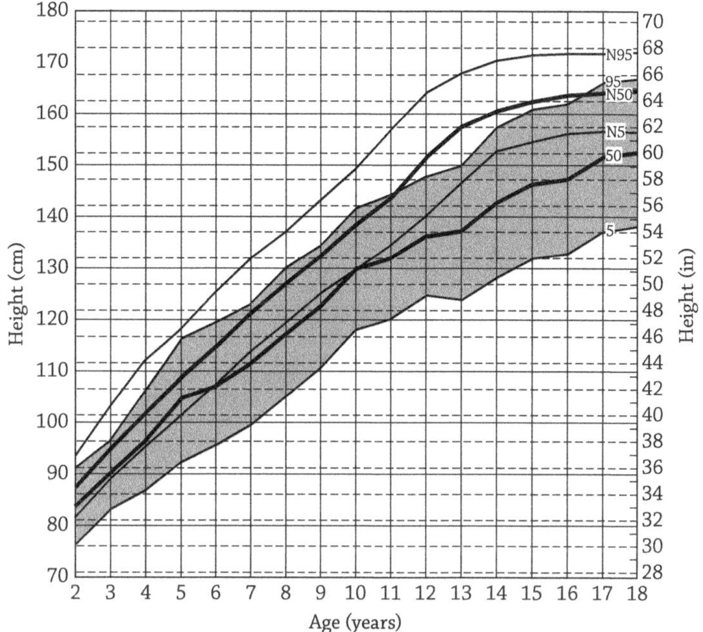

Figure 17.33 Cri-du-chat syndrome, height, females, 2 to 18 years. Normal growth curves (N) are included. Adapted from Marinescu et al. (2000); all Cri-du-chat syndrome graphs were derived from a total of 374 patients.

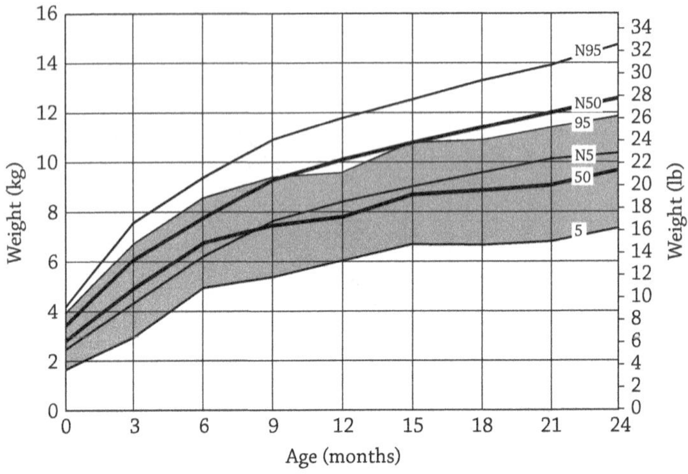

Figure 17.34 Cri-du-chat syndrome, weight, males, birth to 2 years. Normal growth curves (N) are included. Adapted from Marinescu et al. (2000); all Cri-du-chat syndrome graphs were derived from a total of 374 patients.

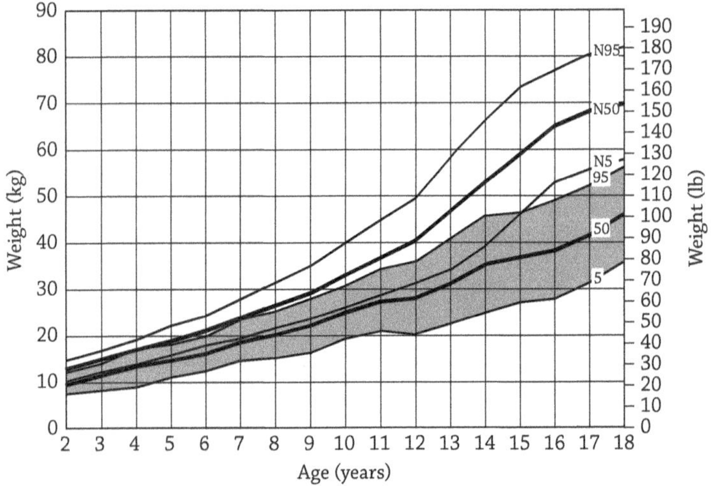

Figure 17.35 Cri-du-chat syndrome, weight, males, 2 to 18 years. Normal growth curves (N) are included. Adapted from Marinescu et al. (2000); all Cri-du-chat syndrome graphs were derived from a total of 374 patients.

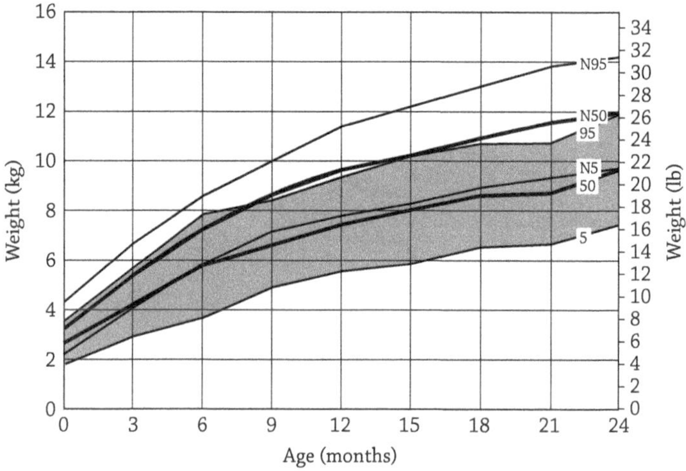

Figure 17.36 Cri-du-chat syndrome, weight, females, birth to 2 years. Normal growth curves (N) are included. Adapted from Marinescu et al. (2000); all Cri-du-chat syndrome graphs were derived from a total of 374 patients.

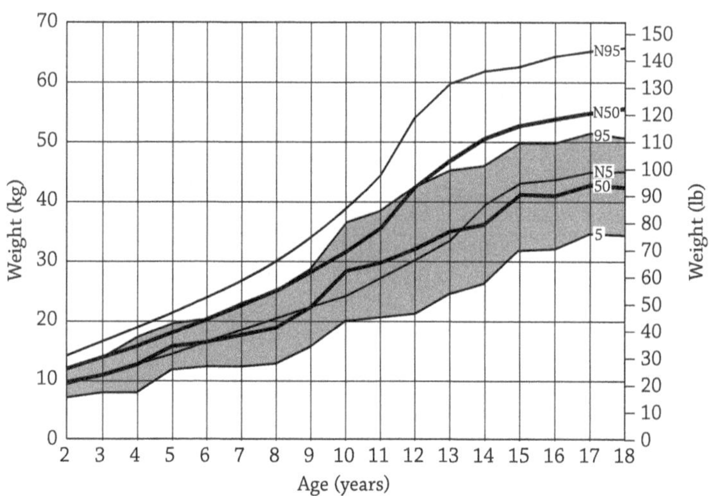

Figure 17.37 Cri-du-chat syndrome, weight, females, 2 to 18 years. Normal growth curves (N) are included. Adapted from Marinescu et al. (2000); all Cri-du-chat syndrome graphs were derived from a total of 374 patients.

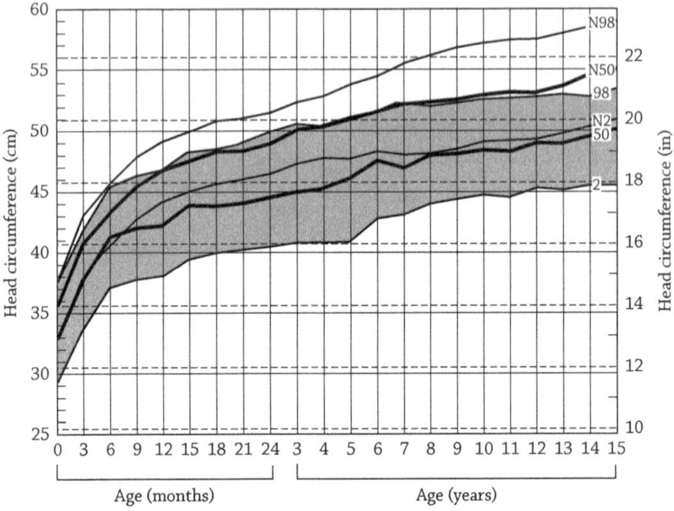

Figure 17.38 Cri-du-chat syndrome, head circumference, males, birth to 15 years. Normal growth curves (N) are included. Adapted from Marinescu et al. (2000); all Cri-du-chat syndrome graphs were derived from a total of 374 patients.

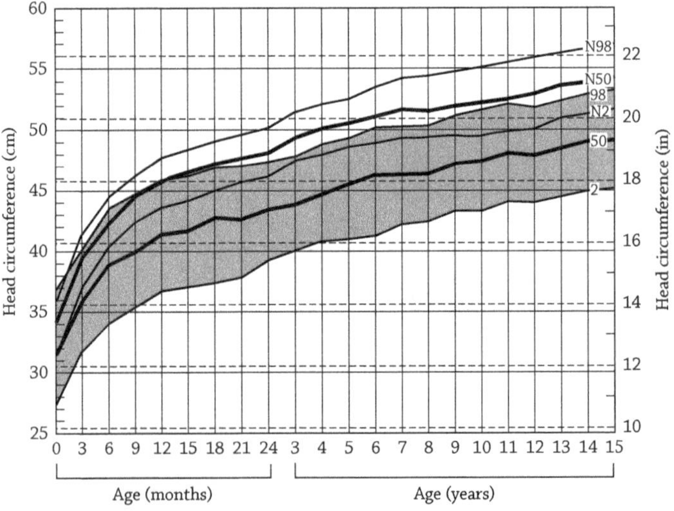

Figure 17.39 Cri-du-chat syndrome, head circumference, females, birth to 15 years. Normal growth curves (N) are included. Adapted from Marinescu et al. (2000); all Cri-du-chat syndrome graphs were derived from a total of 374 patients.

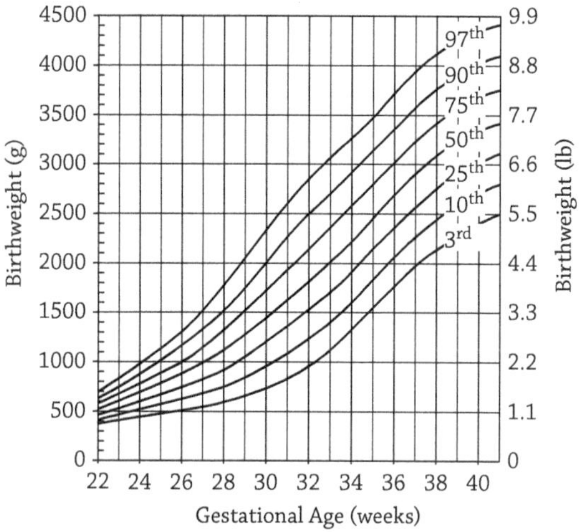

Figure 17.40 Down syndrome, birthweight by gestational age, for North American males. Adapted from Boghossian et al. (2012).

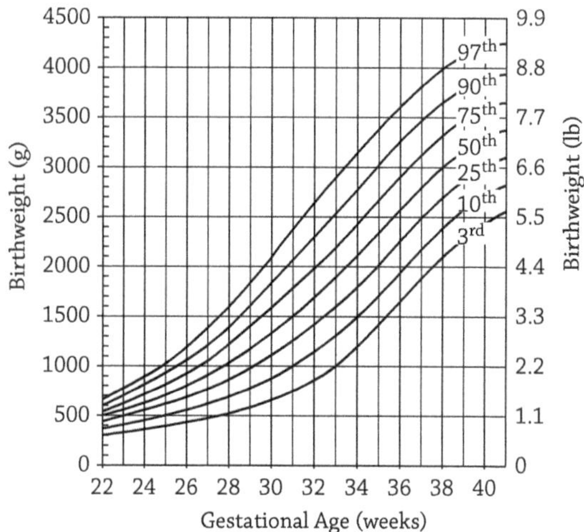

Figure 17.41 Down syndrome, birthweight by gestational age, for North American females. Adapted from Boghossian et al. (2012).

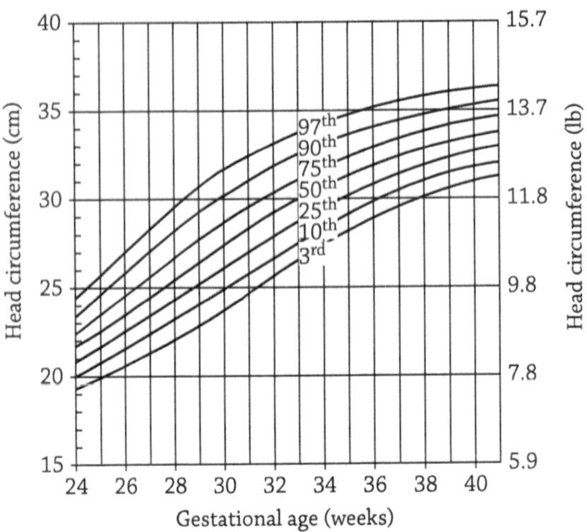

Figure 17.42 Down syndrome, head circumference by gestational age, for North American males. Adapted from Boghossian et al. (2012).

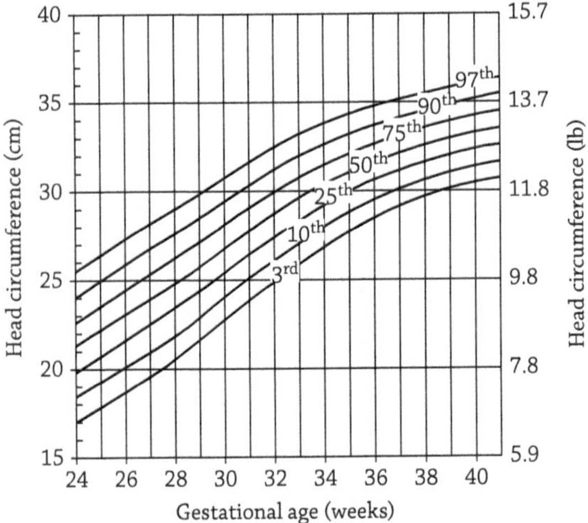

Figure 17.43 Down syndrome, head circumference by gestational age, for North American females. Adapted from Boghossian et al. (2012).

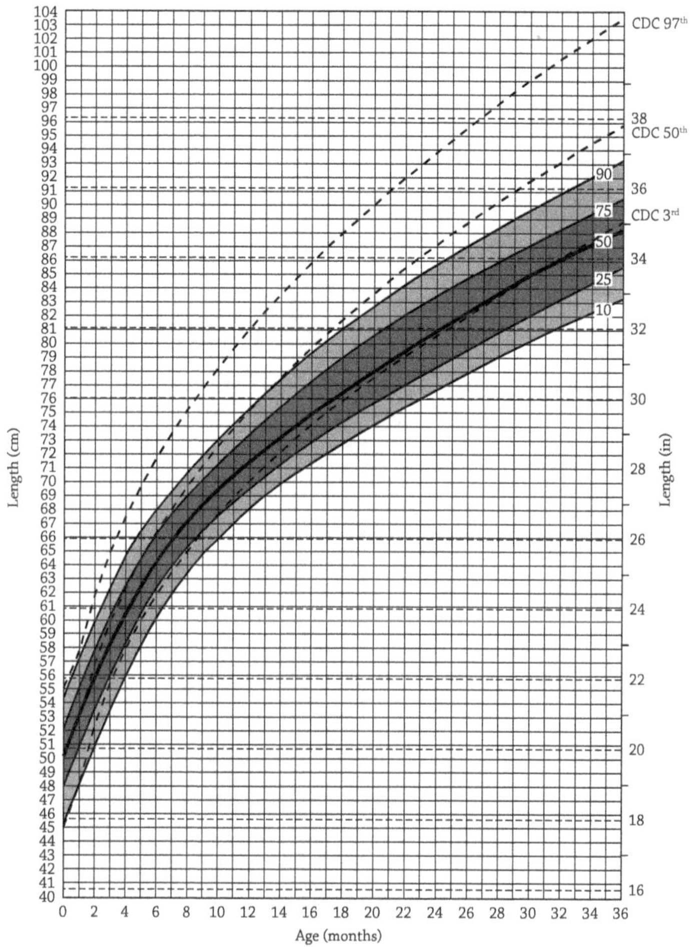

Figure 17.44 Down syndrome, length, North American males, birth to 3 years. CDC 3rd, 50th, and 97th centile curves are provided. Adapted from Cronk et al. (1988) and http://www.growthcharts.com/

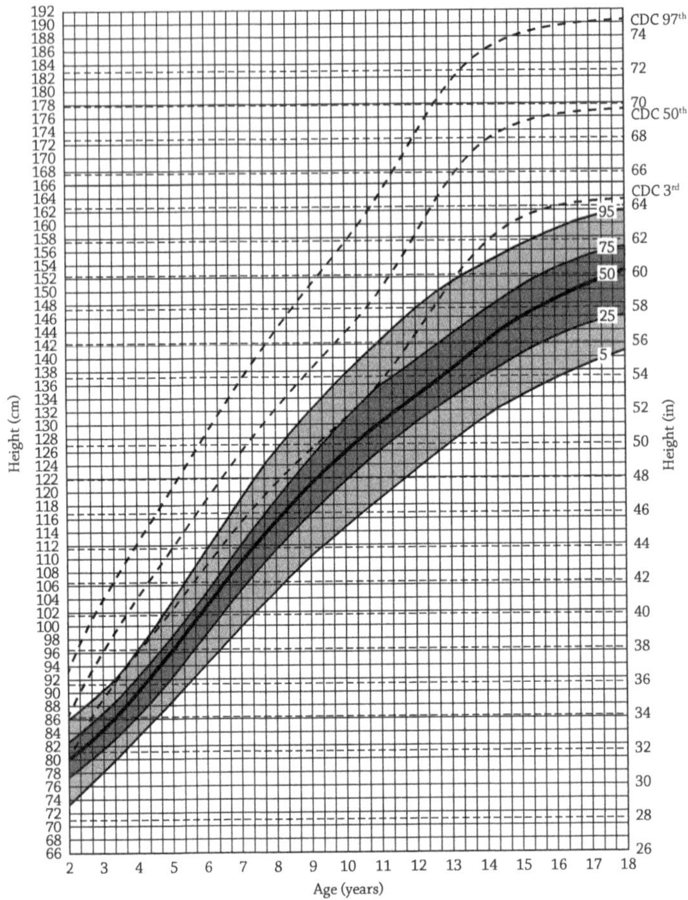

Figure 17.45 Down syndrome, height, North American males, 2 to 18 years. Adapted from Cronk et al. (1988) and http://www.growthcharts.com/. CDC 3rd, 50th, and 97th centile curves are provided.

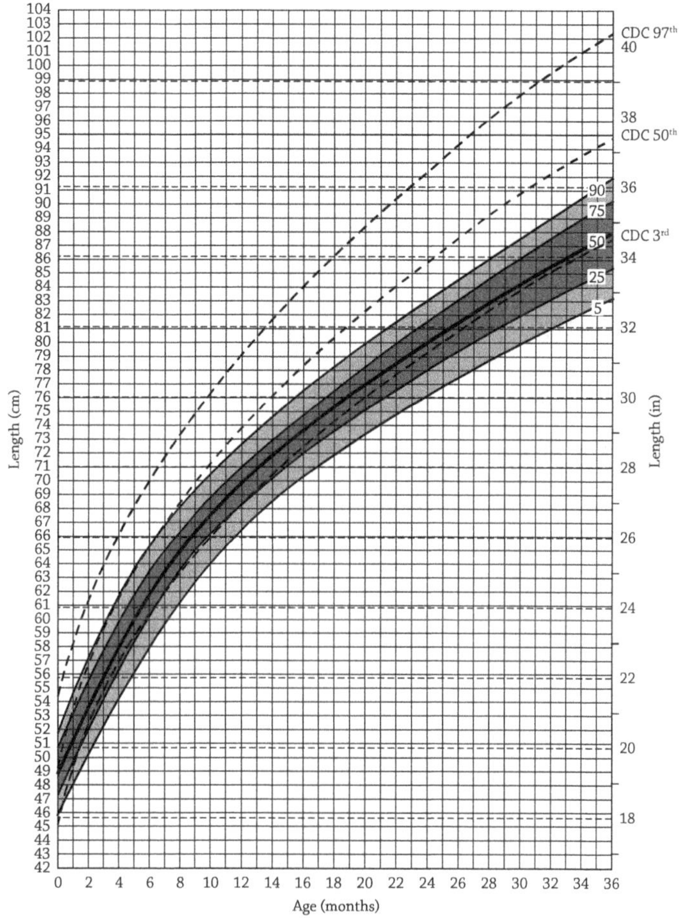

Figure 17.46 Down syndrome, length, North American females, birth to 3 years. Adapted from Cronk et al. (1988) and http://www.growthcharts.com/. CDC 3rd, 50th, and 97th centile curves are provided.

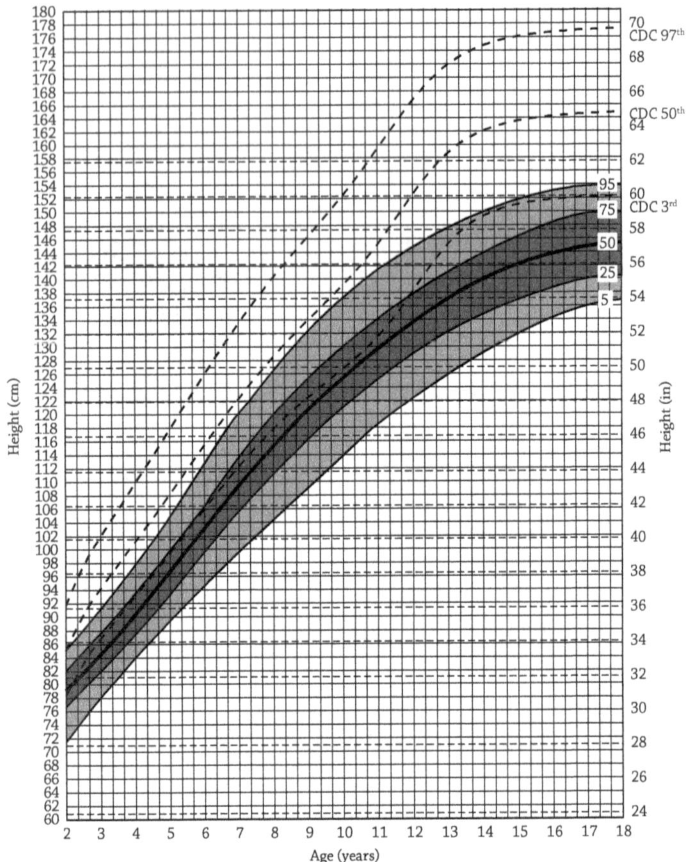

Figure 17.47 Down syndrome, height, North American females, 2 to 18 years. Adapted from Cronk et al. (1988) and http://www.growthcharts.com/. CDC 3rd, 50th, and 97th centile curves are provided.

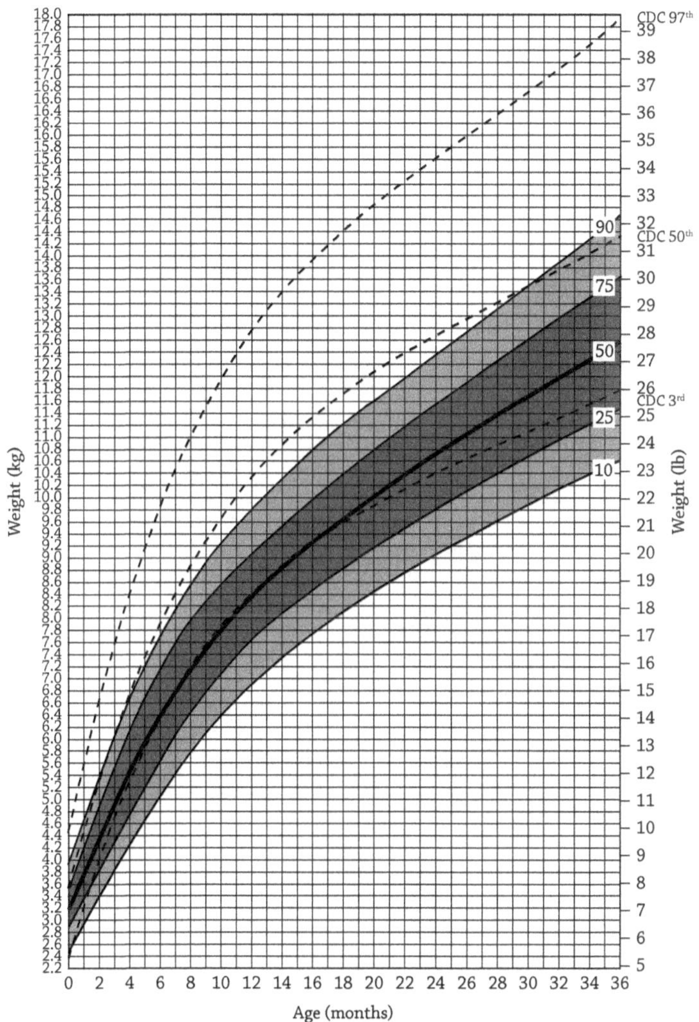

Figure 17.48 Down syndrome, weight, North American males, birth to 3 years. Adapted from Cronk et al. (1988) and http://www.growthcharts.com. CDC 3rd, 50th, and 97th centile curves are provided.

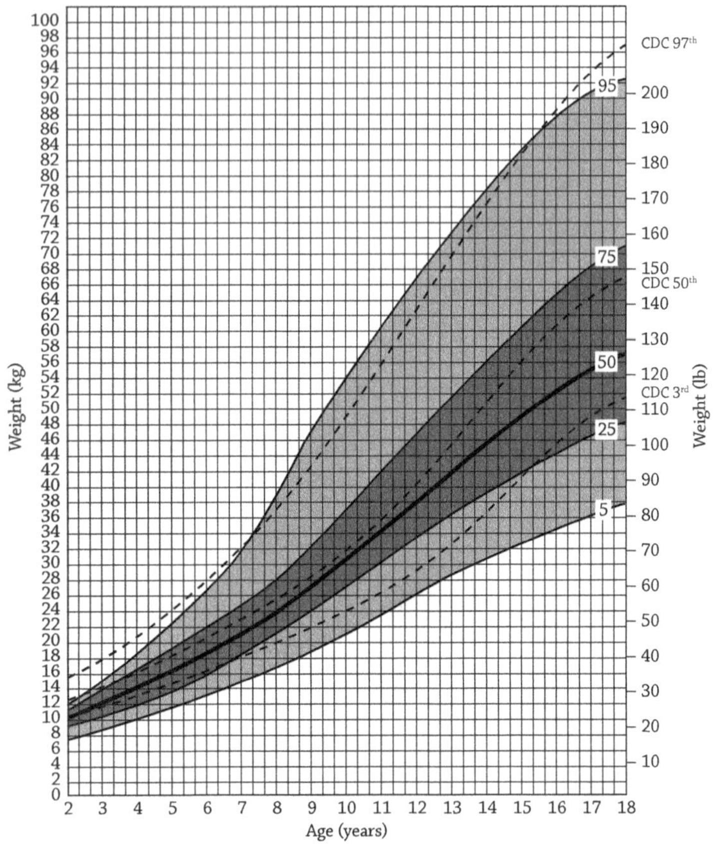

Figure 17.49 Down syndrome, weight, North American males, 2 to 18 years. Adapted from Cronk et al. (1988) and http://www.growthcharts.com/. CDC 3rd, 50th, and 97th centile curves are provided.

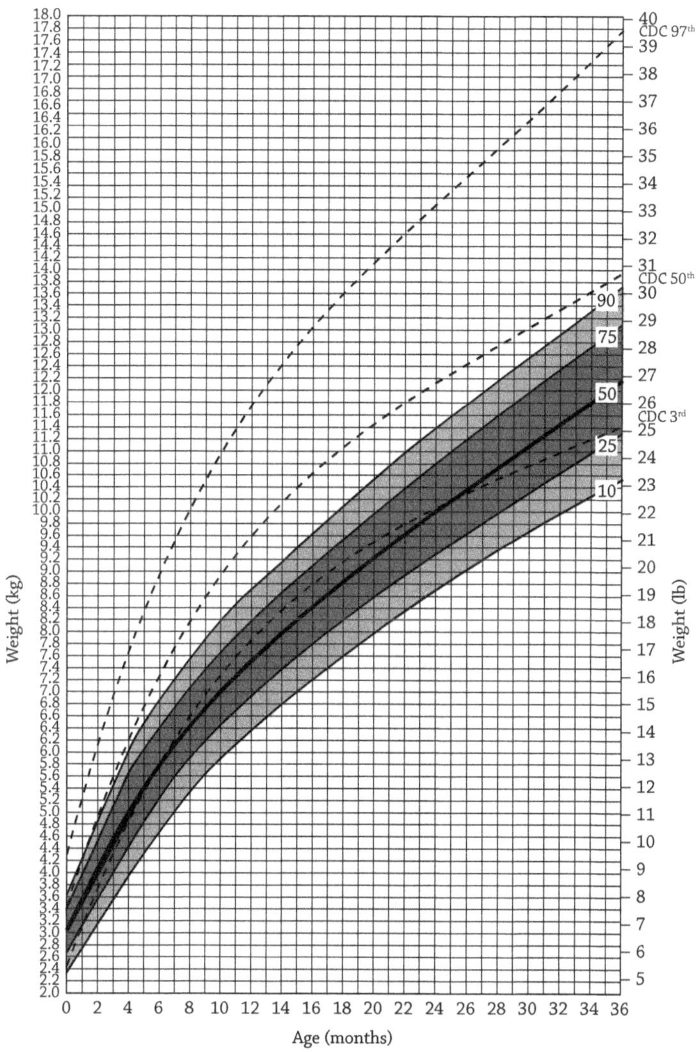

Figure 17.50 Down syndrome, weight, North American females, birth to 3 years. Adapted from Cronk et al. (1988) and http://www.growthcharts.com/. CDC 3rd, 50th, and 97th centile curves are provided.

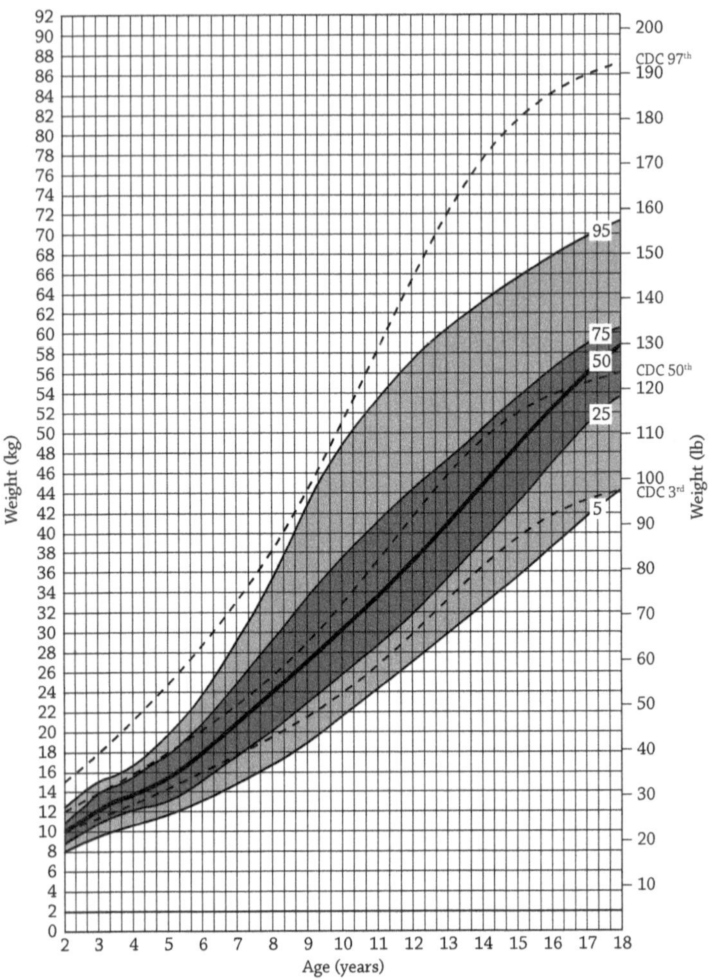

Figure 17.51 Down syndrome, weight, North American females, 2 to 18 years. Adapted from Cronk et al. (1988) and http://www.growthcharts.com/. CDC 3rd, 50th, and 97th centile curves are provided.

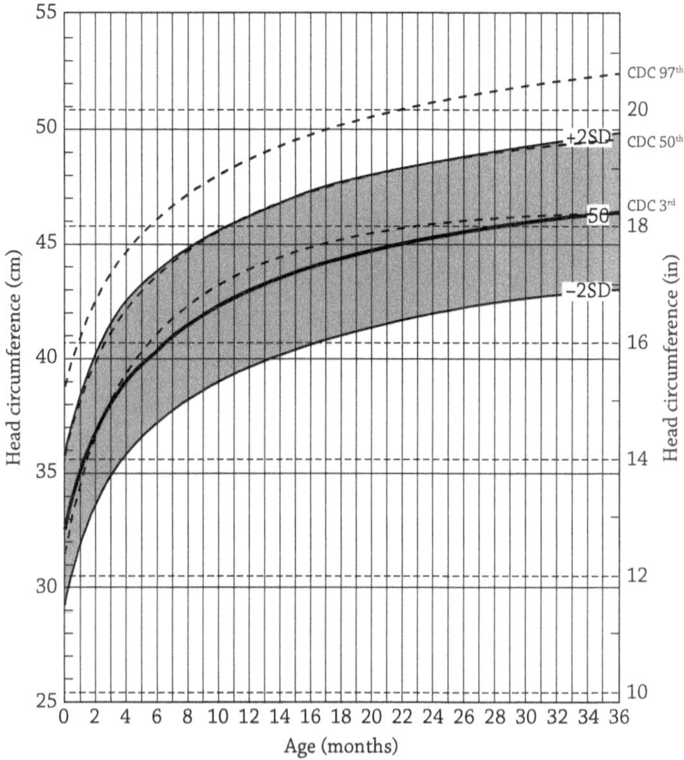

Figure 17.52 Down syndrome, head circumference, North American males, birth to 3 years. Adapted from Palmer et al. (1992) and http://www.growthcharts.com/. CDC 3rd, 50th, and 97th centile curves are provided.

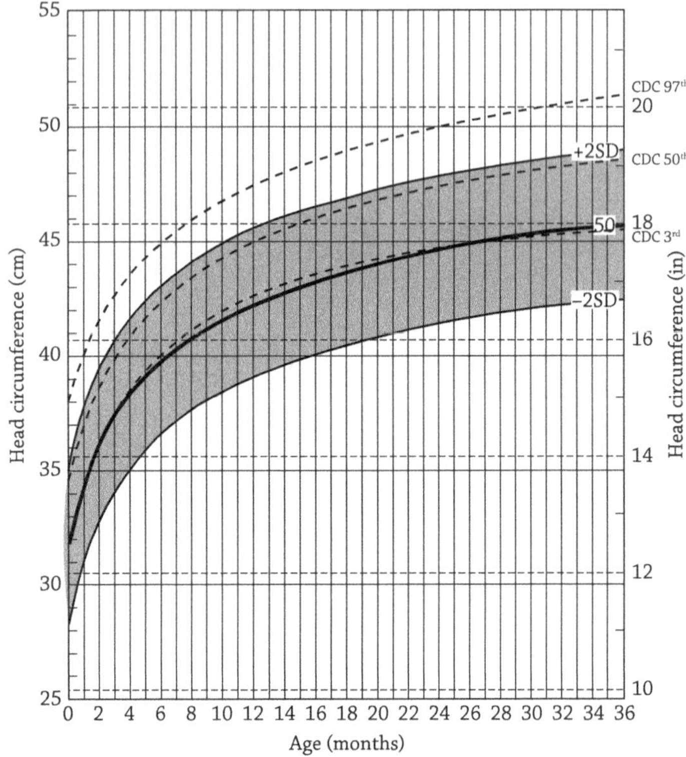

Figure 17.53 Down syndrome, head circumference, North American females, birth to 3 years. Adapted from Palmer et al. (1992) and http://www.growthcharts.com/. CDC 3rd, 50th, and 97th centile curves are provided.

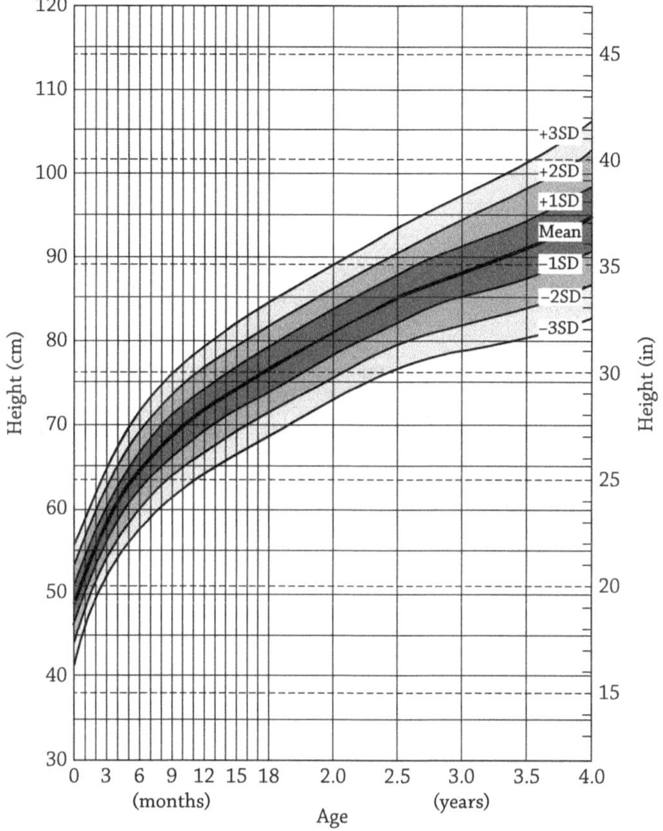

Figure 17.54 Down syndrome, height, North European males, birth to 4 years. Adapted from Myrelid et al. (2000).

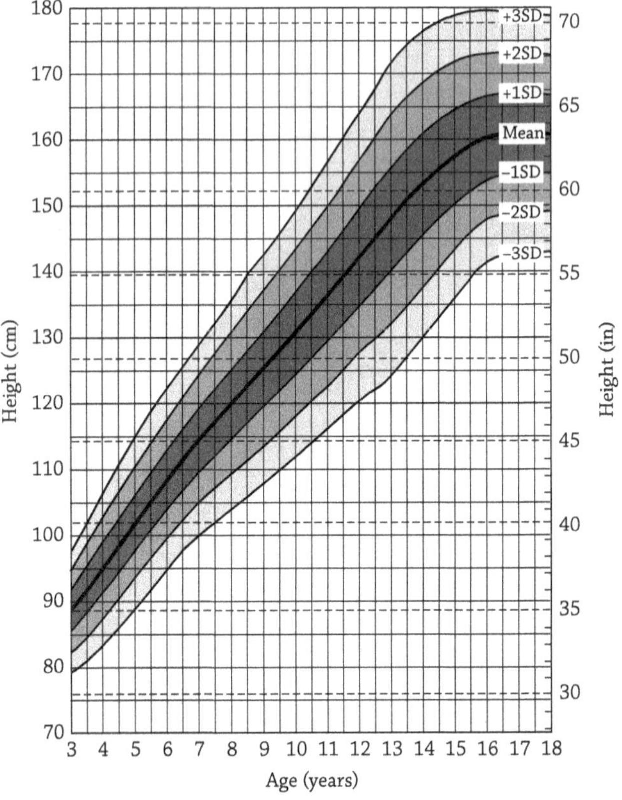

Figure 17.55 Down syndrome, height, North European males, 3 to 18 years. Adapted from Myrelid et al. (2002).

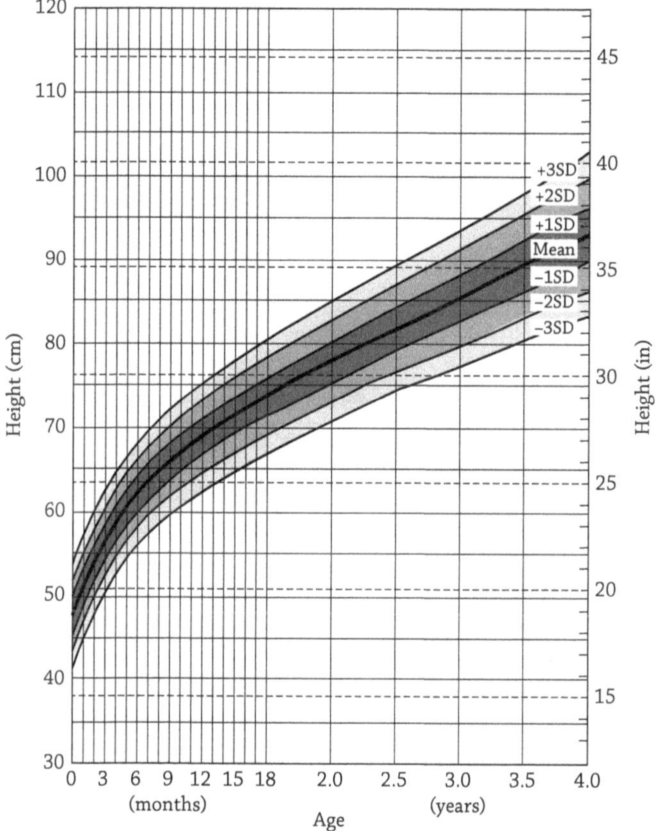

Figure 17.56 Down syndrome, height, North European females, birth to 4 years. Adapted from Myrelid et al. (2002).

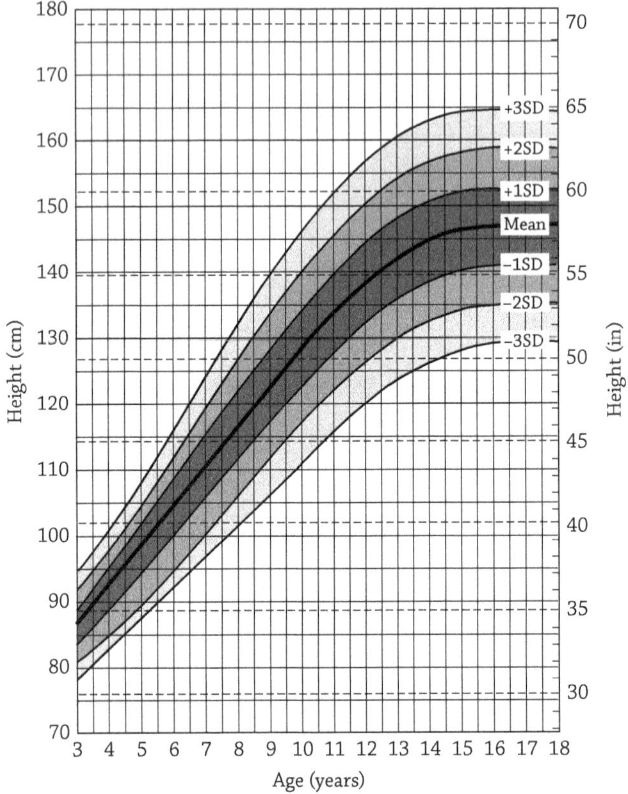

Figure 17.57 Down syndrome, height, North European females, 3 to 18 years. Adapted from Myrelid et al. (2002).

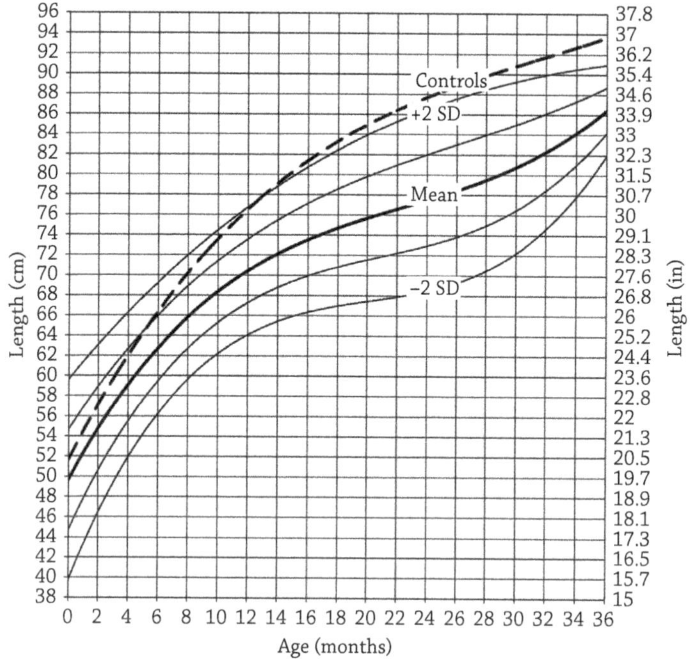

Figure 17.58 Down syndrome, length, Egyptian males, birth to 3 years. Dotted line represents 50th centile for typical Egyptian controls. Adapted from Afifi et al. (2012).

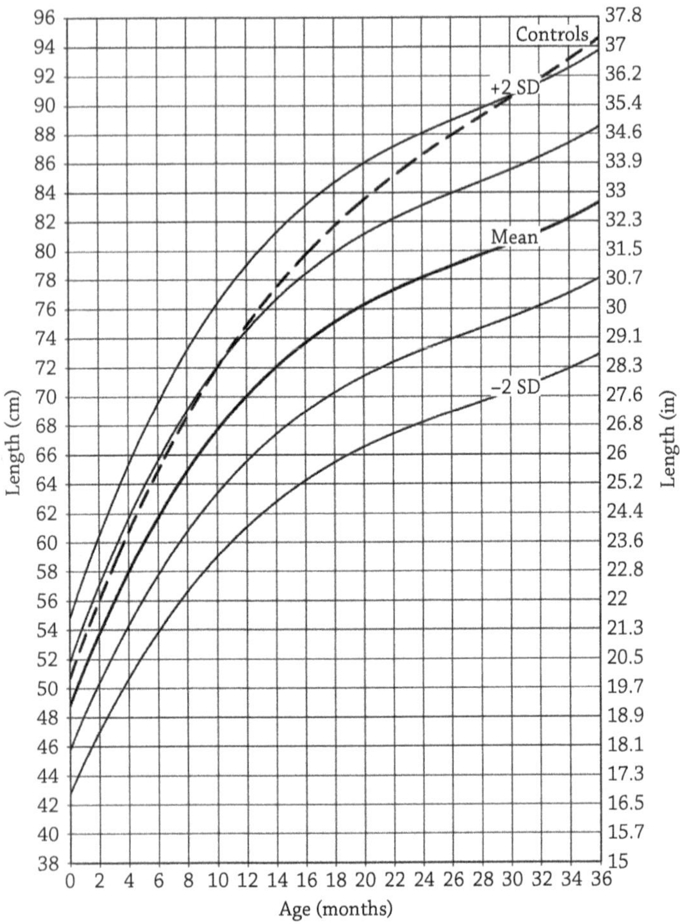

Figure 17.59 Down syndrome, length, Egyptian females, birth to 3 years. Dotted line represents 50th centile for typical Egyptian controls. Adapted from Afifi et al. (2012).

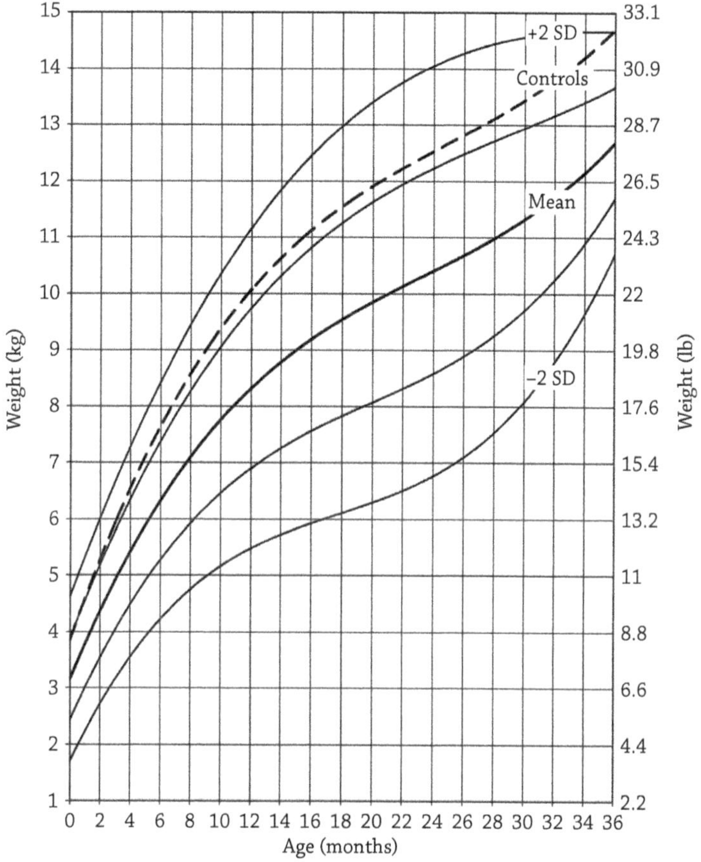

Figure 17.60 Down syndrome, weight, Egyptian males, birth to 3 years. Dotted line represents 50th centile for typical Egyptian controls. Adapted from Afifi et al. (2012).

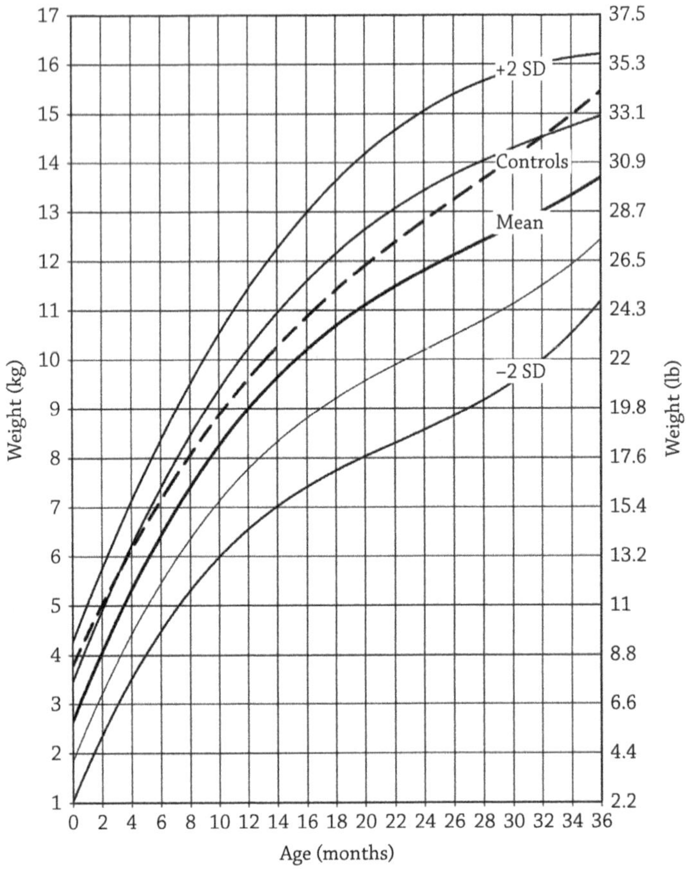

Figure 17.61 Down syndrome, weight, Egyptian females, birth to 3 years. Dotted line represents 50th centile for typical Egyptian controls. Adapted from Afifi et al. (2012).

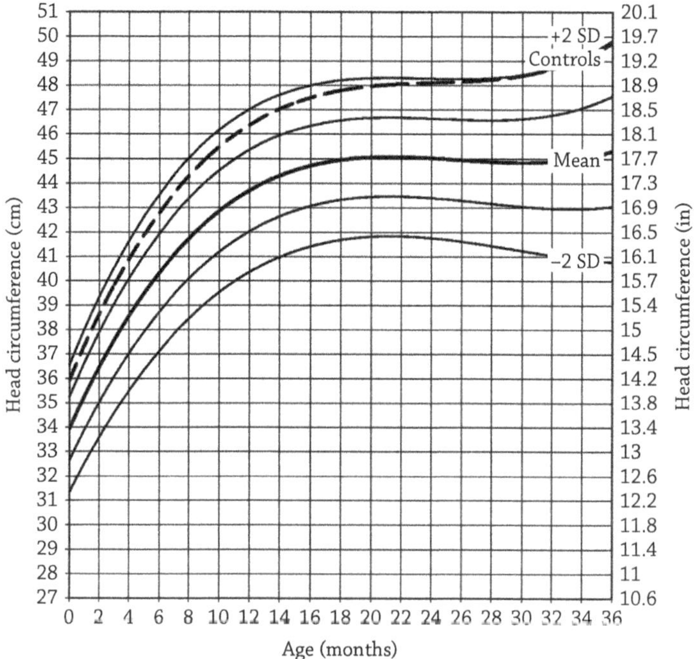

Figure 17.62 Down syndrome, head circumference, Egyptian males, birth to 3 years. Dotted line represents 50th centile for typical Egyptian controls. Adapted from Afifi et al. (2012).

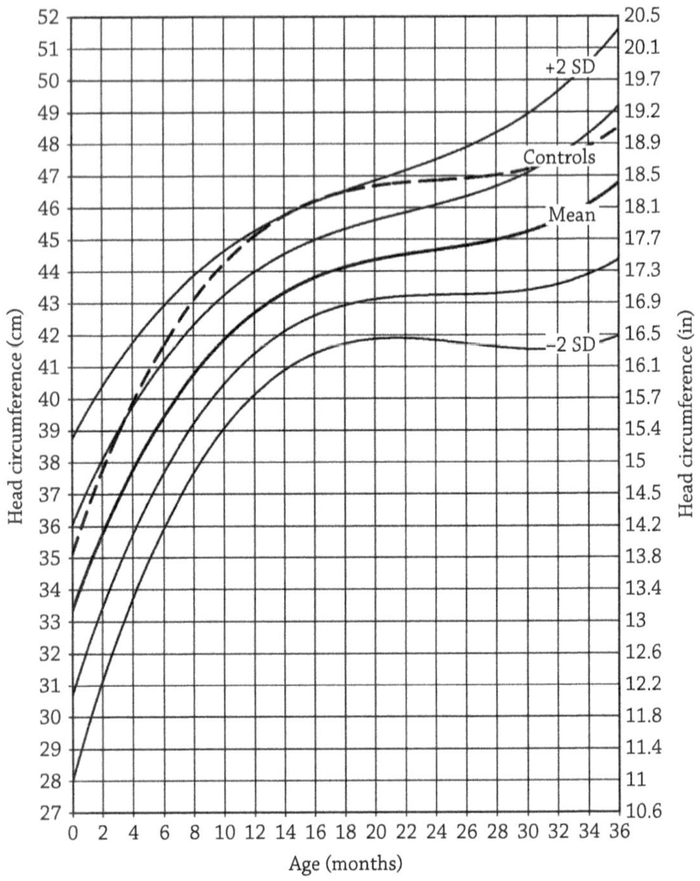

Figure 17.63 Down syndrome, head circumference, Egyptian females, birth to 3 years. Dotted line represents 50th centile for typical Egyptian controls. Adapted from Afifi et al. (2012).

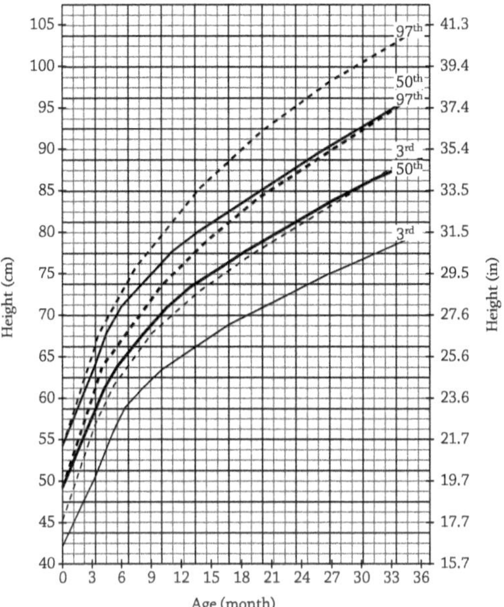

Figure 17.64 Down syndrome, length/height, Turkish males, birth to 3 years. Dotted lines represent 3rd, 50th, and 97th centiles for typical Turkish controls. Adapted from Tüysüz et al. (2012).

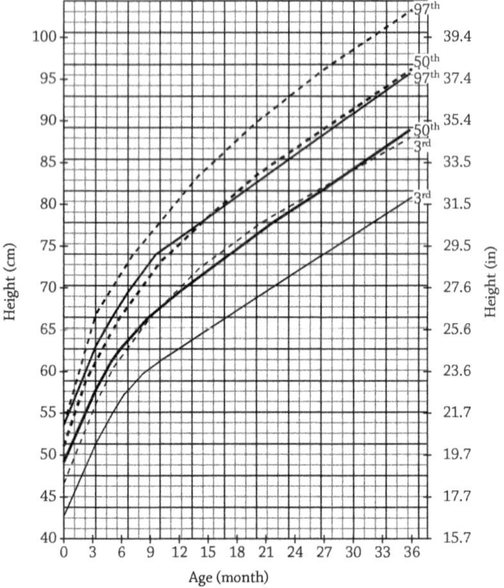

Figure 17.65 Down syndrome, length/height, Turkish females, birth to 3 years. Dotted lines represent 3rd, 50th, and 97th centiles for typical Turkish controls. Adapted from Tüysüz et al. (2012).

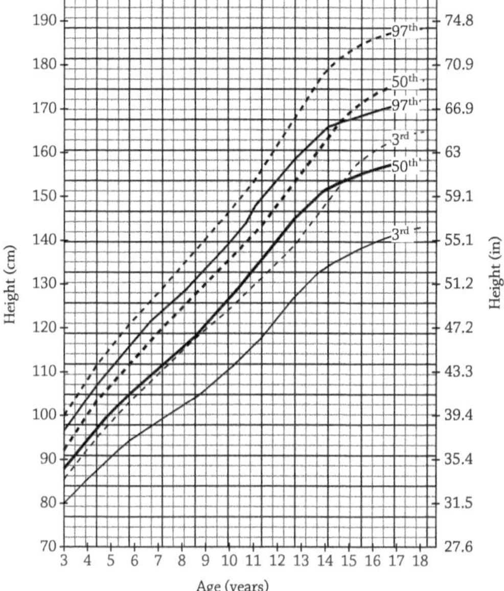

Figure 17.66 Down syndrome, height, Turkish males, from 3 to 18 years. Dotted lines represent 3rd, 50th, and 97th centiles for typical Turkish controls. Adapted from Tüysüz et al. (2012).

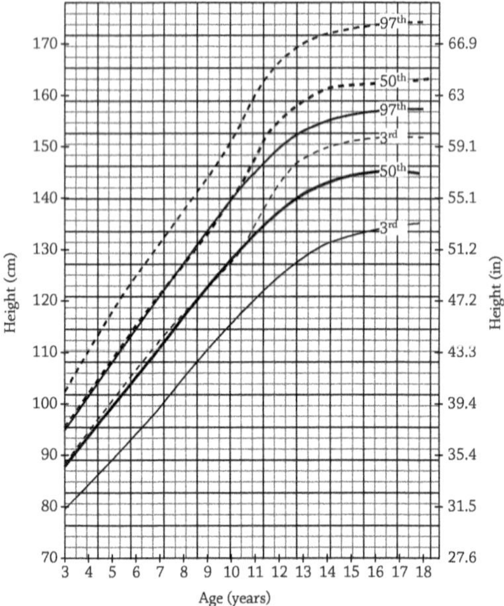

Figure 17.67 Down syndrome, height, Turkish females, from 3 to 18 years. Dotted lines represent 3rd, 50th, and 97th centiles for typical Turkish controls. Adapted from Tüysüz et al. (2012).

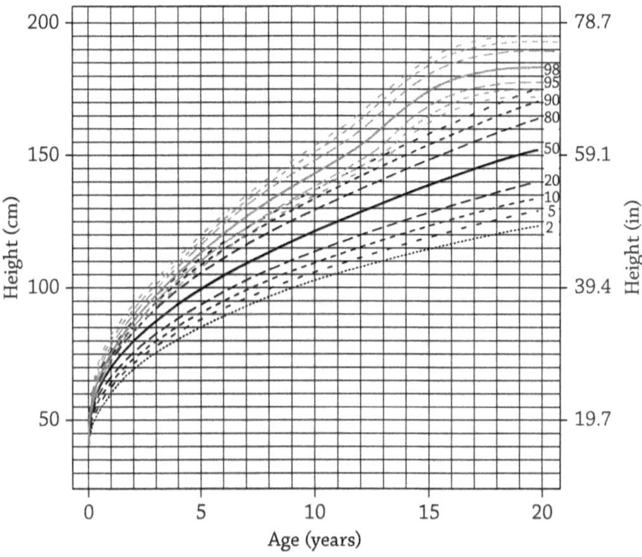

Figure 17.68 Ellis-van Creveld syndrome, height, Dutch males. Adapted from Verbeek et al. (2011).

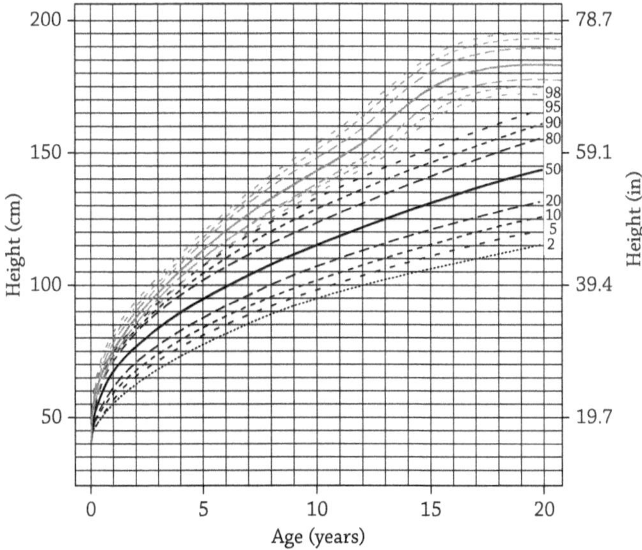

Figure 17.69 Ellis-van Creveld syndrome, height, Dutch females. Adapted from Verbeek et al. (2011).

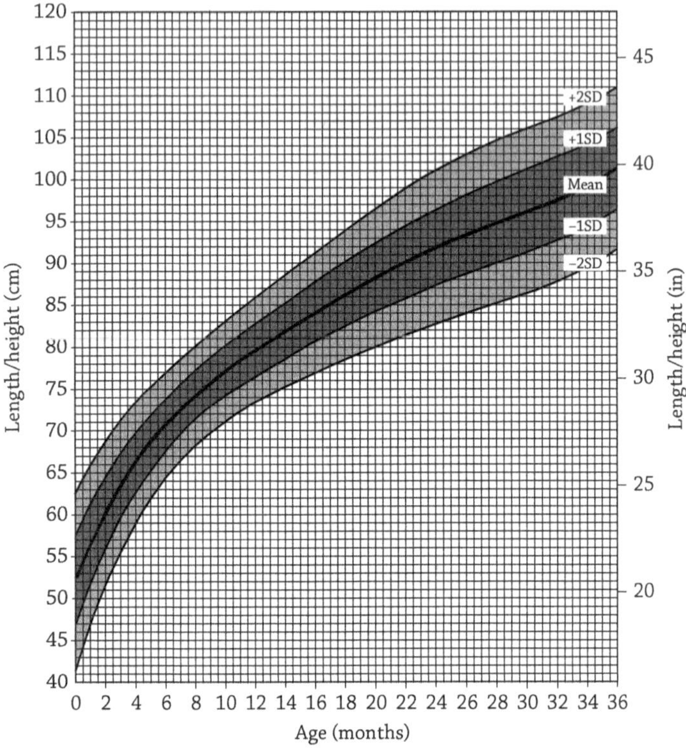

Figure 17.70 Marfan syndrome, length/height, males, birth to 3 years. Adapted from Erkula et al. (2002).

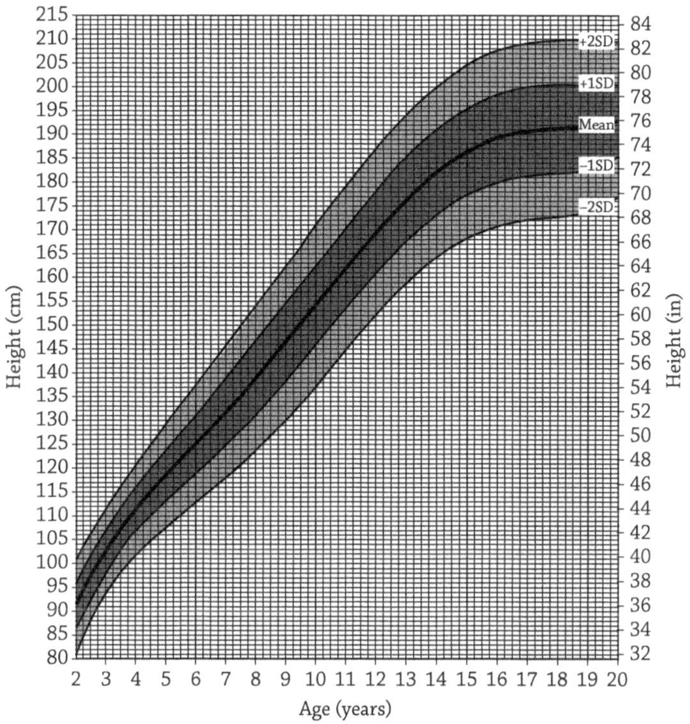

Figure 17.71 Marfan syndrome, height, males, 2 to 20 years. Adapted from Erkula et al. (2002).

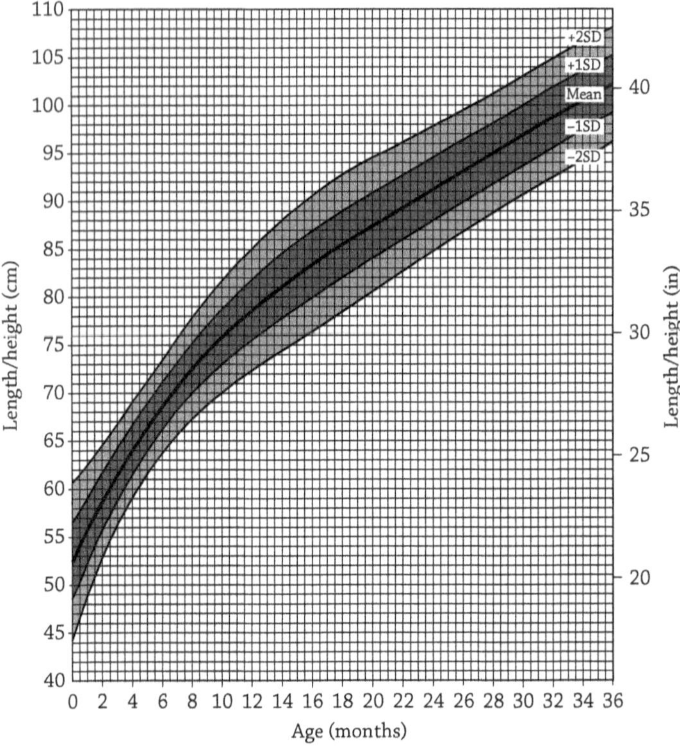

Figure 17.72 Marfan syndrome, length/height, females, birth to 3 years. Adapted from Erkula et al. (2002).

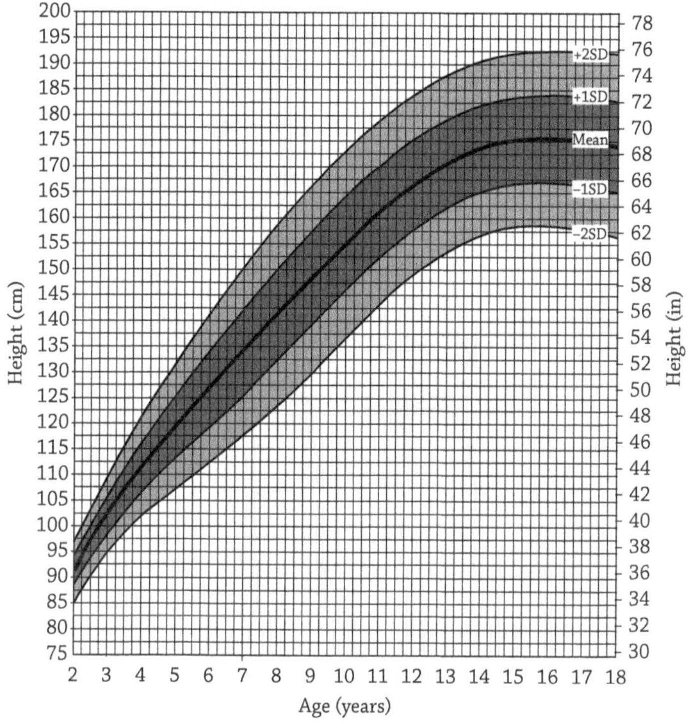

Figure 17.73 Marfan syndrome, height, females, 2 to 20 years. Adapted from Erkula et al. (2002).

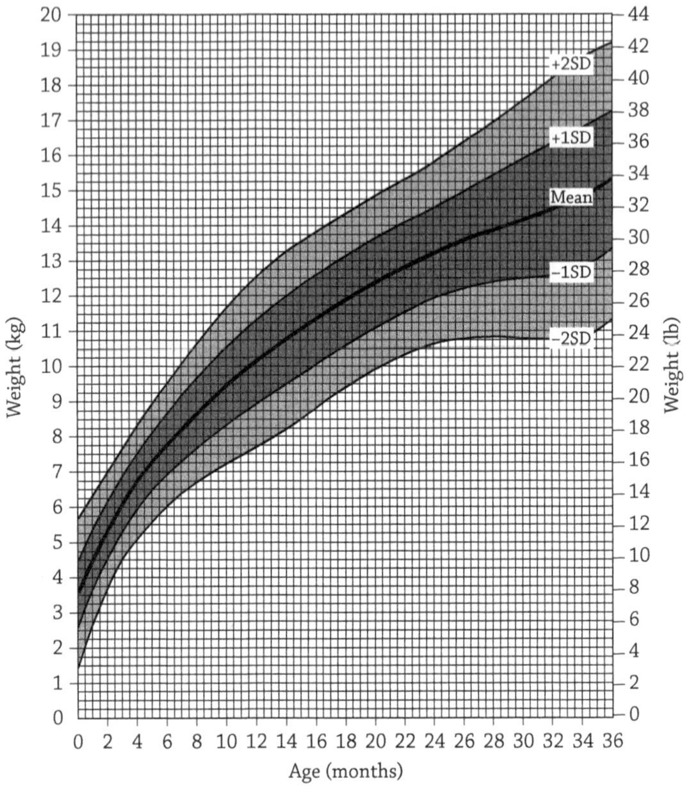

Figure 17.74 Marfan syndrome, weight, males, birth to 3 years. Adapted from Erkula et al. (2002).

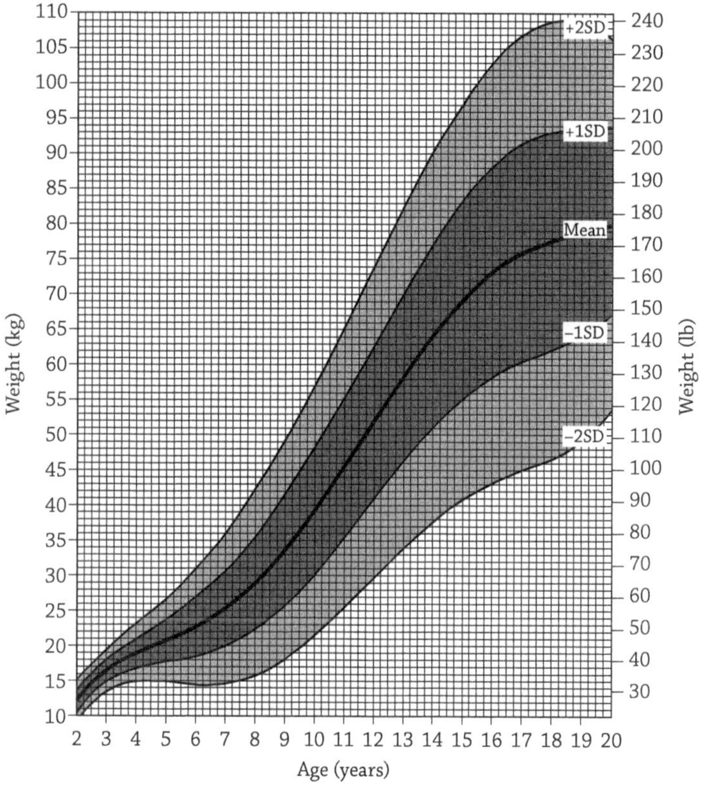

Figure 17.75 Marfan syndrome, weight, males, 2 to 20 years. Adapted from Erkula et al. (2002).

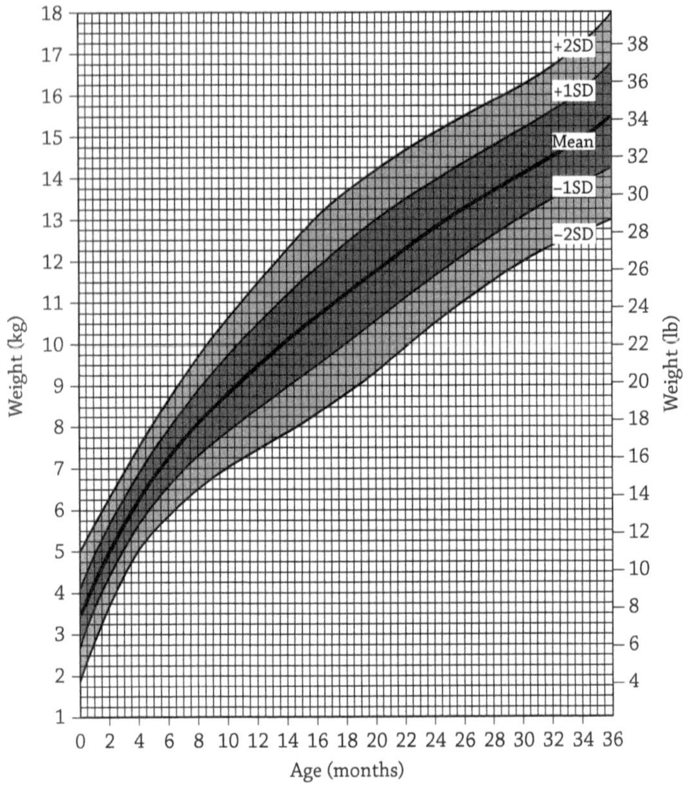

Figure 17.76 Marfan syndrome, weight, females, birth to 3 years. Adapted from Erkula et al. (2002).

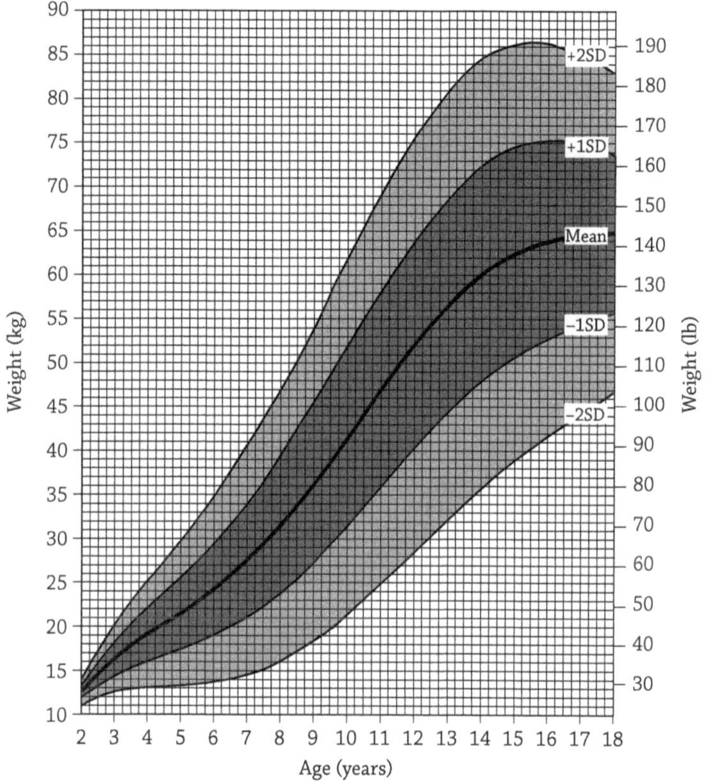

Figure 17.77 Marfan syndrome, weight, females, 2 to 20 years. Adapted from Erkula et al. (2002).

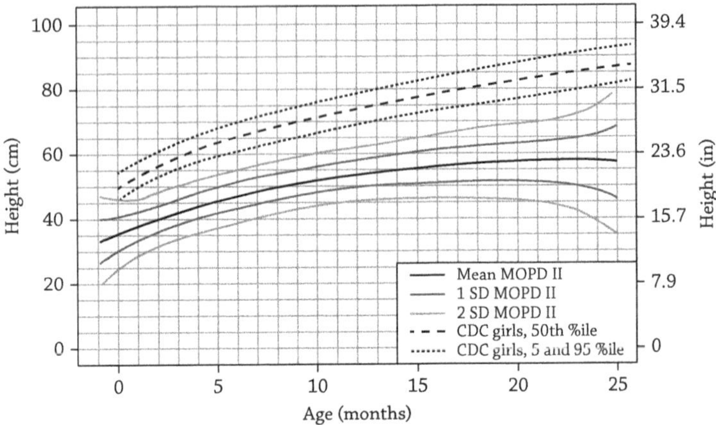

Figure 17.78 Majewski osteodysplastic primordial dwarfism (MOPD) II (Pericentrin mutation positive), length/height in males and females combined, from birth to 2 years. Adapted from Bober et al. (2012).

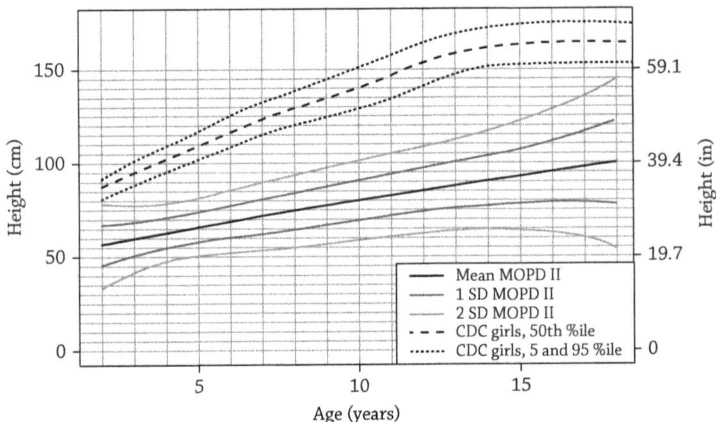

Figure 17.79 Majewski osteodysplastic primordial dwarfism (MOPD) II (Pericentrin mutation positive), length/height in males and females combined, from birth to 18 years. Adapted from Bober et al. (2012).

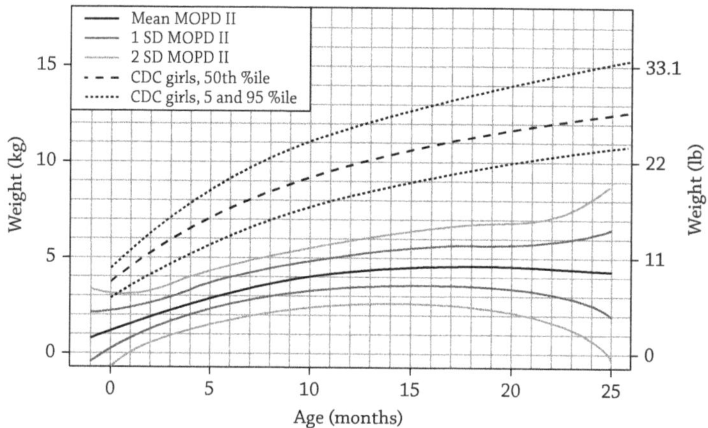

Figure 17.80 Majewski osteodysplastic primordial dwarfism (MOPD) II (Pericentrin mutation positive), weight in males and females combined, from birth to 2 years. Adapted from Bober et al. (2012).

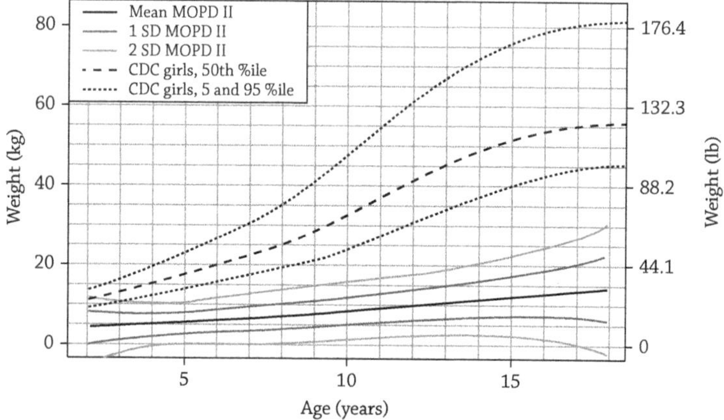

Figure 17.81 Majewski osteodysplastic primordial dwarfism (MOPD) II (Pericentrin mutation positive), weight in males and females combined, from birth to 18 years. Adapted from Bober et al. (2012).

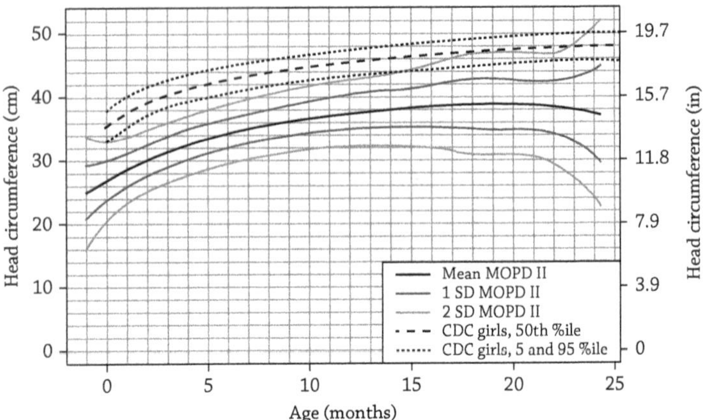

Figure 17.82 Majewski osteodysplastic primordial dwarfism (MOPD) II (Pericentrin mutation positive), head circumference in males and females combined, from birth to 2 years. Adapted from Bober et al. (2012).

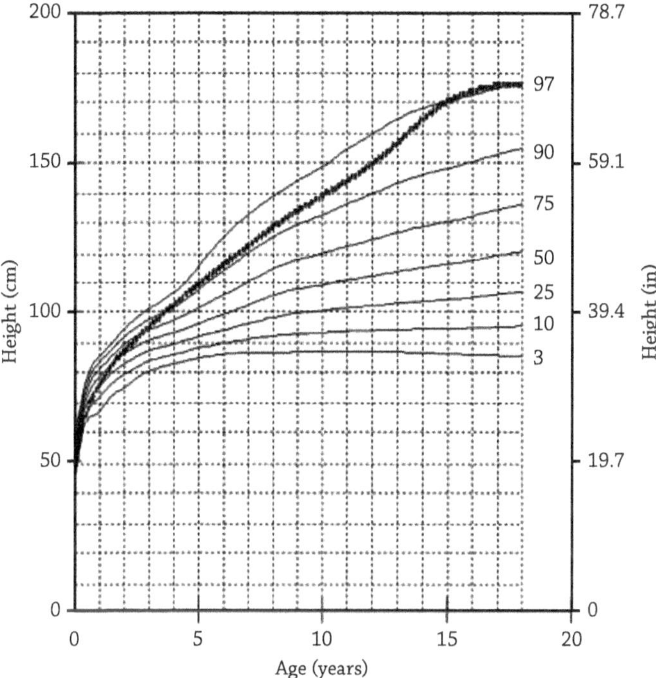

Figure 17.83 Morquio A syndrome, length/height in males, 0 to 18 years. The dotted line shows the 50th centile values for normal males. Adapted from Montaño et al. (2008).

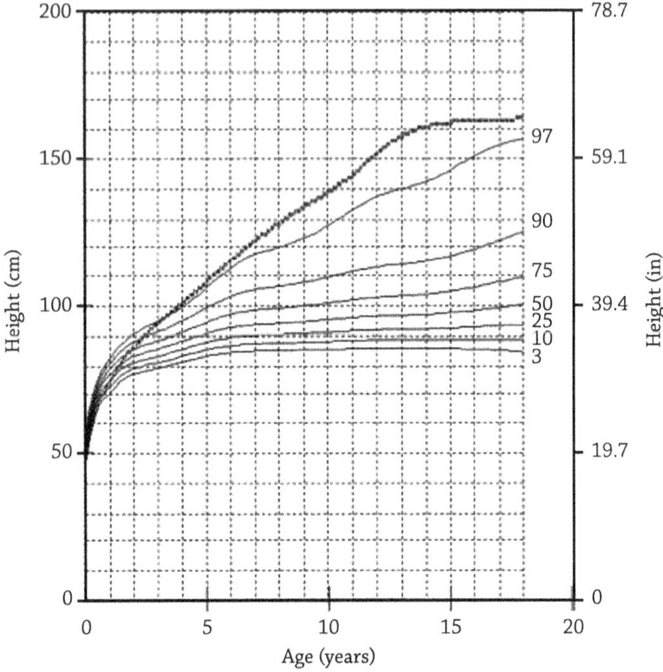

Figure 17.84 Morquio A syndrome, length/height in females, 0 to 18 years. The dotted line shows the 50th centile values for normal females. Adapted from Montaño et al. (2008).

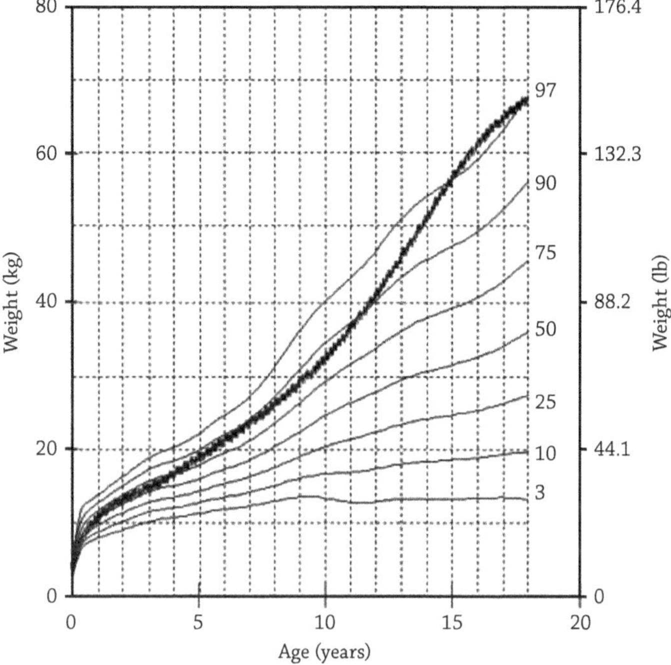

Figure 17.85 Morquio A syndrome, weight in males, 0 to 18 years. The dotted line shows the 50th centile values for normal males. Adapted from Montaño et al. (2008).

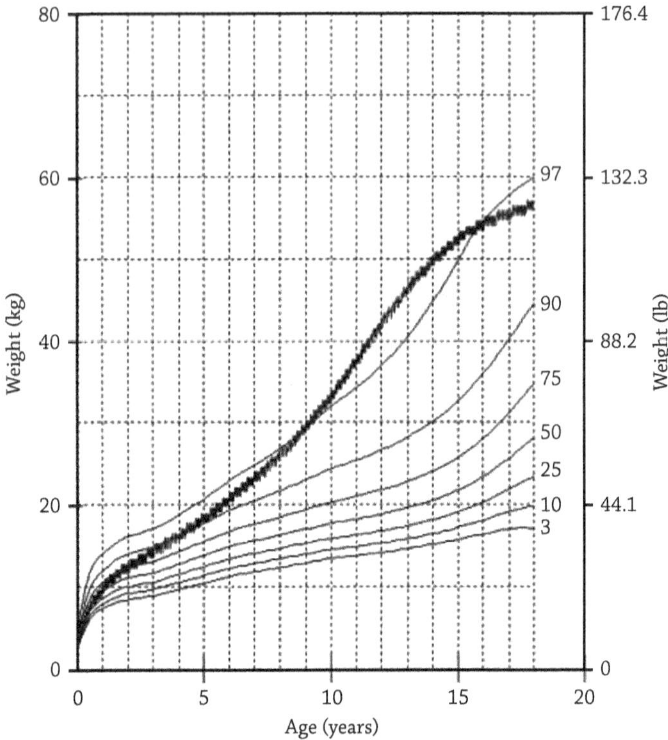

Figure 17.86 Morquio A syndrome, weight in females, 0 to 18 years. The dotted line shows the 50th centile values for normal females. Adapted from Montaño et al. (2008).

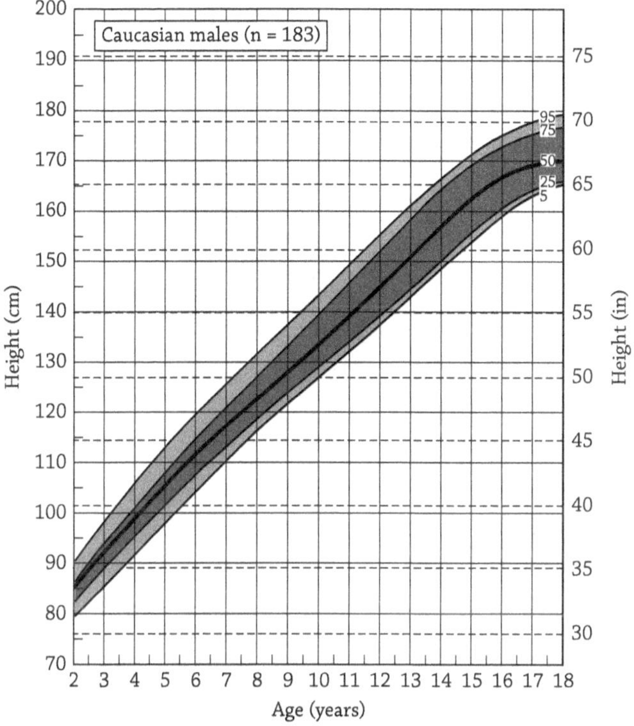

Figure 17.87 Neurofibromatosis, type I, height, North American males, 2 to 18 years. Adapted from Szudek et al. (2000).

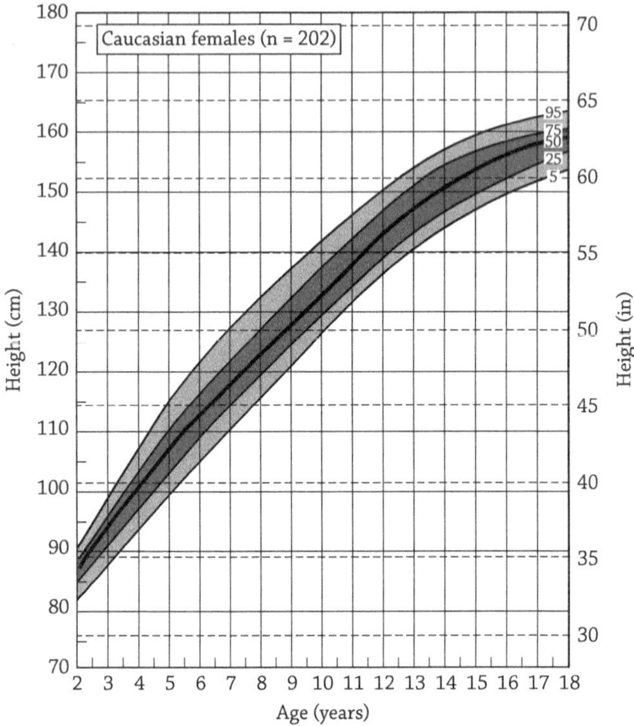

Figure 17.88 Neurofibromatosis, type I, height, North American females, 2 to 18 years. Adapted from Szudek et al. (2000).

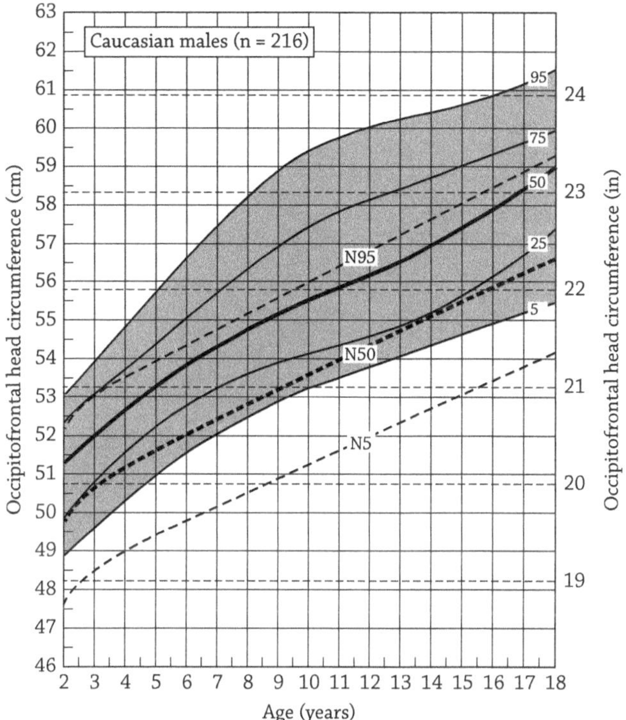

Figure 17.89 Neurofibromatosis, type I, head circumference, North American males, 2 to 18 years. Adapted from Szudek et al. (2000). Dashed lines represent 5th, 50th and 95th centiles for typical population.

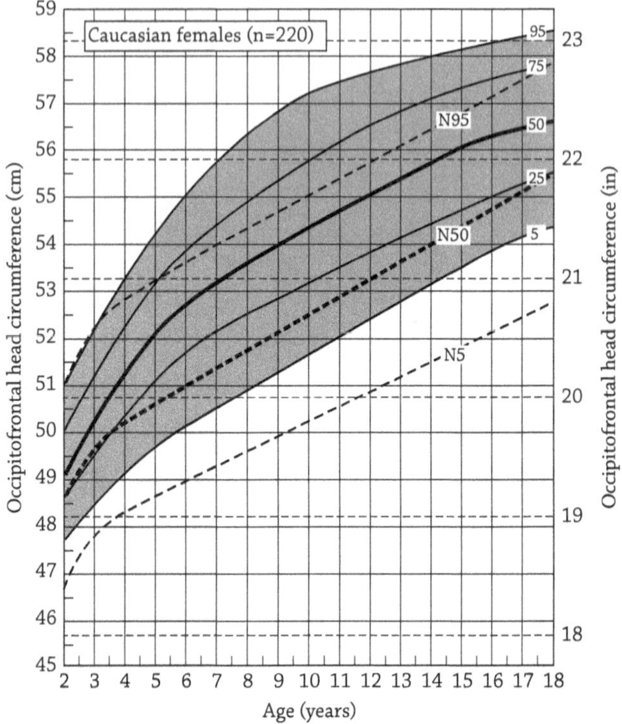

Figure 17.90 Neurofibromatosis, type I, head circumference, North American females, 2 to 18 years. Adapted from Szudek et al. (2000). Dashed lines represent 5th, 50th and 95th centiles for typical population.

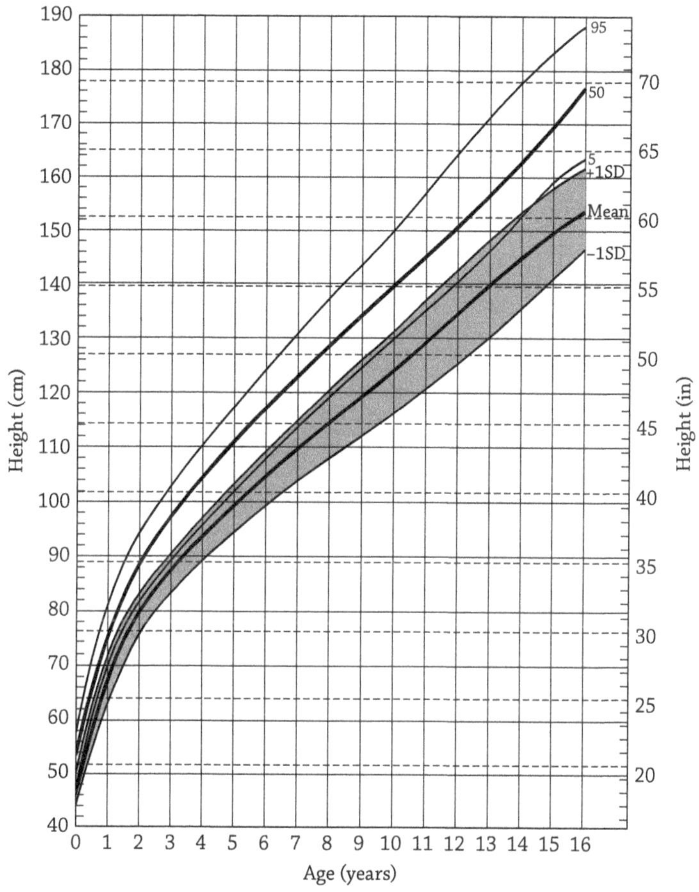

Figure 17.91 Noonan syndrome, height, males, birth to 16 years. From Witt et al. (1986) and Ranke et al. (1988), by permission. 5th, 50th and 95th centiles for typical population are provided.

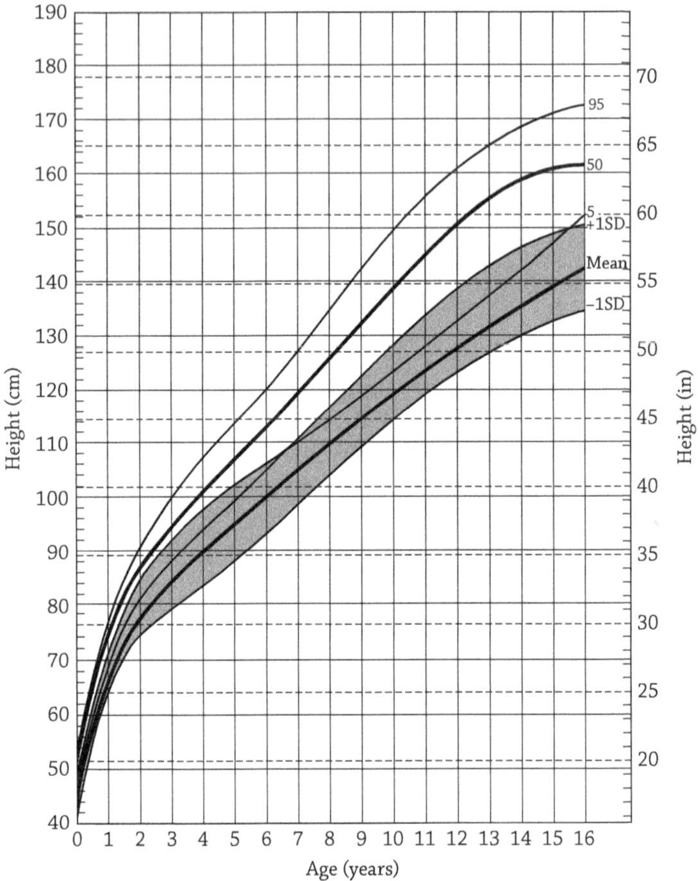

Figure 17.92 Noonan syndrome, height, females, birth to 16 years. From Witt et al. (1986) and Ranke et al. (1988), by permission. 5th, 50th and 95th centiles for typical population are provided.

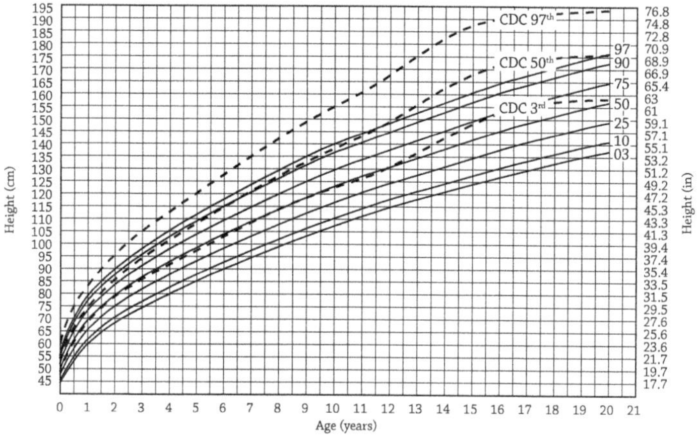

Figure 17.93 Noonan syndrome and related conditions (mutation in *PTPN11, SOS1, RAF1, KRAS, BRAF*, or *SHOC2*), length/height in Brazilian males compared to typical CDC cohort. Adapted from Malaquias et al. (2012).

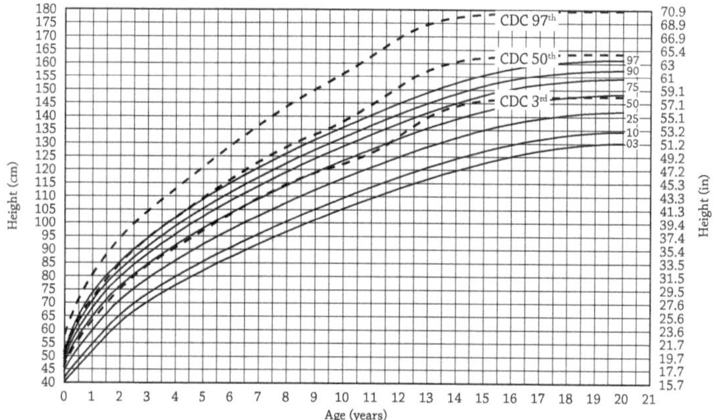

Figure 17.94 Noonan syndrome and related conditions (mutation in *PTPN11, SOS1, RAF1, KRAS, BRAF*, or *SHOC2*), length/height in Brazilian females compared to typical CDC cohort. Adapted from Malaquias et al. (2012).

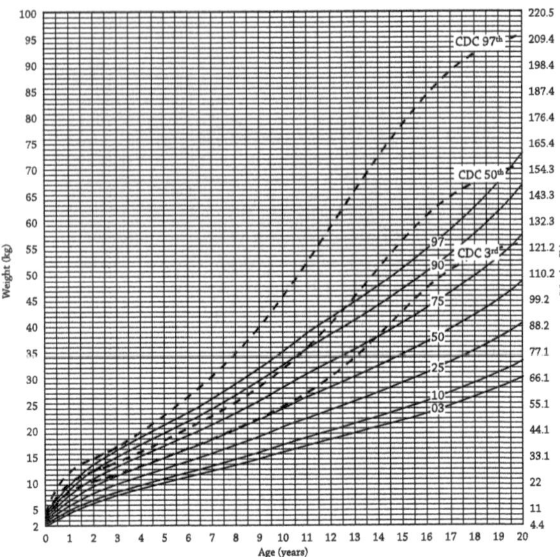

Figure 17.95 Noonan syndrome and related conditions (mutation in *PTPN11, SOS1, RAF1, KRAS, BRAF,* or *SHOC2*), weight in Brazilian males compared to typical CDC cohort. Adapted from Malaquias et al. (2012).

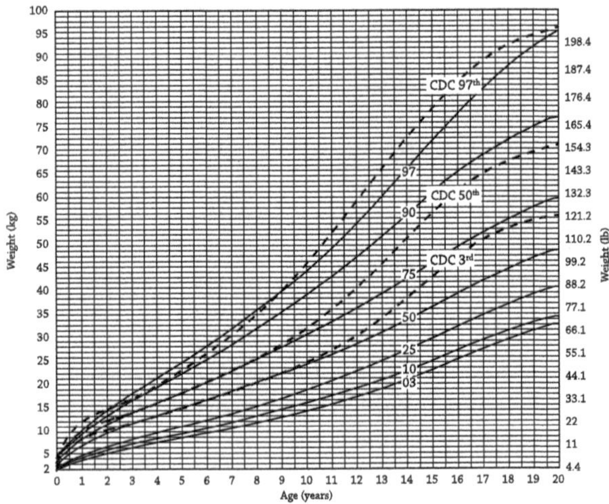

Figure 17.96 Noonan syndrome and related conditions (mutation in *PTPN11, SOS1, RAF1, KRAS, BRAF,* or *SHOC2*), weight in Brazilian females compared to typical CDC cohort. Adapted from Malaquias et al. (2012).

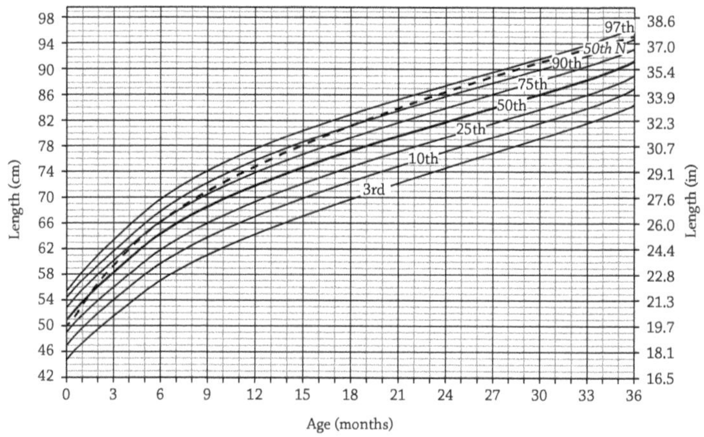

Figure 17.97 Prader-Willi syndrome, length/height, males, birth to 36 months (solid lines). Adapted from Butler et al. (2011).

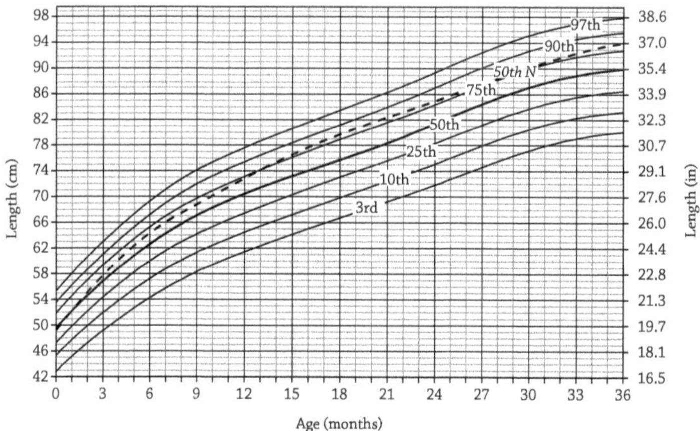

Figure 17.98 Prader-Willi syndrome, length/height, females, birth to 36 months (solid lines). Adapted from Butler et al. (2011).

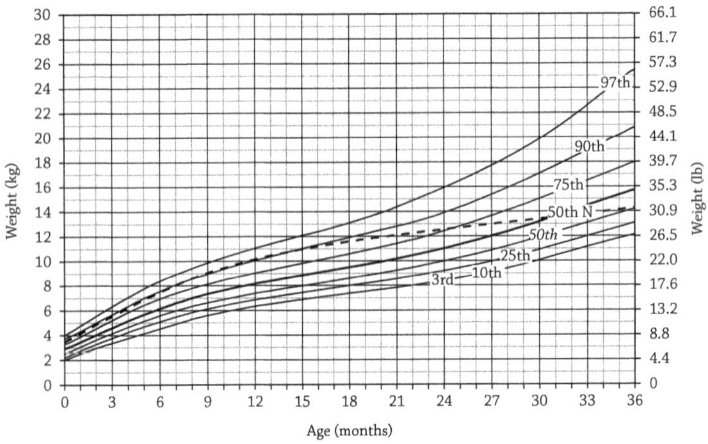

Figure 17.99 Prader-Willi syndrome, weight, males, birth to 36 months (solid lines). Adapted from Butler et al. (2011).

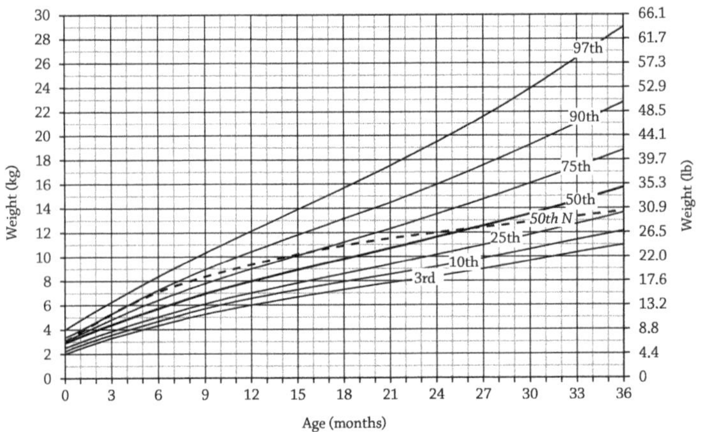

Figure 17.100 Prader-Willi syndrome, weight, females, birth to 36 months (solid lines). Adapted from Butler et al. (2011).

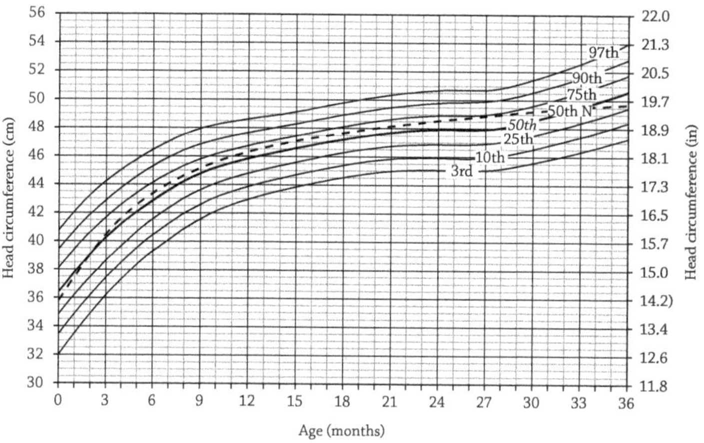

Figure 17.101 Prader-Willi syndrome, head circumference, males, birth to 36 months (solid lines). Adapted from Butler et al. (2011).

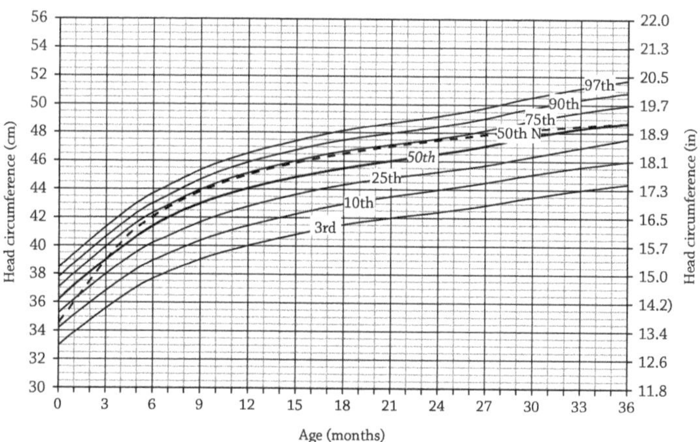

Figure 17.102 Prader-Willi syndrome, head circumference, females, birth to 36 months (solid lines). Adapted from Butler et al. (2011).

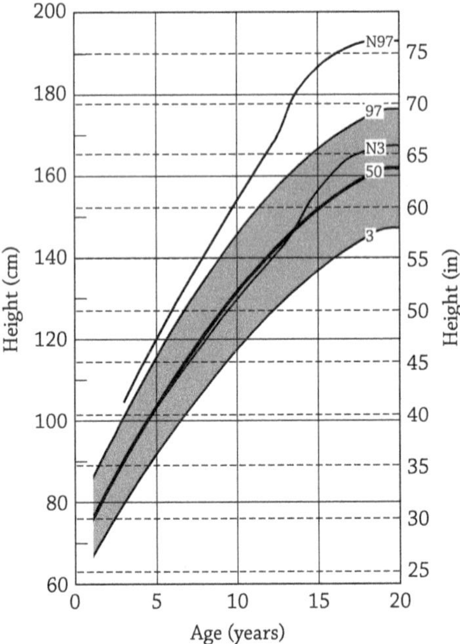

Figure 17.103 Prader-Willi syndrome, height, North European males, 2 to 18 years. Adapted from Wollmann et al. (1998). 3rd and 97th centiles for typical population are provided.

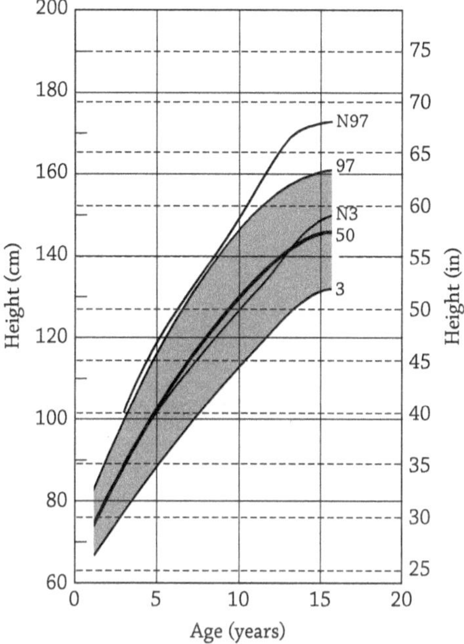

Figure 17.104 Prader-Willi syndrome, height, North European females, 2 to 18 years. Adapted from Wollmann et al. (1998). 3rd and 97th centiles for typical population are provided.

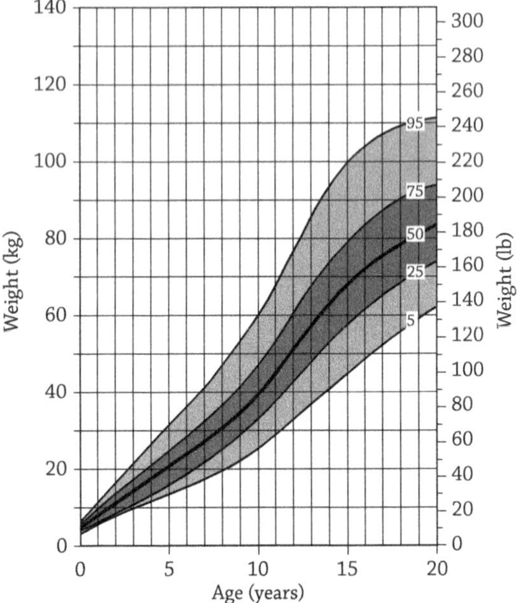

Figure 17.105 Prader-Willi syndrome, weight, North European males, birth to 20 years. Adapted from Hauffa et al. (2000).

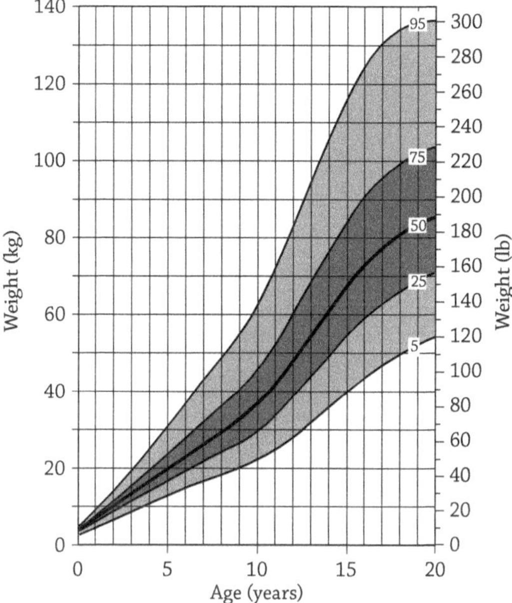

Figure 17.106 Prader-Willi syndrome, weight, North European females, birth to 20 years. Adapted from Hauffa et al. (2000).

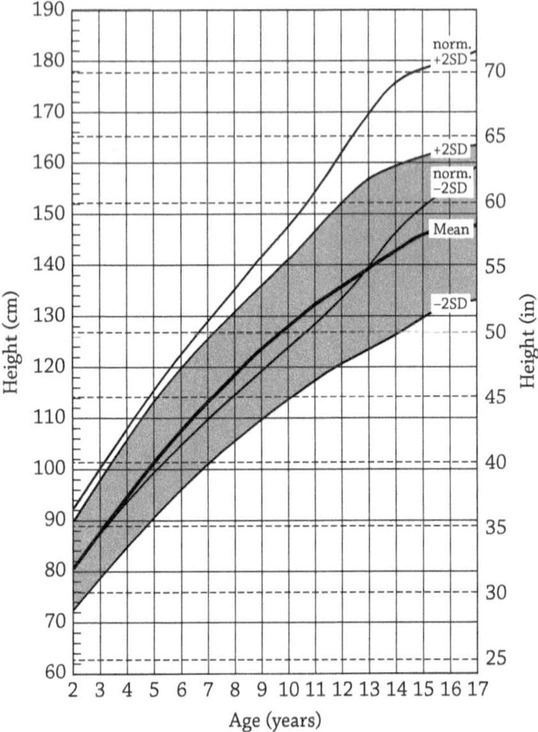

Figure 17.107 Prader-Willi syndrome, height, Asian males, 2 to 17 years. Adapted from Nagai et al. (2000). –2SD and +2SD for typical population are provided.

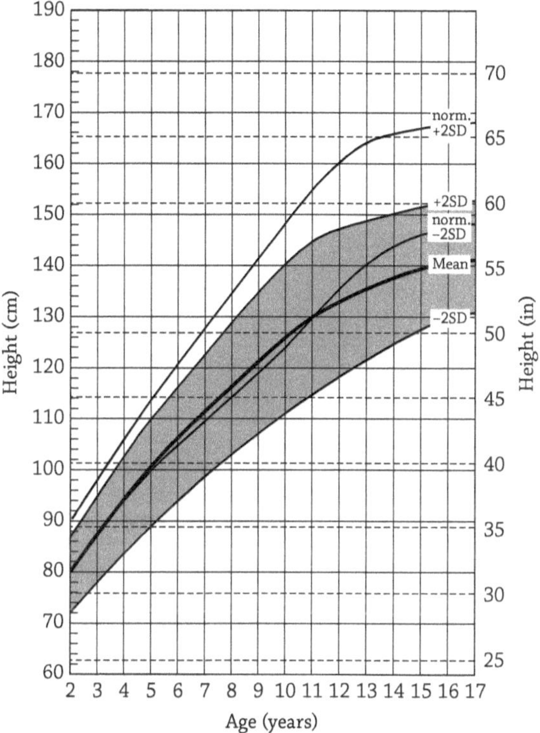

Figure 17.108 Prader-Willi syndrome, height, Asian females, 2 to 17 years. Adapted from Nagai et al. (2000). −2SD and +2SD for typical population are provided.

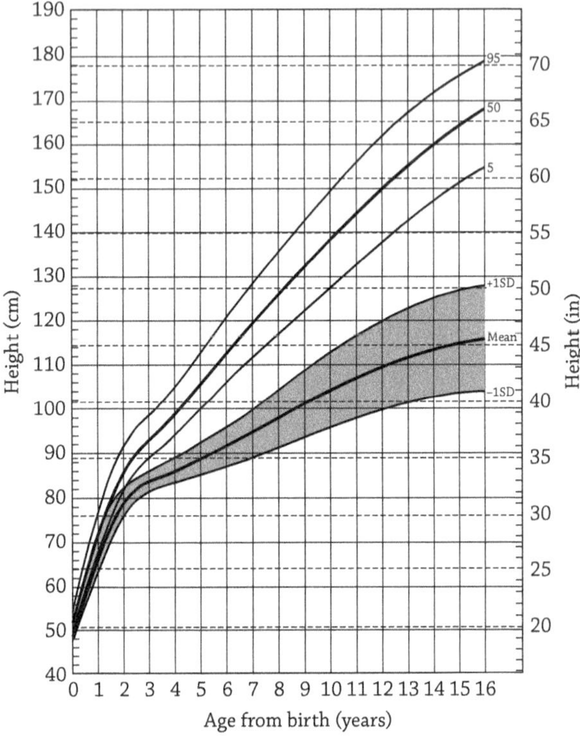

Figure 17.109 Pseudoachondroplasia, height, birth to 16 years. From Horton et al. (1982), by permission. 5th, 50th and 95th centile for typical population are provided.

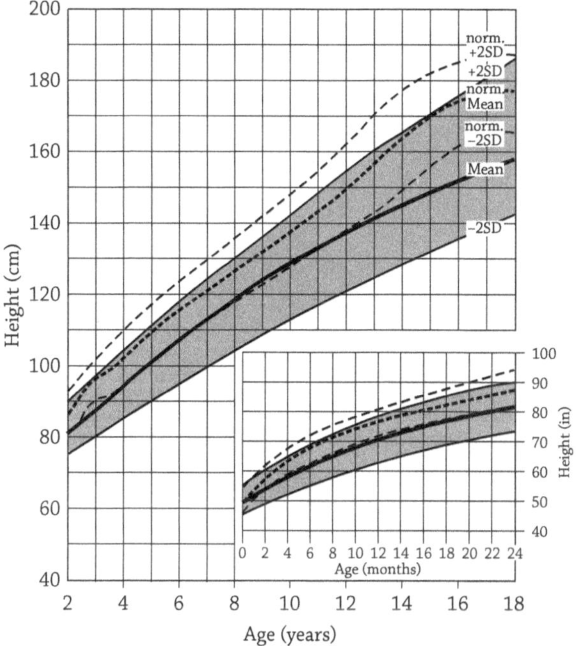

Figure 17.110 Rubinstein-Taybi syndrome, height, North American and North European males, birth to 18 years. From Stevens et al. (1990). –2SD, mean and +2SD for typical population are provided.

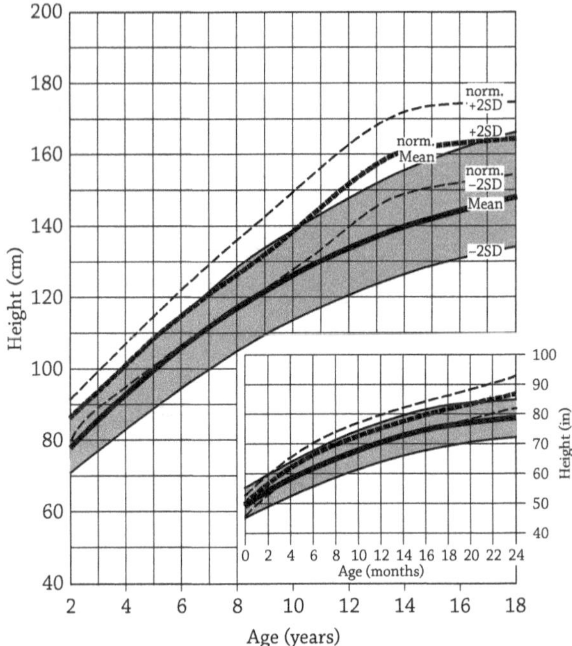

Figure 17.111 Rubinstein-Taybi syndrome, height, North American and North European females, birth to 18 years. From Stevens et al. (1990). –2SD, mean and +2SD for typical population are provided.

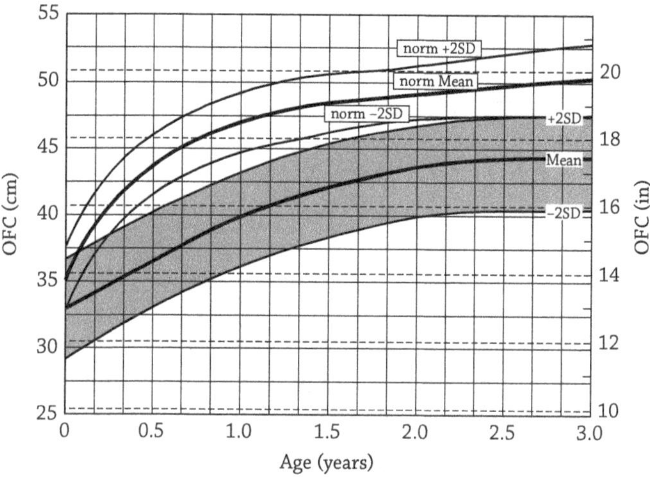

Figure 17.112 Rubinstein-Taybi syndrome, head circumference, North American and North European males, birth to 3 years. From Stevens et al. (1990).

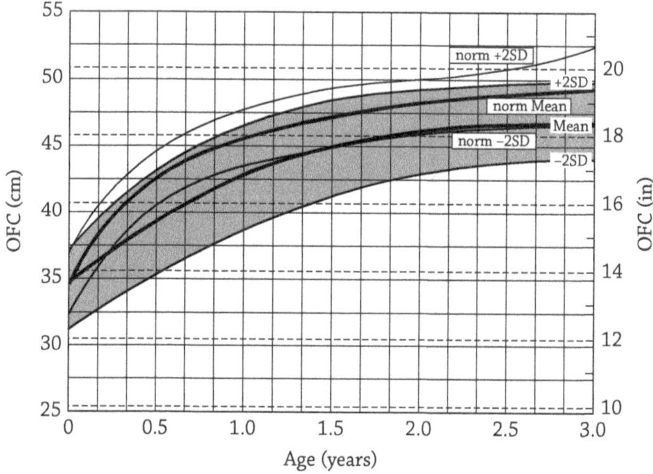

Figure 17.113 Rubinstein-Taybi syndrome, head circumference, North American and North European females, birth to 3 years. From Stevens et al. (1990).

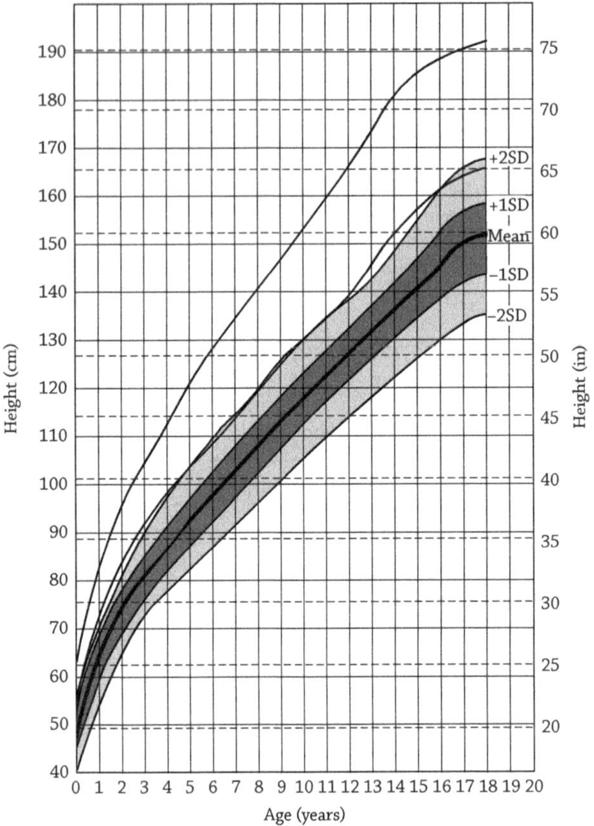

Figure 17.114 Russell-Silver syndrome, height, males, birth to 20 years. From Wollmann et al. (1995). The top two solid lines represent Prader standards from Pankau et al. (1992).

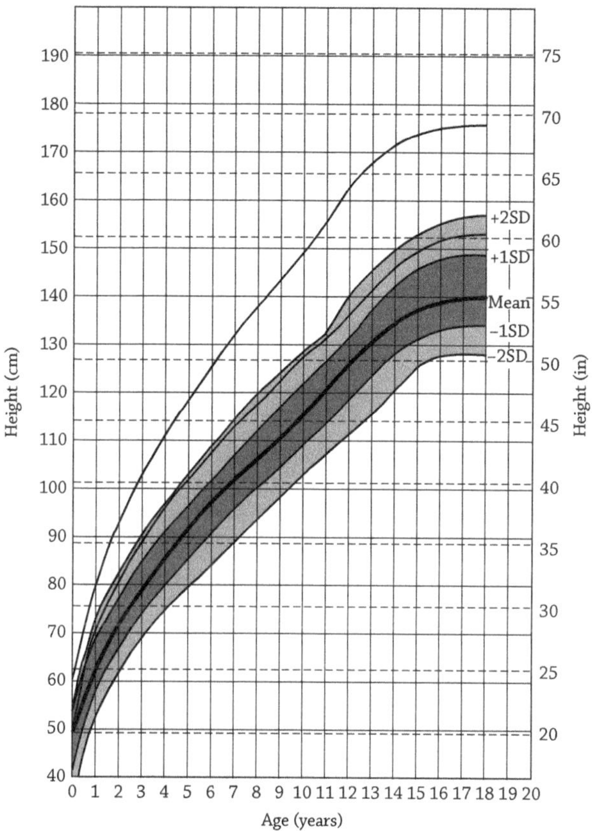

Figure 17.115 Russell-Silver syndrome, height, females, birth to 20 years. From Wollmann et al. (1995). The top two solid lines represent Prader standards from Pankau et al. (1992).

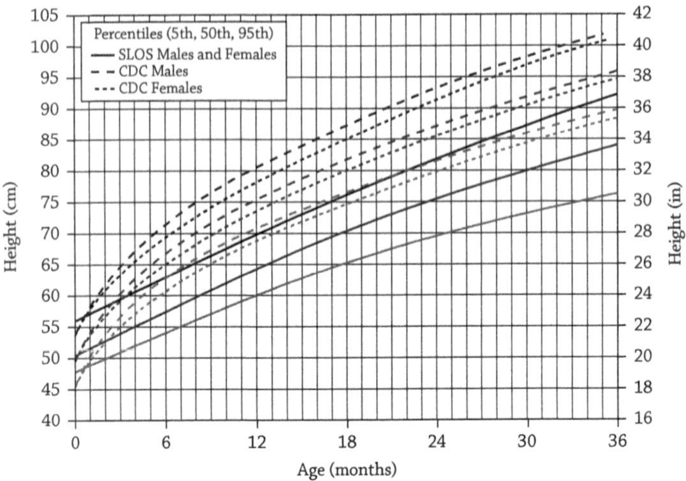

Figure 17.116 Smith-Lemli-Opitz syndrome, height in males and females combined from birth to 36 months (solid lines), compared to CDC centiles for typical males and females (dashed and dotted lines, respectively). Adapted from Lee et al. (2012).

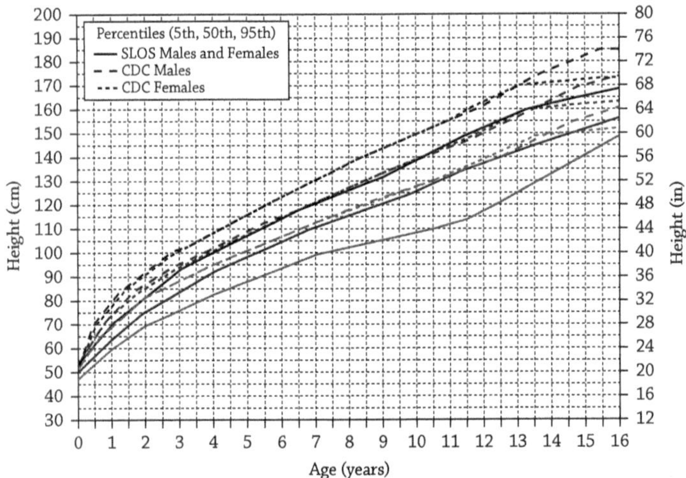

Figure 17.117 Smith-Lemli-Opitz syndrome, height in males and females combined from birth to 16 years (solid lines), compared to CDC centiles for typical males and females (dashed and dotted lines, respectively). Adapted from Lee et al. (2012).

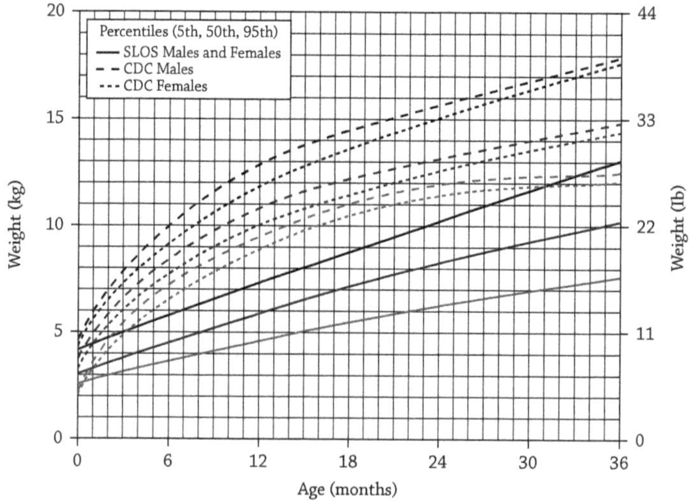

Figure 17.118 Smith-Lemli-Opitz syndrome, weight in males and females combined from birth to 36 months (solid lines), compared to CDC centiles for typical males and females (dashed and dotted lines, respectively). Adapted from Lee et al. (2012).

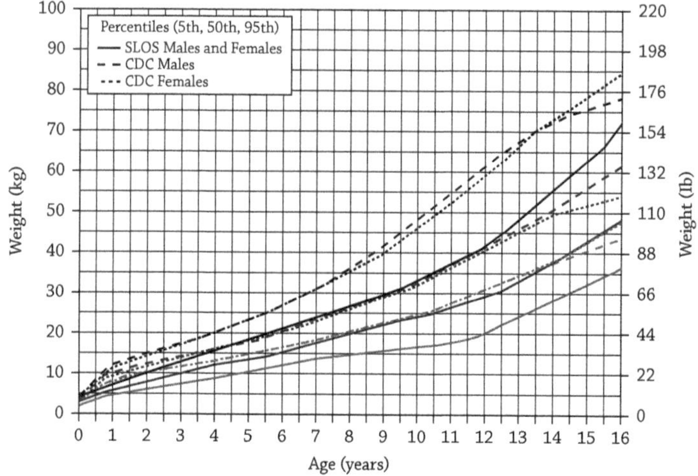

Figure 17.119 Smith-Lemli-Opitz syndrome, weight in males and females combined from birth to 16 years (solid lines), compared to CDC centiles for typical males and females (dashed and dotted lines, respectively). Adapted from Lee et al. (2012).

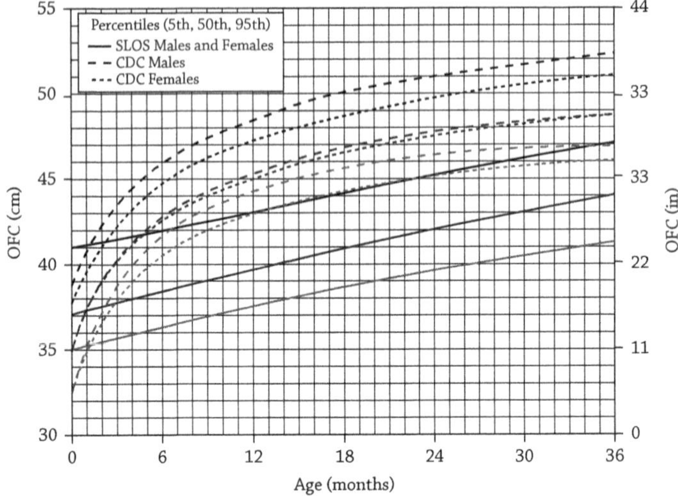

Figure 17.120 Smith-Lemli-Opitz syndrome, head circumference (OFC) in males and females combined from birth to 36 months (solid lines), compared to CDC centiles for typical males and females (dashed and dotted lines, respectively). Adapted from Lee et al. (2012).

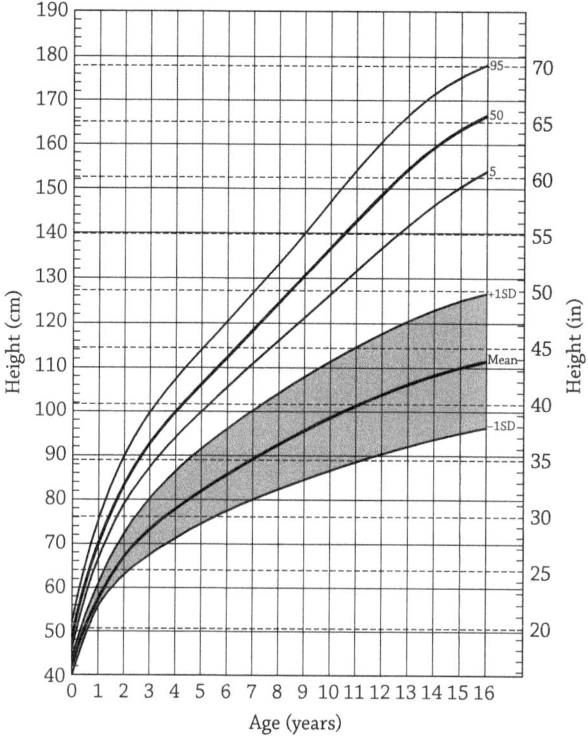

Figure 17.121 Spondyloepiphysial dysplasia congenita, height, birth to 16 years. From Horton et al. (1982), by permission. 5th, 50th and 95th centile for typical population are provided.

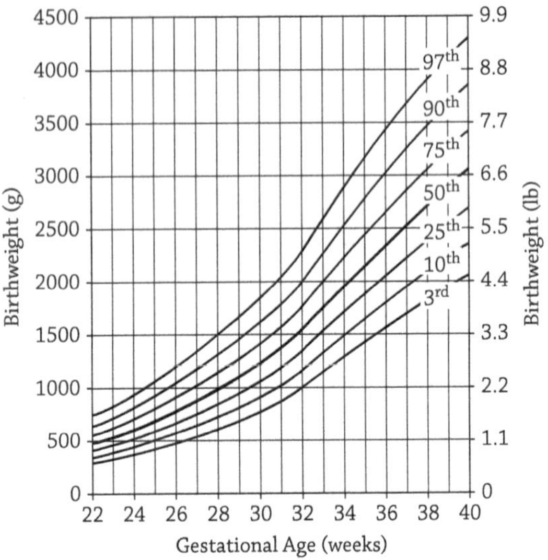

Figure 17.122 Trisomy 13, birthweight by gestational age, for males and females combined. Adapted from Boghossian et al. (2012).

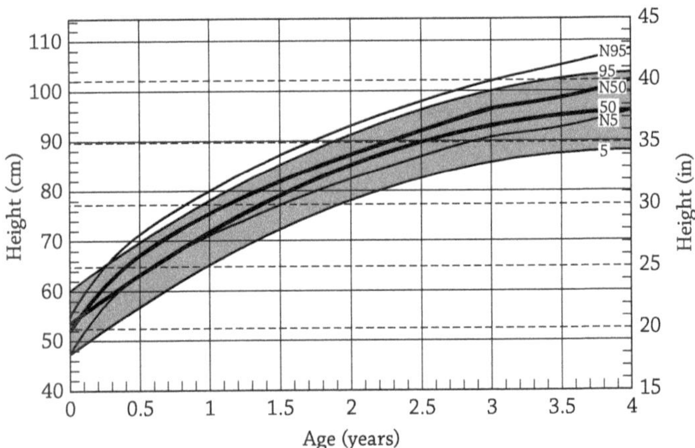

Figure 17.123 Height for males and females with trisomy 13, birth to 4 years. Adapted from Baty et al. (1994).

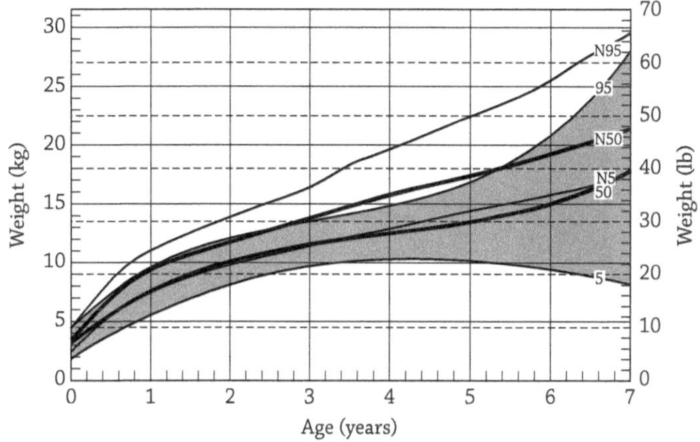

Figure 17.124 Weight for males and females with trisomy 13, birth to 7 years. Adapted from Baty et al. (1994).

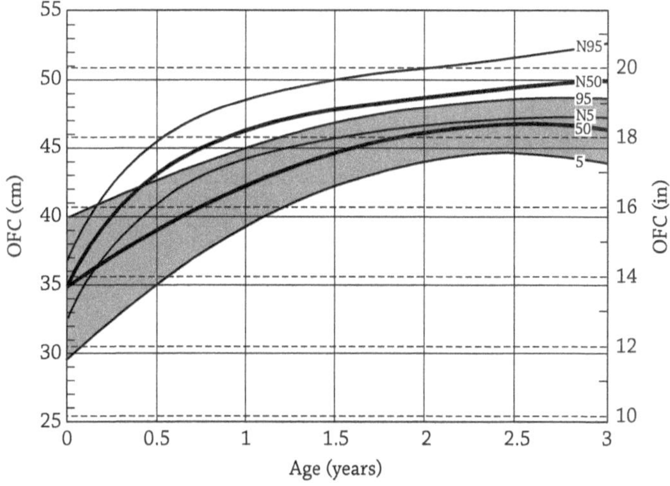

Figure 17.125 Head circumferences for males and females with trisomy 13, birth to 3 years. Adapted from Baty et al. (1994).

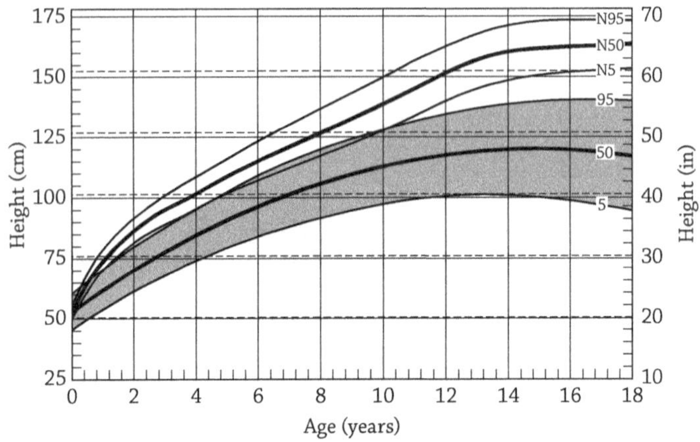

Figure 17.126 Height for males and females with trisomy 18, birth to 18 years. Adapted from Baty et al. (1994).

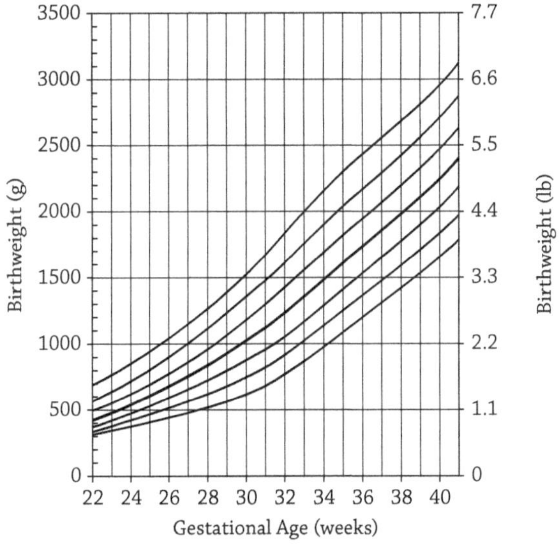

Figure 17.127 Trisomy 18, birthweight by gestational age, for males and females combined. Adapted from Boghossian et al. (2012).

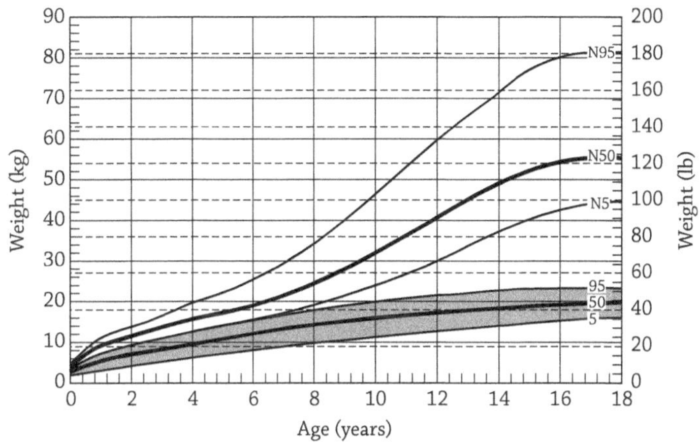

Figure 17.128 Weight for males and females with trisomy 18, birth to 18 years. Adapted from Baty et al. (1994).

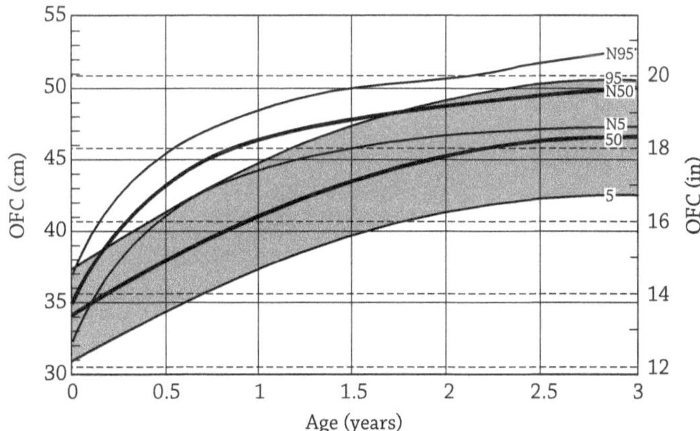

Figure 17.129 Head circumference (OFC) for males and females with trisomy 18, birth to 3 years. Adapted from Baty et al. (1994).

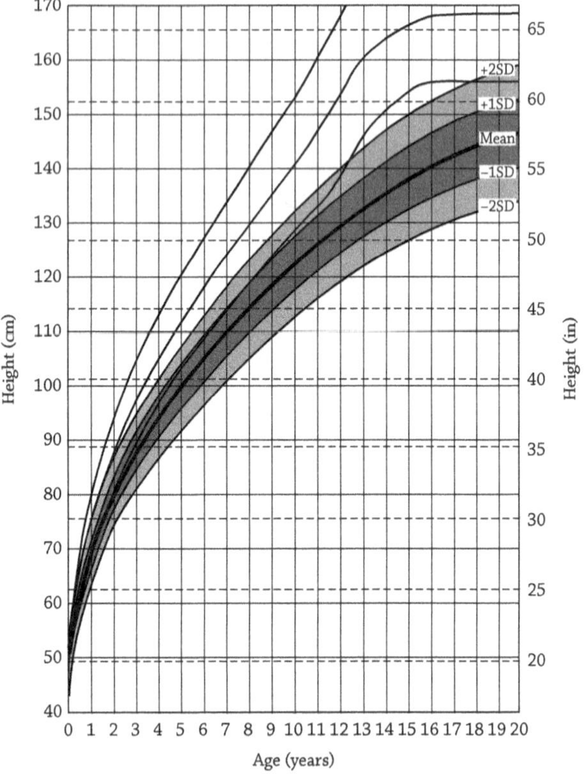

Figure 17.130 Turner syndrome, height, North European females, birth to 20 years. Adapted from Rougen–Weiterlaken et al. (1997).

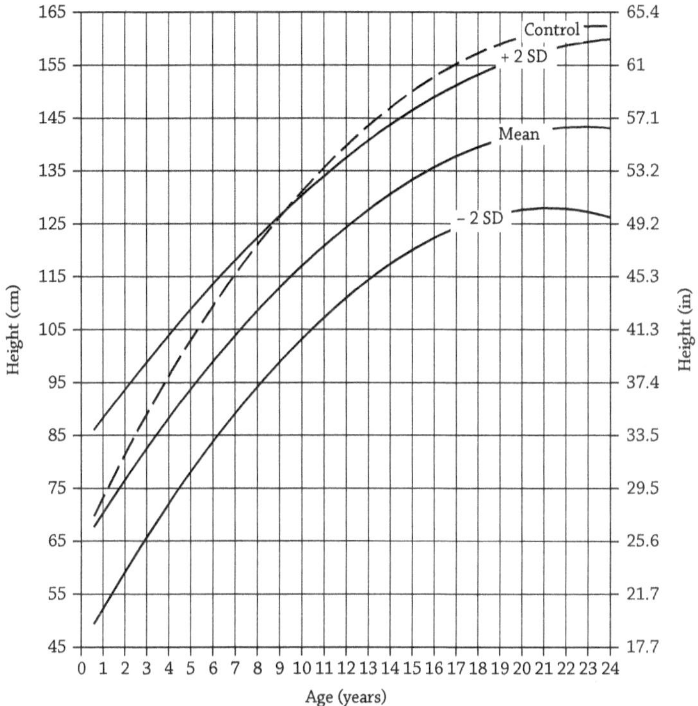

Figure 17.131 Turner syndrome, height in Egyptian individuals (solid lines) and 50th centile for typical Egyptian females (dashed line). Adapted from El-Bassyouni et al. (2012).

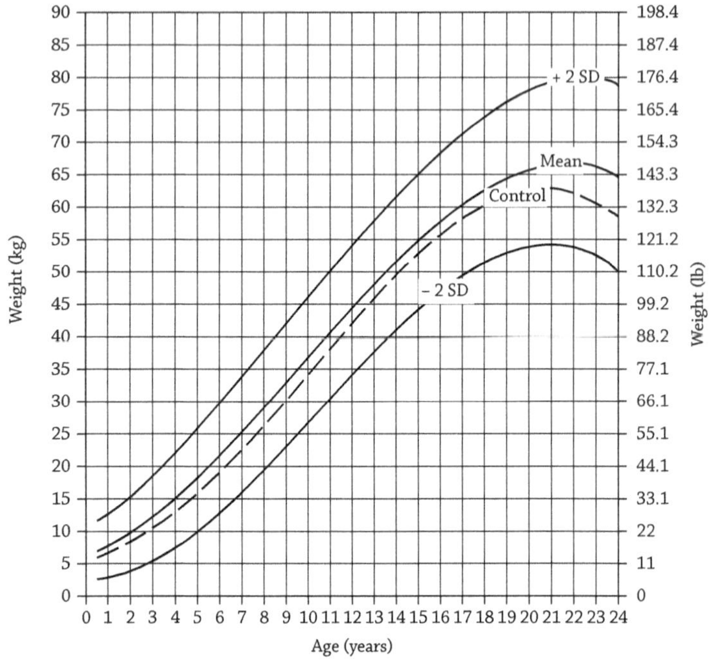

Figure 17.132 Turner syndrome, weight in Egyptian individuals (solid lines) and 50th centile for typical Egyptian females (dashed line). Adapted from El-Bassyouni et al. (2012).

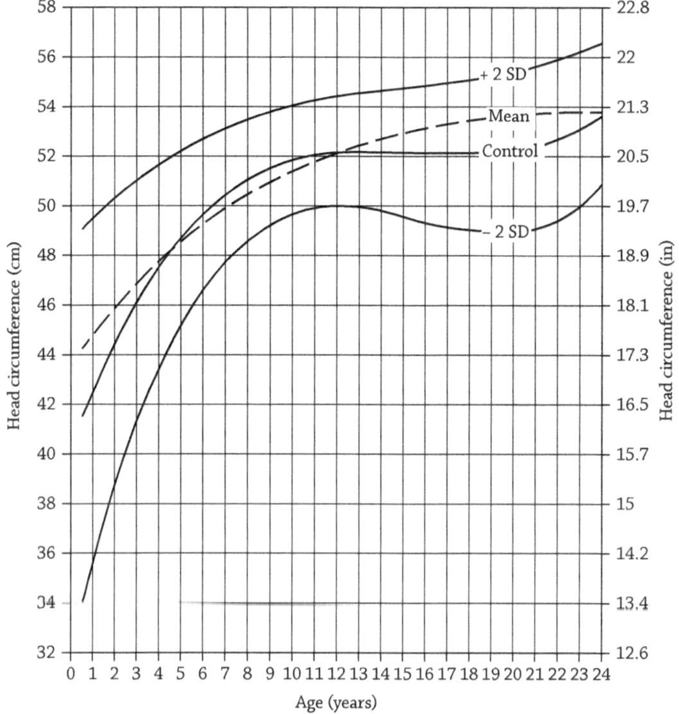

Figure 17.133 Turner syndrome, head circumference in Egyptian individuals (solid lines) and 50th centile for typical Egyptian females (dashed line). Adapted from El-Bassyouni et al. (2012).

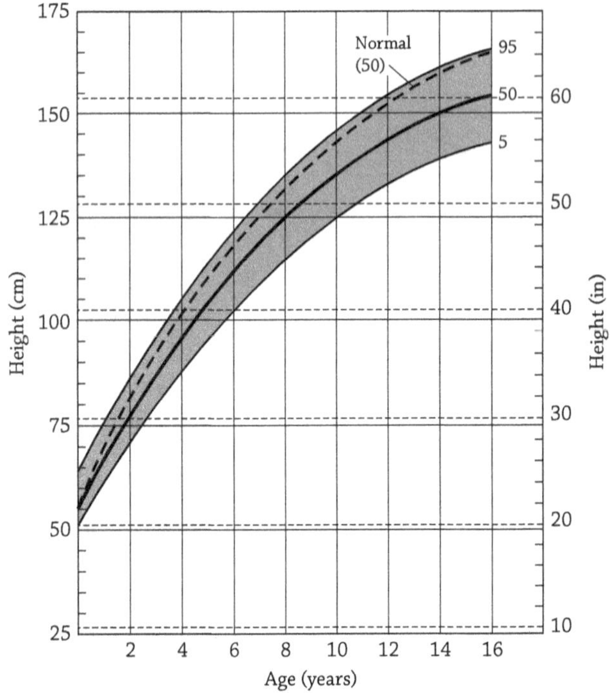

Figure 17.134 Williams syndrome, height, males, birth to 16 years. From Morris et al. (1988), by permission.

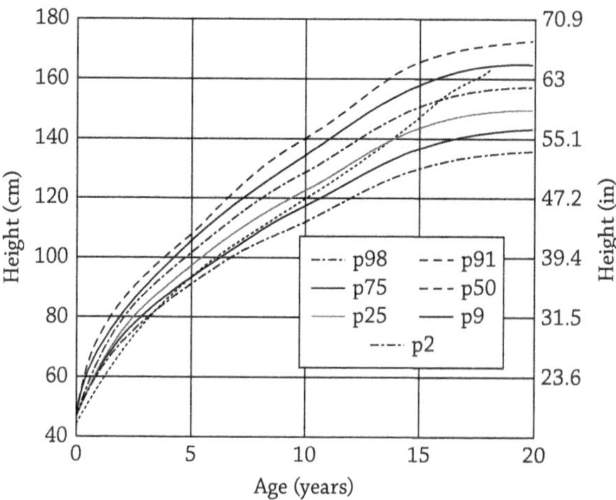

Figure 17.135 Williams syndrome, height in British cohort, males, birth to 20 years. Adapted from Martin et al. (2007).

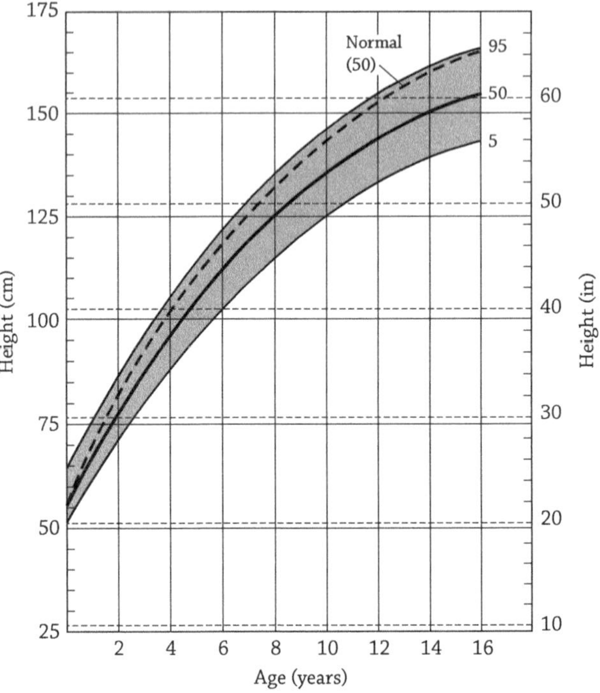

Figure 17.136 Williams syndrome, height, females, birth to 16 years. From Morris et al. (1988), by permission.

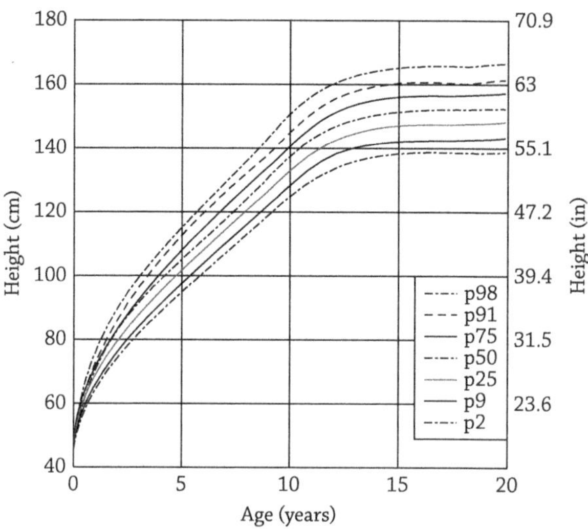

Figure 17.137 Williams syndrome, height in British cohort, females, birth to 20 years. Adapted from Martin et al. (2007).

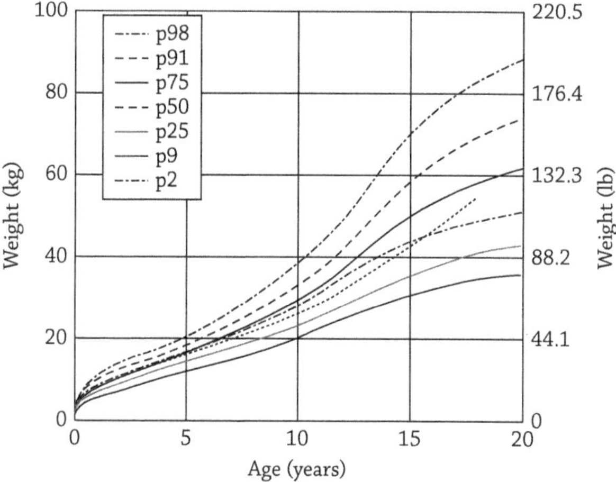

Figure 17.138 Williams syndrome, weight in British cohort, males, birth to 20 years. Adapted from Martin et al. (2007).

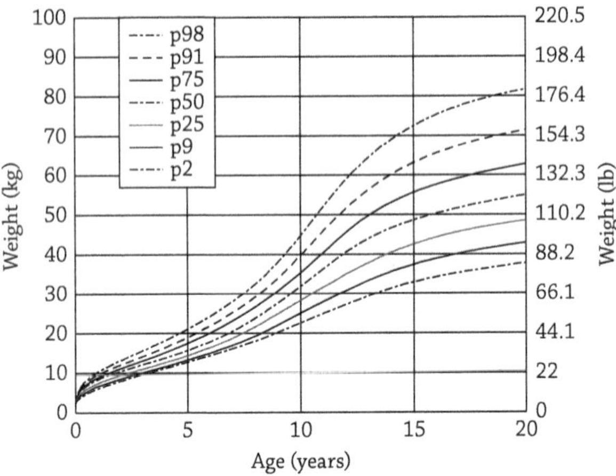

Figure 17.139 Williams syndrome, weight in British cohort, females, birth to 20 years. Adapted from Martin et al. (2007).

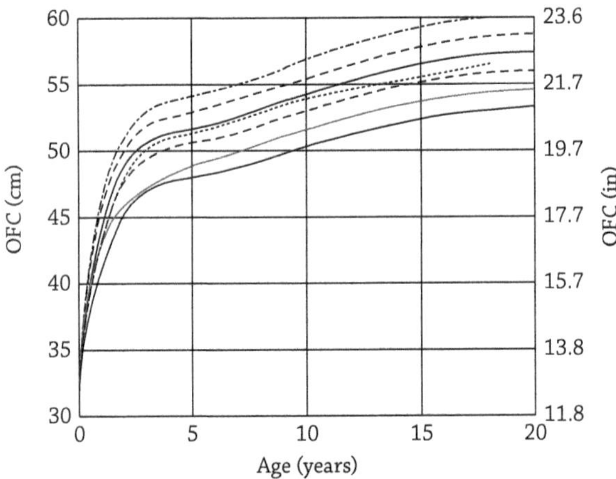

Figure 17.140 Williams syndrome, head circumference in British cohort, males, birth to 20 years. Adapted from Martin et al. (2007).

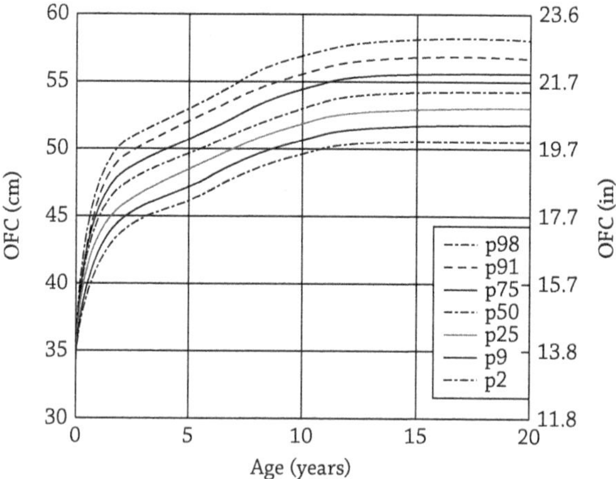

Figure 17.141 Williams syndrome, head circumference in British cohort, females, birth to 20 years. Adapted from Martin et al. (2007).

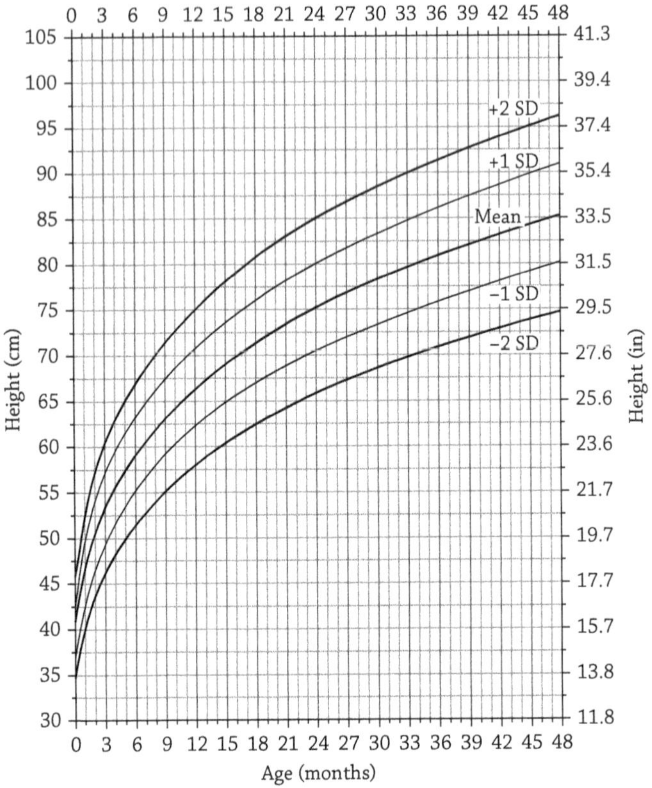

Figure 17.142 Wolf-Hirschhorn syndrome, height in males. Data derived from, respectively, 35 male and 66 female European, North American, and Australian individuals. Adapted from Antonius et al. (2008).

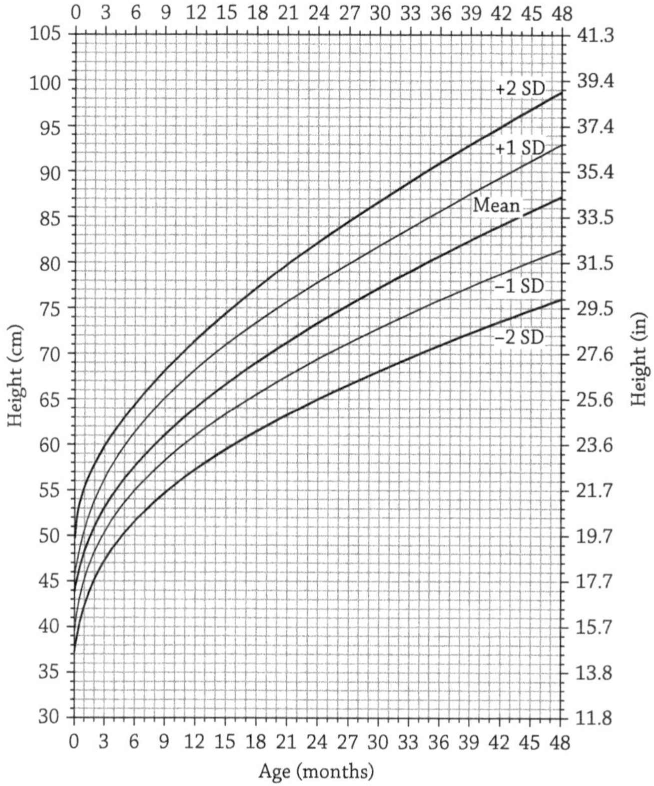

Figure 17.143 Wolf-Hirschhorn syndrome, height in females. Data derived from, respectively, 35 male and 66 female European, North American, and Australian individuals. Adapted from Antonius et al. (2008).

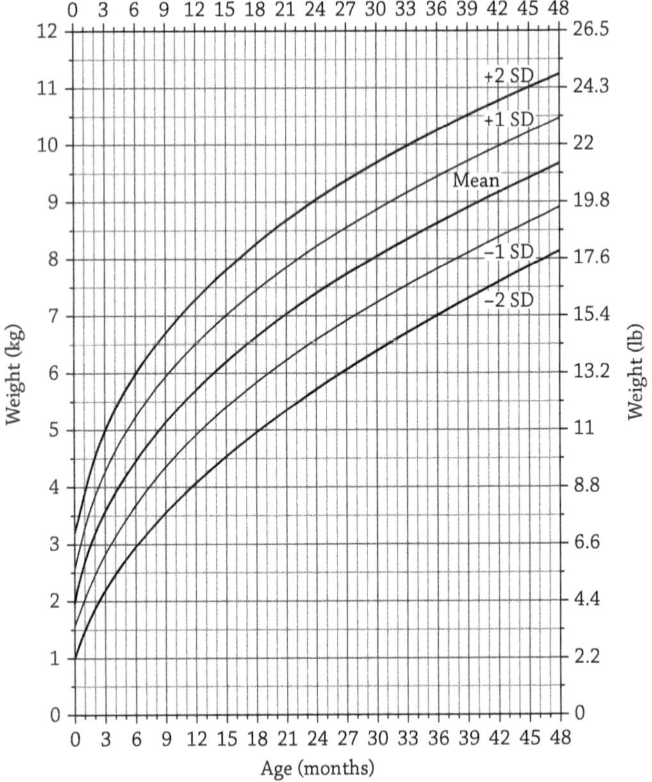

Figure 17.144 Wolf-Hirschhorn syndrome, weight in males. Data derived from, respectively, 35 male and 66 female European, North American, and Australian individuals. Adapted from Antonius et al. (2008).

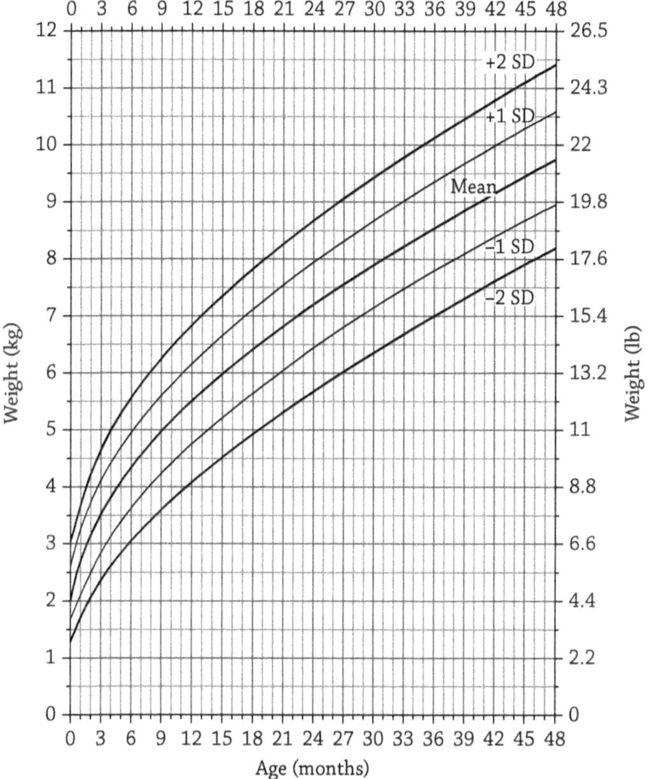

Figure 17.145 Wolf-Hirschhorn syndrome, weight in females. Data derived from, respectively, 35 male and 66 female European, North American, and Australian individuals. Adapted from Antonius et al. (2008).

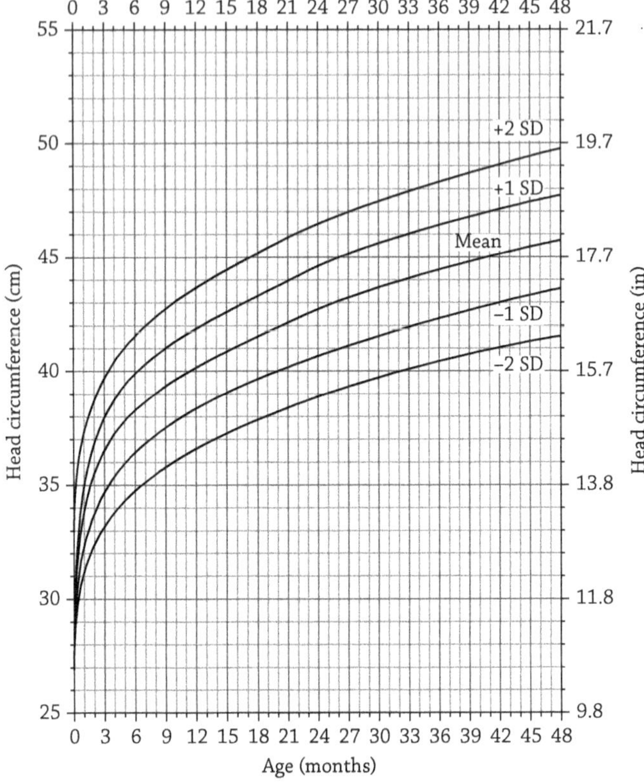

Figure 17.146 Wolf-Hirschhorn syndrome, head circumference in males and females, combined. Data derived from 35 male and 66 female European, North American, and Australian individuals. Adapted from Antonius et al. (2008).

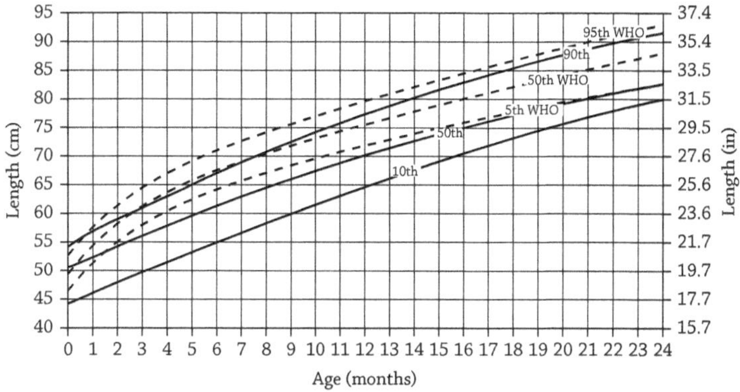

Figure 17.147 22q11.2 microdeletion syndrome, length/height, Chilean males, birth to 24 months. Adapted from Guzman et al. (2012).

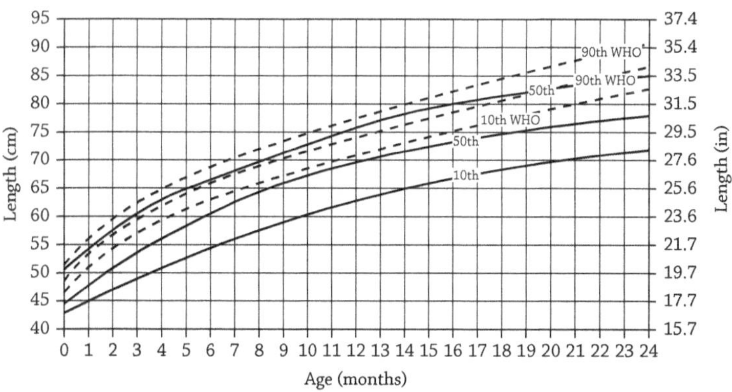

Figure 17.148 22q11.2 microdeletion syndrome, length/height, Chilean females, birth to 24 months. Adapted from Guzman et al. (2012).

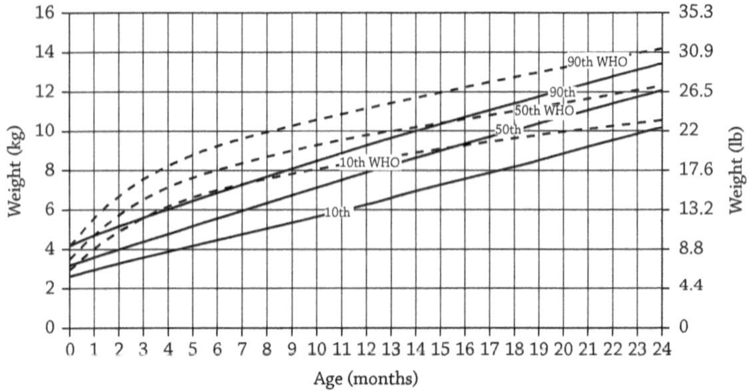

Figure 17.149 22q11.2 microdeletion syndrome, weight, Chilean males, birth to 24 months. Adapted from Guzman et al. (2012).

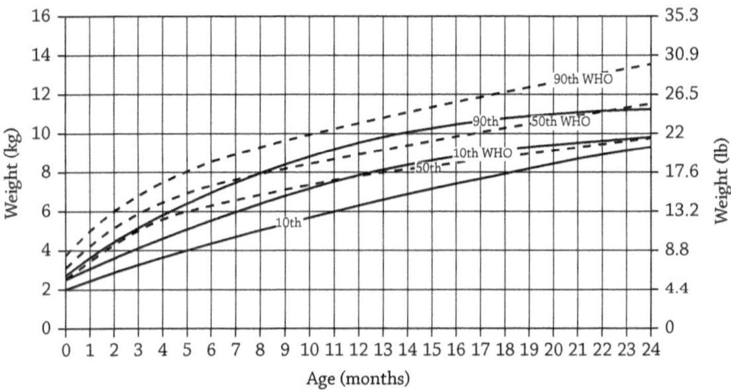

Figure 17.150 22q11.2 microdeletion syndrome, weight, Chilean females, birth to 24 months. Adapted from Guzman et al. (2012).

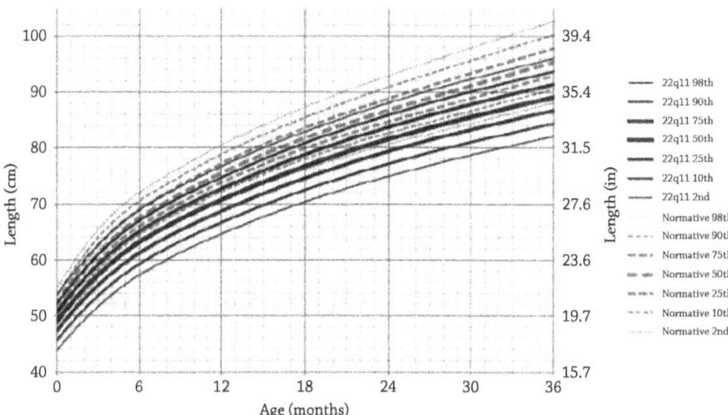

Figure 17.151 22q11.2 microdeletion syndrome, length/height, North American males, birth to 36 months. Adapted from Tarquinio et al. (2012).

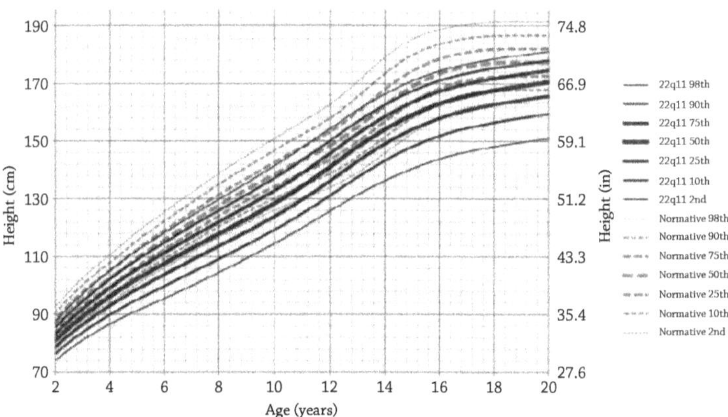

Figure 17.152 22q11.2 microdeletion syndrome, length/height, North American males, birth to 20 years. Adapted from Tarquinio et al. (2012).

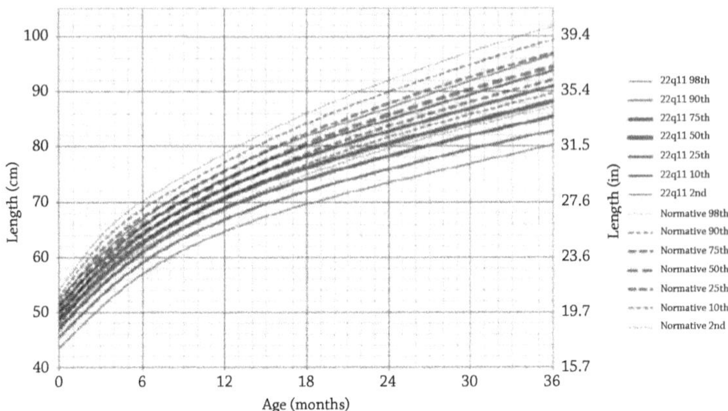

Figure 17.153 22q11.2 microdeletion syndrome, length/height, North American females, birth to 36 months. Adapted from Tarquinio et al. (2012).

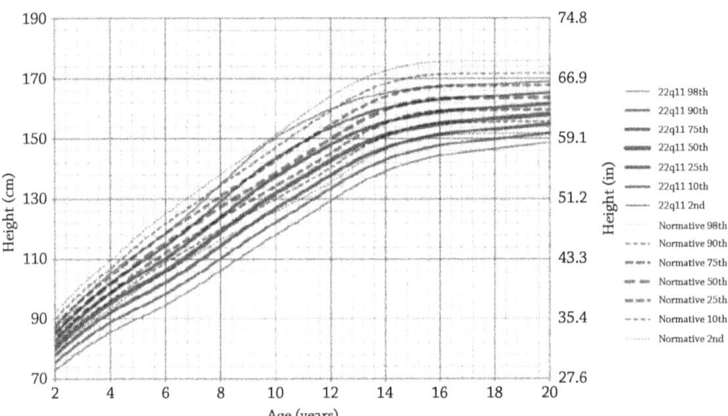

Figure 17.154 22q11.2 microdeletion syndrome, length/height, North American females, birth to 20 years. Adapted from Tarquinio et al. (2012).

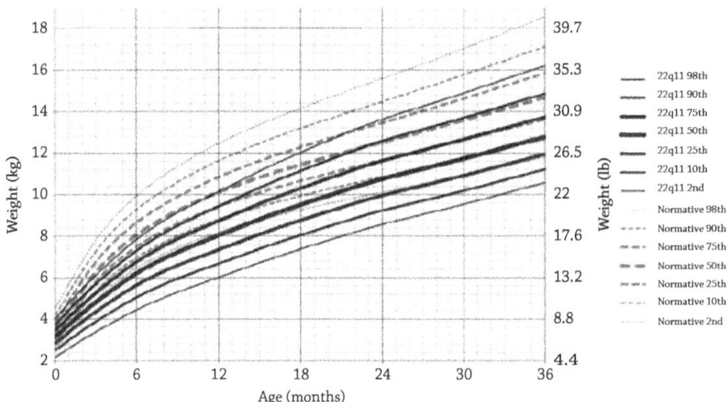

Figure 17.155 22q11.2 microdeletion syndrome, weight, North American males, birth to 36 months. Adapted from Tarquinio et al. (2012).

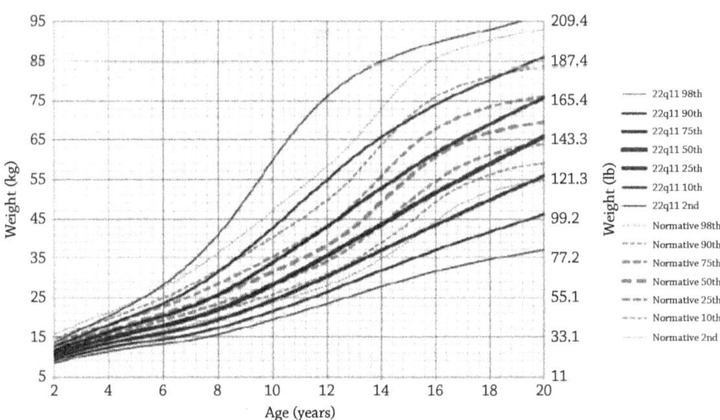

Figure 17.156 22q11.2 microdeletion syndrome, weight, North American males, birth to 20 years. Adapted from Tarquinio et al. (2012).

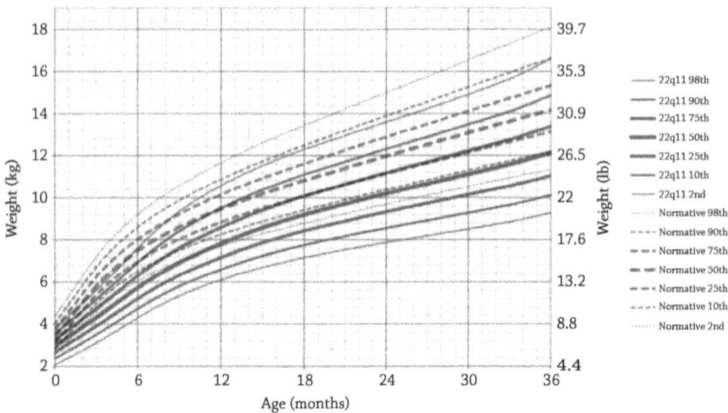

Figure 17.157 22q11.2 microdeletion syndrome, weight, North American females, birth to 36 months. Adapted from Tarquinio et al. (2012).

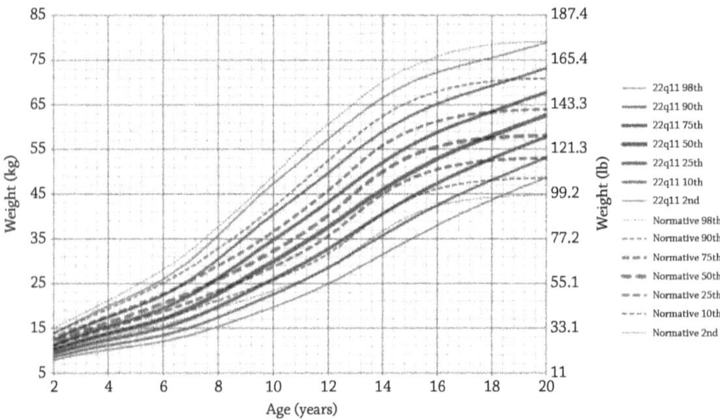

Figure 17.158 22q11.2 microdeletion syndrome, weight, North American females, birth to 20 years. Adapted from Tarquinio et al. (2012).

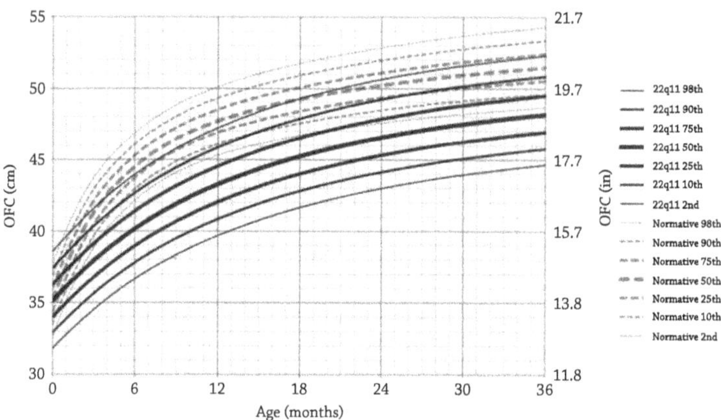

Figure 17.159 22q11.2 microdeletion syndrome, head circumference, North American males, birth to 36 months. Adapted from Tarquinio et al. (2012).

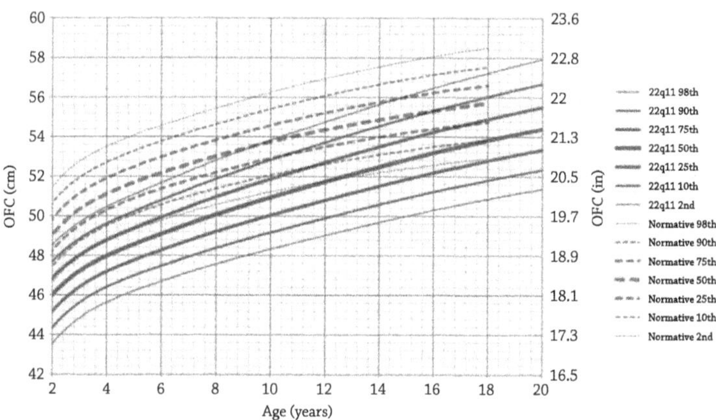

Figure 17.160 22q11.2 microdeletion syndrome, head circumference, North American females, birth to 36 months. Adapted from Tarquinio et al. (2012).

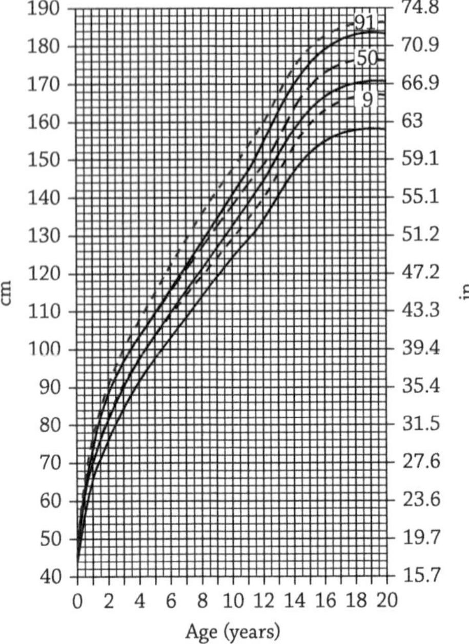

Figure 17.161 22q11.2 microdeletion syndrome, length/height, North American males, birth to 20 years. Dotted lines represent 9th, 50th, and 91st centile in typical individuals. Adapted from Habel et al. (2012).

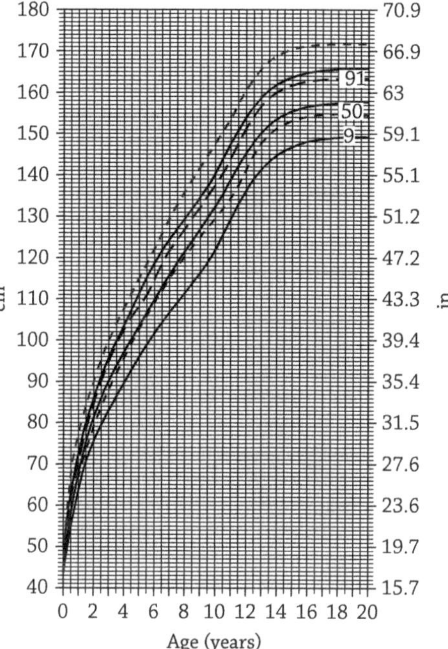

Figure 17.162 22q11.2 microdeletion syndrome, length/height, North American females, birth to 20 years. Dotted lines represent 9th, 50th, and 91st centile in typical individuals. Adapted from Habel et al. (2012).

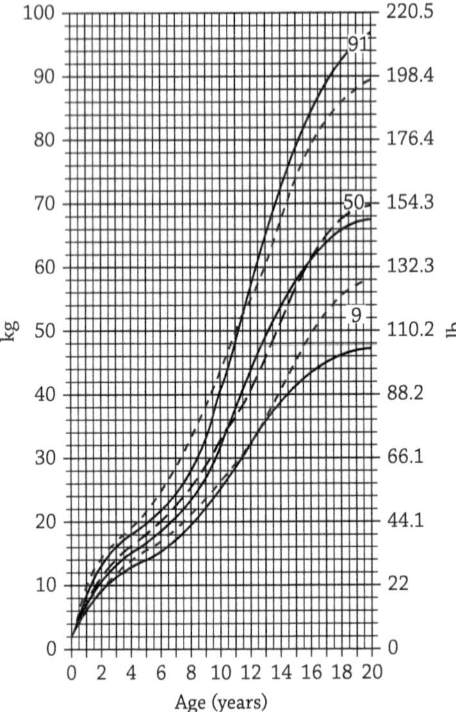

Figure 17.163 22q11.2 microdeletion syndrome, weight, North American males, birth to 20 years. Dotted lines represent 9th, 50th, and 91st centile in typical individuals. Adapted from Habel et al. (2012).

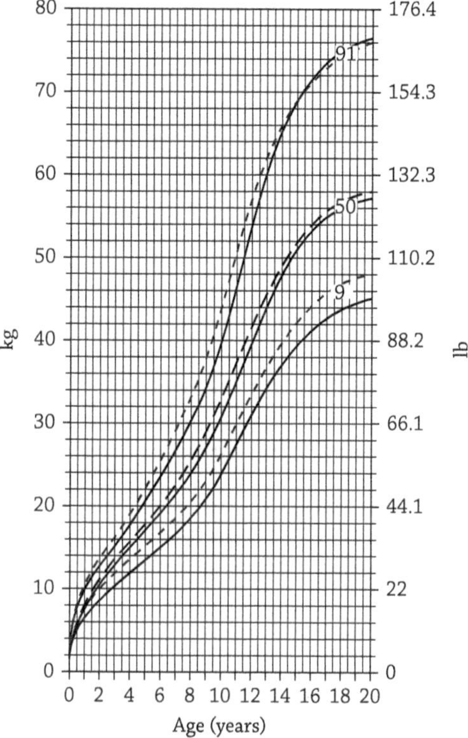

Figure 17.164 22q11.2 microdeletion syndrome, weight, North American females, birth to 20 years. Dotted lines represent 9th, 50th, and 91st centile in typical individuals. Adapted from Habel et al. (2012).

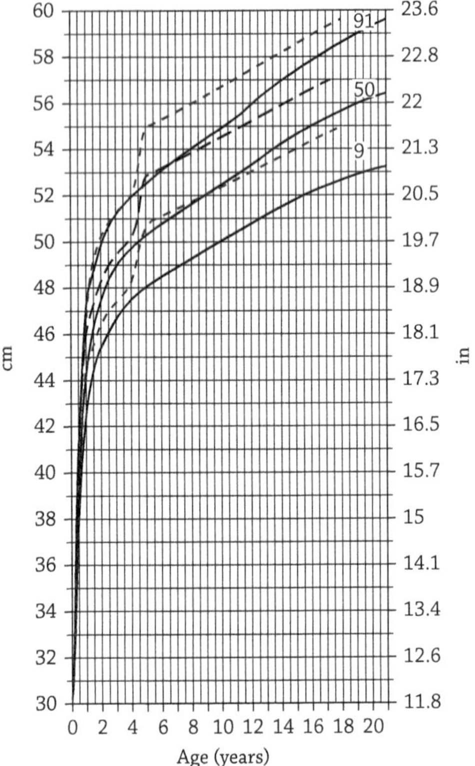

Figure 17.165 22q11.2 microdeletion syndrome, head circumference (OFC), North American males, birth to 20 years. Dotted lines represent 9th, 50th, and 91st centile in typical individuals. Adapted from Habel et al. (2012).

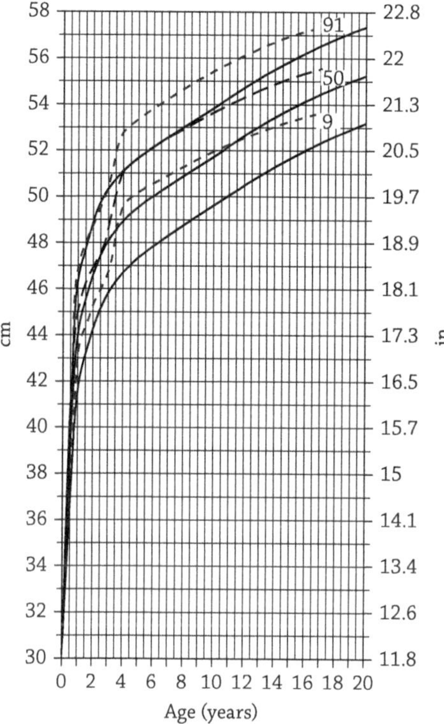

Figure 17.166 22q11.2 microdeletion syndrome, head circumference (OFC), North American females, birth to 20 years. Dotted lines represent 9th, 50th, and 91st centile in typical individuals. Adapted from Habel et al. (2012).

BIBLIOGRAPHY

Afifi, H. H., Aglan, M. S., Zaki, M. E., Thomas, M. M., and Tosson, A. M. S. (2012). Growth charts of Down syndrome in Egypt: A study of 434 children 0–36 months of age. *American Journal Medical Genetics Part A*, 158A, 2647–2655.

Antonius, T., Draaisma, J., Levtchenko, E., Knoers, N., Renier, W., and van Ravenswaaij, C. (2008). Growth charts for Wolf-Hirschhorn syndrome (0–4 years of age). *European Journal of Pediatrics*, 167, 807–810.

Baty, B. J., Blackburn, B. L., and Carey, J. C. (1994). Natural history of trisomy 18 and trisomy 13: I. Growth, physical assessment, medical histories, survival, and recurrence risk. *American Journal of Medical Genetics*, 49, 175–188.

Bober, M. B., Niiler, T., Duker, A. L., Murray, J. E., Ketterer, T., Harley, M. E., Alvi, S., Flora, C., Rustad, C., Bongers, E. M. H. F., Bicknell, L. S., Wise, C., and Jackson, A. P. (2012). Growth in individuals with Majewski osteodysplastic primordial dwarfism type II caused by pericentrin mutations. *American Journal of Medical Genetics Part A*, 158A, 2719–2725.

Boghossian, N. S., Horbar, J. D., Murray, J. C., and Carpenter, J. H., for the Vermont Oxford Network. (2012). Anthropometric charts for infants with trisomies 21, 18, or 13 born between 22 weeks gestation and term: The VON charts. *American Journal of Medical Genetics Part A*, 158A, 322–332.

Butler, M. G., Sturich, J., Lee, J., Myers, S. E., Whitman, B. Y., Gold, J-A., Kimonis, V., Scheimann, A., Terrazas, N., and Driscoll, D. J. (2011). Growth standards of infants with Prader-Willi syndrome. *Pediatrics*, 127, 687–695.

Cronk, C., Crocker, A. C., Pueschel, S. M., Shea, A. M., Zackai, E., Pickens, G., and Reed, R. B. (1988). Growth charts for children with Down syndrome: 1 month to 18 years of age. (1988). *Pediatrics*, 81, 102–110.

El-Bassyouni, H. T., Afifi, H. H., Aglan, M. S., Mahmoud, W. M., and Zaki, M. E. (2012). Growth curves of Egyptian patients with Turner syndrome. *American Journal of Medical Genetics Part A*, 158A, 2687–2691.

Erkula, G., Jones, K. B., Sponseller, P. D., Diele, H. C., and Pyeritz, R. E. (2002). Growth and maturation in Marfan syndrome. *American Journal of Medical Genetics*, 109, 100–115.

Guzman, M. L., Delgado, I., Lay-Son, G., Willans, E., Alonso, P., and Repetto, G. M. (2012). Growth in Chilean infants with chromosome 22q11 microdeletion syndrome. *American Journal of Medical Genetics Part A*, 158A, 2682–2686.

Habel, A., McGinn, M-J., Zackai, E. H., Unanue, N., and McDonald-McGinn, D. M. (2012). Syndrome specific growth charts for 22q11.2 deletion syndrome in Caucasian children. *American Journal of Medical Genetics Part A*, 158A, 2665–2671.

Hall, J. G. (1985). A study of individuals with arthrogryposis. *Endocrine Genetics and Genetics of Growth*, pp. 155–162. New York: Alan R. Liss.

Hauffa, B. P., Schlippe, G., Roos, M., Gillessen-Kaesbach, G., and Gasser, T. (2000). Spontaneous growth in German children and adolescents with genetically confirmed Prader-Willi Syndrome. *Acta Paediatrica*, 89, 1302–1311.

Holm, V. A., and Nugent, J. K. (1982). Growth in the Prader-Willi syndrome. *Birth Defects: Original Article Series*, 18(3B), 93–100.

Hoover-Fong, J. E., McGready, J., Schulze, K. J., Barnes, H., and Scott, C. I. (2007). Weight for age charts for children with achondroplasia. *American Journal of Medical Genetics Part A*, 143A, 2227–2235.

Horton, W. A., Hall, J. G., Scott, C. I., Pyeritz, R. E., and Rimoin, D. L. (1982). Growth curves for height for diastrophic dysplasia, spondyloepiphyseal dysplasia congenita, and pseudoachondroplasia. *American Journal of Diseases in Children*, 136, 316–319.

Horton, W. A., Rotter, J. I., Rimoin, D. L., Scott, C. I., and Hall, J. G. (1978). Standard growth curves for achondroplasia. *Journal of Pediatrics*, 93, 435–438.

Hunter, A. G. W., Hecht, J. T., and Scott, C. I. Jr. (1996a). Standard weight for height curves in achondroplasia. *American Journal of Medical Genetics*, 62, 255–261.

Hunter, A. G. W., Reid, C. S., Pauli, R. M., and Scott, I. Jr. (1996b). Standard curves of chest circumference in achondroplasia and the relationship of chest circumference to respiratory problems. *American Journal of Medical Genetics*, 62, 91–97.

Ikeda, Y., Higurashi, M., Egi, S., Ohzeki, N., and Hoshina, H. (1982). An anthropometric study of girls with the Ullrich–Turner syndrome. *American Journal of Medical Genetics*, 12, 271–280.

Kline, A. D., Barr, M., and Jackson, L. G. (1993). Growth manifestations in the Brachmann–de Lange syndrome. *American Journal of Medical Genetics*, 47, 1042–1049.

Lee, R. W. Y., McGready, J., Conley, S. K., Yanjanin, N. M., Nowaczyk, M. J. M., and Porter, F. D. (2012). Growth charts for individuals with Smith–Lemli–Opitz syndrome. *American Journal of Medical Genetics Part A*, 158, 2707–2713.

Malaquias, A. C., Brasil, A. S., Pereira, A. C., Arnhold, I. J. P., Mendonca, B. B., Bertola, D. R., and Jorge, A. A. L. (2012). Growth standards of patients with Noonan and Noonan-like syndromes with mutations in the RAS/MAPK pathway. *American Journal of Medical Genetics Part A*, 158A, 2700–2706.

Marinescu, R. C., Mainardi, P. C., Collins, M. R., Kouahou, M., Coueourde, G., Pastore, G., Eaton-Evans, J., and Overhauser, J. (2000). Growth charts for Cri-du-chat syndrome: An international collaborative study. *American Journal of Medical Genetics*, 94, 153–162.

Martin, N. D. T., Smith, W. R., Cole, T. J., and Preece, M. A. (2007). New height, weight and head circumference charts for British children with Williams syndrome. *Archives of Disease in Childhood,* 92, 598–601.

Meaney, F. J., and Farrer, L. A. (1986). Clinical anthropometry and medical genetics: a compilation of body measurements in genetic and congenital disorders. *American Journal of Medical Genetics*, 25, 343–359.

Montano, A. M., Tomatsu, S., Brusius, A., Smith, M., and Orii, T. (2008). Growth charts for patients affected with Morquio A disease. *American Journal of Medical Genetics Part A,* 146A,1286–1295.

Morris, C. A., Derusey, S. A., Leonard, C. O., Dilts, C., and Blackburn, B. L. (1988). Natural history of Williams syndrome: physical characteristic. *Journal of Pediatrics*, 113, 318–326.

Myrelid, A., Gustafsson, J., Ollars, B., and Anneren, G. (2002). Growth charts for Down's syndrome for birth to 18 years of age. *Archives of Disease in Childhood*, 87, 97–103.

Nagai, T., Matsuo, N., Kayanuma, Y., Tonoki, H., Fukushima, Y., Ohashi, H., Murai, T., Hasegawa, T., Kuroki, Y., and Niikawa, N. (2000). Standard growth curves for Japanese patients with Prader-Willi syndrome. *American Journal of Medical Genetics*, 95, 130–134.

Palmer, C. G., Cronk, C., Pureschel, S. M., Wisniewski, K. E., Laxova, R., Crocker, A. C., and Pauli, R. M. (1992). Head circumference of children with Down syndrome (0–36 months). *American Journal of Medical Genetics*, 42, 61–67.

Pankau R, Partsch, C.J., Gosch A, Oppermann H. C., Wessel A. (1992). Statural growth in Williams-Beuren syndrome. *Eur J Pediatr*, 151:751–755.

Park, E., Bailey, J. D., and Cowell, C.A. (1983). Growth and maturation of patients with Turner's syndrome. *Pediatric Research*, 7, 1–7.

Pelz, V. L., Sussmann, S., Timm, D., and Rostock, I. (1981). Ullrich-Turner syndrome. *Kinderarztliche Praxis*, 49, 206–212.

Pyeritz, R. E. (1985). Growth and anthropometrics in the Marfan syndrome. In *Endocrine genetics and genetics of growth*, pp. 135–140. New York: Alan R. Liss.

Ranke, M. B., Heidemann, P., Knupfer, C., Enders, H., Schmaltz, A., and Bierich, J. R. (1988). Noonan syndrome: Growth and clinical manifestations in 144 cases. *European Journal of Paediatrics*, 48, 220–227.

Richards, G. (2006). Growth charts for children with Down syndrome. Available at http://www.growthcharts.com/. Accessed March 30, 2006.

Roberts, A. E., Nixon, C., Steward, C. G., Gauvreau, K., Maisenbacher, M., Fletcher, M., Geva, J., Byrne, B. J., and Spencer, C. T. (2012). The Barth

Syndrome Registry: Distinguishing disease characteristics and growth data from a longitudinal study. *American Journal of Medical Genetics Part A*, 158A, 2726–2732.

Sammon, M. R., Doyle, D., Hopkins, E., Sol-Church, K., Stabley, D. L., McGready, J., Schulze, K., Alade, Y., Hoover-Fong, J., and Gripp, K. W. (2012). Normative growth charts for individuals with Costello syndrome. *American Journal of Medical Genetics Part A*, 158A, 2692–2699.

Stevens, C. A., Hennekan, R. C. M., and Blackburn, B. L. (1990). Growth in the Rubinstein-Taybi syndrome. *American Journal of Medical Genetics Supplement*, 6, 51–55.

Szudek, J., Birch, P., Friedman, J. M. (2000). Growth in North American white children with neurofibromatosis 1 (NF1). *Journal of Medical Genetics*, 37, 933–938.

Tarquinio, D. C., Jones, M. C., Jones, K. L., and Bird, L. M. (2012). Growth charts for 22q11 deletion syndrome. *American Journal of Medical Genetics Part A, 158A*, 933–938.

Tüysüz, B., Göknar, N. T., and Öztürk, B. (2012). Growth charts of Turkish children with down syndrome. *American Journal of Medical Genetics Part A*, 158A, 2656–2664.

Verbeek, S., Eilers, P. H. C., Lawrence, K., Hennekam, R. C. M., and Versteegh, F. G. A. (2011). Growth charts for children with Ellis-van Creveld syndrome. *European Journal of Pediatrics*, 170, 207–211.

Witt, D. R., Keena, B. A., Hall, J. G., and Allanson, J. E. (1986). Growth curves for height in Noonan syndrome. *Clinical Genetics*, 30, 150–153.

Wollmann, H. A., Kirchner, T., Enders, H., Preece, M. A., and Ranke, M. B. (1995). Growth and symptoms in Silver-Russell syndrome: Review on the basis of 386 patients. *European Journal of Pediatrics*, 154, 958–968.

Wollmann, H. A., Schultz, U., Grauer, M. L., and Ranke, M. B. (1998). Reference values for height and weight in Prader-Willi syndrome based on 315 patients. *European Journal of Pediatrics*, 157, 634–642.

Chapter 18

An Approach to the Child with Dysmorphic Features

The approach to the child with unusual physical features, multiple congenital anomalies, or a dysmorphic syndrome is a complex one. Careful physical measurements are not only important for determining the child's condition and present status but are also important for establishing baseline measurements in order to follow the affected individual over time and to define the natural history of the condition. If a child is seen repeatedly, careful serial measurements are invaluable for demonstrating the disproportionate growth of different parts of the body and the changing proportions that may occur with time.

As stated earlier in the book, a measurement has meaning only in comparison with other measurements; therefore, all measurements need to be taken and recorded in a way that allows comparisons with norms for chronological age, the norms for height age, the bone age–related norms, or the age-related measurement of some other part of the body. In each area of the body, there is a standard against which other measurements should be compared. For example, in the craniofacial area, the age-related head circumference (OFC) is used for the comparison with other measurements. Are the ears small or large for the age that corresponds to the head size? For example a 6-year-old boy, who is 50th percentile for height with a head size that is 50th percentile for a 2-year-old and an ear size that is 50th percentile for a 4-year-old will appear to have large ears even though they are small for his age.

It is a general rule of thumb that any measurements that deviate more than two standard deviations from each other are considered to be outside the range of normal and need an explanation. Thus, if height is at the 10th percentile and weight is at the 90th percentile, although both measurements are normal, the child will be relatively overweight, and the physician should ask why. Similarly, if head circumference is at the 10th percentile and inner canthal distance is at the 90th percentile, the child will appear to have relative ocular hypertelorism, and the physician should ask why.

Similar to any other medical evaluation, a careful prenatal, medical, developmental, and family history; a thorough general physical examination; and appropriate laboratory evaluations should be obtained on a child with dysmorphic features or congenital anomalies. This book is aimed at providing data that allow the physician to describe and quantify physical anomalies as a meaningful and useful part of the evaluation. Most chapters deal with particular parts of the body. They outline the ways to describe and measure that area and provide graphs of normal values for frequently used measurements. There are about 36 measurements that should be performed on all children who are evaluated for dysmorphic features. These 36 measurements take less than 10 minutes to record. If a particular area seems to be disproportionate or abnormal, additional measurements or studies that can be performed. Photographs should be taken with parental permission.

Figure 18.1 gives an example of an outline form for recording measurements. If the child is quiet, they can be done in a logical way. If the child is crying or agitated, it can be helpful to obtain distal measurements such as hands, feet, and OFC first, before moving in toward the face and chest.

After the measurements are obtained, they should be compared with the normal age- and sex-related standards. Percentiles for the individual are generated. The measurements are then analyzed and deviating percentiles can be evaluated. The next step is to compare the measurements with the norms for height age of that child. For example, if the chronological age of the child is 4 years but the child's

Patient name ______________ **Date of birth** ______________ **Hospital no.** ______________

Paternal ethnic origin ______________ **Height** ______________ **Date of examination** ______________

Maternal ethnic origin ______________ **Height** ______________ **Examiner** ______________

Patient age ______________ **Height age** ______________ **Bone age** ______________

	Percentile						Other anomalies
	Right	**Left**	**Chron-ologic age**	**Height age**	**Bone age**		
Body							
Length/height							
Weight							
Span							
Lower segment							
Upper segment (crown–rump or sitting height)							
U/L segment ratio							
Chest circumference							
Internipple distance							
Sternal length							
Craniofacies							
Head circumference (OFC)							
Anterior fontanelle							
Facial width							
Facial height							
Outer canthal distance							
Inner canthal distance							
Interpupillary distance							
Palpebral fissure length							
Nasal height							
Nasal protrusion							
Nasal width							
Ear length							
Ear width							
Ear position							
Ear rotation							
Philtrum length							
Mouth width							
Limbs							
Hand length							
Palm length							
Palm width							
Finger length							
Elbow angle							
Foot length							
Foot width							
Genitalia							
Labial size							
Testicle size							
Penile length							

Development assessment ______________

____

Summary of unusual/abnormal measurements ______________

____

Any special techniques or instruments for measuring ______________

Dermatoglyphics done Yes/No **Photographs done** Yes/No **X-ray done** Yes/No **Bone age done** Yes/No

Figure 18.1. An example of an easy-to-use outline form for recording measurements.

height is that of an average (e.g., 50th percentile) 2-year-old, the other body measurements need to be compared to the 2-year-old standards. They may be completely normal for 2 years, suggesting that the child is growing like a 2-year-old, or there may be marked disproportion. It may then be useful to compare particular parts of the body, such as comparing hand and foot measurements to the "age-related" or "height-related" hand and foot standards. These comparisons allow the physician to define better which body area, if any, is disproportionate. Finally, the child's measurements should be compared to bone age–related norms. If the bone age was advanced in the 4-year-old described earlier, the disparity between chronological age and height would be even greater.

In subsequent examinations, repeated measurements may be taken in the same way, allowing the construction of a longitudinal growth curve for various areas of the body. In many syndromes with disproportionate growth, the growth curves have not yet been defined. The definition of disproportionate growth in various body areas in these conditions should allow better understanding of the pathogenetic mechanisms leading to the disproportionate growth.

GLOSSARY

accessory nipple Additional nipple, unilateral or bilateral, on the trunk, lying on the "milk line," which runs caudally from the normal position of the nipples and cranially toward the axilla.

acrocephaly Tall or high skull; the top of the head is pointed, peaked, or conical in shape; usually involving premature closure of the lambdoid and coronal sutures, with a vertical index above 77; also referred to as *oxycephaly*, *turricephaly*, and *tower skull*.

acromelic Referring to the distal portion of the limb.

ala nasi The most lateral part of the nose: the flaring cartilaginous area forming the outer side of each naris (nostril).

albinism Deficiency or absence of pigment in the hair, skin, and/or eyes.

alopecia Absence, loss, or deficiency of hair; may be patchy or total; transient or congenital, natural or abnormal.

aniridia Absence of the iris.

anisocoria Unequal pupil size.

anisomastia Asymmetric or irregular size of the breasts.

ankyloblepharon Adhesion of the ciliary edges of the eyelids to each other.

anodontia Absence of teeth.

anonychia Absence of nails.

anophthalmia Congenital absence or hypoplasia of one or both eyes.

anthropometrics The study of comparative measurements of the human body.

aphakia Absence of the lens of the eye.

arachnodactyly Long slender hands, feet, fingers, and toes; spider fingers, dolichostenomelia.

areola Pigmented skin surrounding the nipple.

arrhinencephaly Congenital absence of the rhinencephalon (hind brain).

arrhinia Congenital absence of the nose.

bathrocephaly A step-like posterior projection of the skull, caused by bulging of the squamous portion of the occipital bone.

biacromial distance Maximum distance between the right and left acromion (shoulder width).

bigonial distance Distance between the lateral aspect of the angle of the jaw on the right and the same point on the left (mandible width).

bi-iliac distance Distance between the most prominent lateral points of the iliac crest.

birth mark Regionally limited alteration of skin color caused by vascular or pigment-distribution anomalies.

bizygomatic distance Maximal distance between the most lateral points on the zygomatic arches (zygion) (facial width).

Blaschko line Streak of pigmented skin reflecting embryonic migration of pigment-producing cells.

blepharochalasis Relaxation or redundancy of the skin of the upper eyelid, so that a fold of skin hangs down, often concealing the corner of the eye.

blue nevus Bluish macular area, mostly over the sacrum and back. More frequent in African, American, Hispanic, and Asian people.

bone age Radiological assessment of physiological age relating growth and skeletal maturation; stage of development of the skeleton as judged by X-rays and compared with chronological age.

bony interorbital distance The distance between the medial margins of the bony orbit, measured radiographically.

brachycephaly Shortening of the length of the skull; the cephalic index is 81.0 to 85.4.

brachydactyly Short finger.

brachyturricephaly Combination of shortening of the skull (brachycephaly) along with towering of the skull (turricephaly, oxycephaly, or acrocephaly).

Brushfield spot Mottled, marbled, or speckled elevation of the iris due to increased density of the anterior border layer of the iris; white or light yellow iris nodule caused by deposition or aggregation of stromal fibrocytes; observed in 85% of patients with Down syndrome. Can be noted in the normal population (about 25%).

buphthalmos Congenital glaucoma; keratoglobus, or enlargement of the eye.

café-au-lait macule Macular area of increased pigment greater than 0.5 cm in diameter. More than five café-au-lait spots of 1.5 cm or greater can be a sign of neurofibromatosis.

calipers Instrument used for measuring distance or thickness.

calvarium Upper, dome-like portion of the skull.

camptodactyly Flexion contracture of a finger or toe; permanent flexion of one or both interphalangeal joints of one or more fingers; bent fingers.

canthal distance, inner Distance between the inner canthi (inner corners) of the two eyes.

canthal distance, outer Distance between the outer canthi (outer corners) of the two eyes.

capillary hemangioma Pink macular mark, localized over the forehead, face, or nape of the neck in the newborn (angel's kiss, salmon patch, stork bite, nevus simplex, erythema nuchae). Represents the fetal circulatory pattern in the skin and will resolve spontaneously.

carpal angle Angle made by the carpal bones at the wrist.

carrying angle Angle subtended by the forearm on the humerus; the deviation of the forearm relative to the humerus; the angle at the elbow joint.

cavernous hemangioma Elevated vascular nevus or strawberry nevus of solid red color.

cebocephaly Form of holoprosencephaly with ocular hypotelorism and a centrally placed nose with a single blind-ended nostril.

cephalic index The ratio of head width, expressed as a percentage of head length:

$$CI = \frac{\text{head width} \times 100}{\text{head length}}$$

cephalometrics The science of precise measurement of bones of the cranium and face, using fixed reproducible positions.

cheilion Most lateral point of the corner of the mouth.

chest circumference Circumference of the chest at the level of the nipples.

chordee Abnormal position of the penis caused by a band of tissue that holds the penis in a ventral or lateral curvature.

clinodactyly Permanent lateral or medial curve (deflection) of one or more fingers or toes.

coloboma Fissuring defect especially of the eye; may involve several layers (i.e., iris, retina, lid), usually congenital but may be of traumatic origin.

columella Fleshy inferior border of the septum of the nose.

concha Structure resembling a shell in shape (e.g., hollow of the external ear, turbinate bone).

cornea, transverse diameter Distance between the medial and lateral border of the iris.

craniorachischisis Congenital failure of closure of the skull and spinal column.

crown–rump length Distance from the top of the head to the bottom of the buttock, with hips in flexion.

cubitus valgus Increased carrying angle at elbow.

cuticle Remnant of the eponychium at the base of a fingernail.

cutis aplasia Absence of skin in specific area; commonly of the scalp at the vertex.

cryptophthalmos Complete congenital adhesion of the eyelid; fused eyelid.

cryptorchidism Failure of the testis to descend into the scrotum.

cystic hygroma Sac, distended with lymphatic fluid, found usually in the neck.

dental age Physiological age of teeth as determined by the number and type of teeth that have erupted or been shed.

Denver Developmental Screening Test A screening test for gross motor, fine motor-adaptive, language, and personal–social skills.

depigmentation Area of absent or reduced pigment due to lack of functional melanocytes. Leaf-shaped area of depigmentation can be a sign of tuberous sclerosis.

dermal ridge count Number of dermal ridges in a particular dermal ridge pattern.

dermatoglyphics Pattern of ridges and grooves of the skin, best seen on the palms and soles.

dermatome Segmental area of skin defined by the distribution of sensory innervation.

dermis Underlying layer of the skin.

developmental delay Delay in acquisition of developmental milestones in comparison with age-related cohort.

dimple Indentation of the skin where the skin is deficient or attached to underlying structures, especially bone.

dolichocephaly Elongation of the skull; with narrowing from side to side. Cephalic index is 75.9 or less (*see also* scaphocephaly).

dystopia canthorum Lateral displacement of the inner canthi of the eye.

ear length Maximum distance from the superior aspect to the inferior aspect of the external ear (pinna).

ear position Location of the superior attachment of the pinna. Note that the size and rotation of the external ear are not relevant.

ear protrusion Protrusion of each ear, measured by the angle subtended from the posterior aspect of the pinna to the mastoid plane of the skull.

ear rotation/angulation Rotation of the longitudinal axis of the external ear (pinna).

ear width Width of the external ear (pinna), from just anterior to the tragus to the lateral margin of the helix.

ectopia Misplaced structure.

ectopia lentis Displacement of the crystalline lens of the eye.

ectopia pupillaris Abnormal eccentric location of the pupil.

ectropion Eversion or turning out of an edge (e.g., of an eyelid or of the lip).

encephalocele Herniation of the brain, manifested by protrusion through a congenital or traumatic opening of the skull; can be frontal or occipital.

enophthalmus Abnormal retraction of the eye into the orbit, producing a deeply set eye.

entropion Inversion of an edge (e.g., of the eyelid).

epicanthal fold Congenital fold of tissue medial to the eye consisting of a vertical fold of skin lateral to the nose, sometimes covering the inner canthus.

epidermis Superficial layer of the skin.

epiphora Abnormal overflow of tears down the cheek; mainly caused by stricture of the nasolacrimal duct.

epispadias Abnormal location of the urethra on the dorsal surface of the penis.

eponychium Epidermal layer which covers the developing fingernail prenatally.

esotropia Inward deviation of an eye when both eyes are open and uncovered; convergent strabismus.

ethmocephaly Form of holoprosencephaly in which there are two separate but hypoteloric eyes and a supraorbital proboscis.

eurion Most prominent lateral point on each side of the skull in the area of the parietal and temporal bones.

exophthalmos Abnormal protrusion of the eyeball.

exotropia Outward deviation of an eye when both eyes are opened and uncovered; divergent strabismus.

facial height Distance from the root of the nose (nasion) to the lowest median landmark on the lower border of the mandible (menton or gnathion); lower two-thirds of the craniofacies.

facial height, lower Distance from the base of the nose (subnasion) to the lowest median landmark on the lower border of the mandible (menton or gnathion); length of the lower one-third of the craniofacies.

facial height, upper Distance from the root of the nose (nasion) to the base of the nose (subnasion); middle one-third of the craniofacies.

facial index Ratio of facial height (nasion to menton) to facial width (bizygomatic distance) used to assess a long, narrow face as compared with a short, wide face.

facial width *See* bizygomatic distance.

finger clubbing Enlargement of the distal part of the finger and nail, with abnormally curved nail and loss of the angle at the nail fold.

flexion crease Crease in skin overlying a joint; secondary to movement at that joint.

fontanelle (fontanel) Membrane-covered space remaining in the incompletely ossified skull of a fetus or infant.

fontanelle size, anterior Sum of the longitudinal and transverse diameters of the anterior fontanella along the sagittal and coronal sutures.

fontanelle size, posterior Length of the posterior fontanelle.

forehead height *See* skull height.

Frankfort plane (FP) Eye–ear plane that is a standard horizontal cephalometric reference. The Frankfort plane or Frankfort horizontal is established when the head is held erect, with the eyes forward, so that the lowest margin of the lower bony orbit (orbitale) and the upper margin of the external auditory meatus (porion) are in the same horizontal plane (the Frankfort plane).

frenulum Small fold of integument or of mucous membrane that may limit the movement of an organ or part (e.g., beneath the tongue).

frontal bossing Prominence of the anterior portion of the frontal bone of the skull.

gastroschisis Congenital fissure of the abdominal wall not involving the site of insertion of the umbilical cord, and usually accompanied by protrusion of the small and part of the large intestine.

genu recurvatum Hyperextension of the knee.

genu valgum Outward bowing of knee; bow-leg.

genu varum Inward deviation of the knee; knock-knee.

gibbus Extreme kyphosis or hump; deformity of the spine in which there is a sharply angulated segment, the apex of the angle being posterior.

glabella The most prominent midline point between the eyebrows.

glossoptosis Downward displacement or retraction of the tongue; sometimes held by a frenulum.

gnathion The lowest median point on the inferior border of the mandible; *see* menton.

gonion The most lateral point of the posteroinferior angle of the mandible.

head circumference Distance around the head at its largest part.

head length Maximum dimension of the sagittal axis of the skull.

head width Maximal biparietal diameter.

height Distance from the top of the head to the sole of the foot in a standing position.

heterochromia Unequal color, usually used in reference to the iris.

holoprosencephaly Impaired midline cleavage of the embryonic forebrain, the most extreme form being cyclopia; a less severe form is arrhinencephaly.

hydrocephaly Abnormal increase in the amount of cerebrospinal fluid accompanied by dilatation of the cerebral ventricles.

hyperextensibility Excessive capability of the skin to stretch; excessive range of movement at a joint.

hypertelorism Abnormal distance between two organs or parts; commonly used to describe increased interpupillary distance (ocular hypertelorism).

hypoacusis Decreased perception of sound.

hypodontia Reduced number of teeth (*see* also oligodontia).

hyponychia Small dysplastic nails.

hypospadias Abnormal location of the urethra on the ventral surface of the penis; may be glandular (1°), penile (2°), scrotal (3°), or perineal (4°).

hypotelorism Abnormally decreased distance between two organs or parts, commonly used to describe decreased interpupillary distance (ocular hypotelorism).

imperforate anus Absence of the normal anal opening.

intelligence quotient (IQ) General intellectual functioning as assessed by special tests.

interalar distance (nasal width) Distance between the most lateral aspects of the alae nasi.

intercommissural distance Mouth width at rest; the distance between the two outer corners of the mouth (cheilion).

internipple distance Distance between the centers of both nipples.

interpupillary distance Distance between the centers of the pupils of the two eyes.

inverted nipple Inwardly directed tip of the nipple; nipple does not protrude from the areola.

iridodonesis Tremor of the iris on movement; usually due to dislocation of the lens.

Kayser–Fleischer ring Greenish-brownish pigment ring due to the deposition of copper at the outer edge of the cornea; as noted in Wilson disease.

keratoconus Conical protrusion of the cornea.

koilonychia Spoon-shaped nails.

kyphoscoliosis Abnormal curvature of the spinal column, both anteroposteriorly and laterally.

kyphosis Curvature of the spine in the anteroposterior plane. A normal kyphosis exists in the shoulder area.

lagophthalmos Condition in which the eyelid cannot be completely closed.

lanugo Embryonic or fetal hair; fine, soft, unmedullated.

length Distance between the top of the head and the sole of the foot when the individual is lying down (height).

lentigo Round or oval, flat, brown, pigmented skin spot caused by increased deposition of melanin, in association with an increased number of melanocytes at the epidermodermal junction.

leukoma Dense white opacity of the cornea.

leukonychia White spots or stripes on the nails.

lingua plicata Fissured tongue.

Lisch nodule Hamartomatous iris structure, usually visible only by slit lamp.

lordosis Curvature of the spinal column with a forward (ventral) convexity. A normal lordosis exists in the lumbar area.

lower segment Distance from the pubic bone to the sole of the foot.

lymphangioma Overgrowth of lymphatic vessels.

macrocephaly Abnormally large head.

macrocranium Abnormally large skull.

macrodactyly Abnormally large digit.

macrocheilia Abnormal or excessive size of the lip.

macroglossia Abnormally large or hypertrophic tongue.

macromastia Abnormally large breast.

macronychia Abnormally large nail.

macrophthalmia Abnormally large eye.

macrostomia Abnormally large mouth.

mandible width *See* bigonial distance.

mandibular length, effective Effective length and prominence of the mandible (cephalometric).

manubrium Cranial portion of the sternum that articulates with the clavicles and the first two pairs of ribs.

maxillomandibular differential Measurement determined by subtracting the effective midfacial length from the effective mandibular length (cephalometric).

megalocephaly Abnormally large head.

melanocyte Pigment cell in the skin.

menton The lowest medial landmark on the lower border of the mandible, identified by palpation, and identical to the bony gnathion.

mesomelic Referring to the middle segment of the limb.

microcephaly Abnormally small head.

microcranium Abnormally small skull.

microgenia Abnormally small chin; an alternative term for *micrognathia.*

microglossia Abnormally small tongue.

micrognathia Abnormally small jaw, especially with lower jaw recession (small chin).

micronychia Abnormally small nail.

microphallus Abnormally small penis; micropenis.

microphthalmia Abnormally small eye.

microstomia Abnormally small opening of the mouth.

midfacial length, effective Size and prominence of the maxilla (cephalometric).

mid-parental height Sum of parents' heights divided by two.

miosis Small, contracted pupil.

mole Circumscribed area of dark pigment that is often raised.

monilethrix Hair exhibiting marked multiple constrictions, with a beading effect and increased brittleness.

mouth width *See* intercommissural distance.

mydriasis Large, dilated pupil.

nasal height The distance from the nasal root (nasion) to base (subnasion).

nasal width *See* interalar distance.

nasion Midline point at the nasal root over the nasofrontal suture.

nevus sebaceous Raised waxy patch, with a mostly linear distribution.

nipple Papilla of the breast.

nystagmus Involuntary rapid movement of the eyeball that may be horizontal, vertical, rotatory, or mixed.

obliquity (slant) of the palpebral fissure Slant of the palpebral fissure from the horizontal.

occipitofrontal circumference (OFC) Distance around the head, the largest obtainable measurement (head circumference).

oligodontia Less than the normal number of teeth (*see* hypodontia).

omphalocele Protrusion, at birth, of part of the intestine through a defect in the abdominal wall at the umbilicus. Protruding bowel is covered only by a thin transparent membrane composed of amnion and peritoneum.

ONO angle Angle subtended from the base of the nose in the midline to the outer canthi of the eyes.

ophthalmoplegia Paralysis of the eye muscles.

opisthocranion Most posterior portion of the occipital bone in the midline.

orbital protrusion Degree of protrusion of the eye (exophthalmos).

orbitale The lowest point of the inferior bony margin of the orbit, identified by palpation.

orchidometer Measuring device for quantifying testicular size.

oxycephaly *See* acrocephaly.

pachyonychia Long thickened nails.

palpebral fissure length Distance between the inner and outer canthus of one eye.

pattern profile Analysis of hand bone length, used to recognize particular syndromes.

pectus carinatum Undue prominence of the sternum, often referred to as pigeon chest.

pectus excavatum Undue depression of the sternum, often referred to as funnel chest.

pes calcaneovalgus Dorsiflexion of the foot due to a contracture of foot (rocker bottom foot).

pes cavus High arched foot with metatarsal heads pushed down (claw foot).

pes equinovarus Planter flexion with internal rotation of ankle joint (club foot).

pes valgus External rotation at ankle joint.

philtrum Ventrical groove in the midline of the upper lip, extending from beneath the nose to the vermilion border of the upper lip.

pili annulati Defect of keratin synthesis resulting in an irregular distribution of air-filled cavities along the hairshaft, which reflects the light differently and appears as alternating bands of white.

pili torti Hair twisted by 180-degree angle.

plagiocephaly Asymmetric head shape.

Poland anomaly Absent or hypoplastic nipple and/or breast tissue in association with aberrant or hypoplastic pectoral development and limb deficiency.

polydactyly Extra digit.

polysyndactyly Extra digit with fused digits.

polythelia Occurrence of more than one nipple on a breast.

porion Highest point on the upper margin of the cutaneous external auditory meatus.

portwine nevus Dark angioma, which can be purple in color and raised.

postaxial Posterior or lateral to the axis (as in postaxial polydactyly, where the extra finger is lateral to the fifth finger).

preaxial Anterior or medial to the axis (as in preaxial polydactyly, where the extra digit is medial to the thumb).

prognathism Protrusion of the jaw.

prolabium Prominent central part of the upper lip, in its full thickness, which overlies the premaxilla.

pronasale Most protruded point of the tip of the nose.

pterygium Wing-shaped web; with regard to the eye, a patch of thickened conjunctiva extending over a part of the cornea. The membrane is usually fan-shaped, with the apex toward the pupil and the base toward the inner canthus. With regard to the limbs, a skin web across a joint.

pterygium colli Thick fold or web of skin on the lateral aspect of the neck, extending from the mastoid region to the acromion.

ptosis Falling or sinking down of any organ (e.g., a drooping of the upper eyelid or breast).

range of movement Range of place or position through which a particular joint can move.

retrognathia Retrusion of the jaw back from the frontal plane of the forehead.

rhizomelic Referring to the proximal portion of the limb.

saddle nose Nose with a sunken bridge.

scaphocephaly Abnormally long and narrow skull as a result of premature closure of the sagittal suture (*see also* dolichocephaly).

scoliosis Appreciable lateral deviation from the normally straight vertical line of the spine.

shawl scrotum Congenital ventral insertion of the scrotum.

single palmar crease Single crease extending across palm.

sitting height Distance from the top of the head to the buttocks when in sitting position.

skinfold thickness Thickness of skin in designated areas (triceps, subscapular, suprailiac), used to assess subcutaneous fat and nutrition.

skull height (forehead height) Distance from the root of the nose (nasion) to the highest point of the head (vertex).

span Distance between the tips of the middle fingers of each hand when the arms are stretched out horizontally from the body.

Sprengel deformity Congenital upward displacement of the scapula.

stadiometer Upright measuring device.

sternal length Length of the sternum from the top of the manubrium to the inferior border of the xiphisternum.

stellate iris Iris pattern (star-like) with prominent iris stroma radiating out from the pupil.

strabismus Deviation of the eye; the visual axes assume a position relative to each other different from that required by physiological conditions.

The various forms of strabismus are spoken of as tropias, their direction being indicated by the appropriate prefix, as in esotropia, exotropia, and so on.

subalare Point at the inferior border of each alar base, where the alar base disappears into the skin of the upper lip.

submental Situated below the chin.

subnasale Midpoint of the columella base at the apex of the angle where the lower border of the nasal septum and the surface of the upper lip meet.

symblepharon Adhesion of the eyelid to the eyeball.

symphalangy Extension contracture of a finger or toe with fusion of the joint.

syndactyly Webbing or fusion of fingers or toes.

synechia Adhesion of parts; especially, adhesion of the iris to the cornea or to the lens.

syngnathia Intraoral bands, possibly remnants of the buccopharyngeal membrane, extending between the jaws.

synophrys Confluent eyebrow growth across the glabella.

talipes/clubfoot Fixed abnormal position of foot due to contracture at ankle; equinovarus, calcaneovalgus.

Tanner stages Grading system to establish visual standards for the stages of puberty.

telangiectasis Prominence of blood vessels on the surface of the skin.

telecanthus Increased distance between the inner canthi of the eyes.

testicular volume Volume of the testis established by an orchidometer, or calculated from measurement or ultrasound.

thoracic index Ratio of the anteroposterior diameter of the chest to the chest width.

torso length Distance from the top of the sternum to the symphysis pubis.

torticollis Contracted state of the cervical muscles, producing twisting of the neck, resulting in an unnatural position of the head. The most common causes for this condition are trauma, inflammation, or congenital malformation involving the cervical vertebrae and/or the sternocleidomastoid muscle on one side.

tragion Superior margin of the tragus of the ear.

trichoglyphics Pattern of hair follicles.

trichorrhexis Nodular swelling of the hair. The hair is light colored and breaks easily.

trigonocephaly Triangular-shaped head and skull resulting from premature synostosis of the portions of the frontal bone with prominence of the metopic suture.

triphalangeal thumb Thumb with three phalanges.

triradius Dermatoglyphic pattern where three sets of ridges converge.

turricephaly *See* acrocephaly.

umbilical cord length Length of the umbilical cord from the insertion at the placenta to the abdominal wall of the neonate.

upper segment Distance from the top of the head to the pubic bone.

vermillion border Red-colored edge of the lip where it meets the normal skin of the face.

vertex Highest point of the head in the midsagittal plane, when the head is held erect.

weight Heaviness of an object or individual.

widow's peak Pointed frontal hairline in the midline that may be seen with ocular hypertelorism.

wormian bone Small, irregular bone in the suture between the bones of the skull.

xiphoid process Most caudal bone of the sternum that articulates with the manubrium and the lowermost ribs.

zygion Most lateral point of each zygomatic arch.

INDEX

Accessory fontanelles, 112, 115
Achenbach behavior checklist, 370
Achondroplasia
  chest circumference, 417
  head circumference, 415–416
  height, 409–410
  weight, 411–414
Acromion of scapula, 201, 204, 278, 351
Adams-Oliver syndrome, 318
Adaptive functioning assessment, 370–371
Adolescence
  breast/nipple development, 304
  craniofacies growth, 91
  growth peak, 11
  height velocity growth, 44–48
  hyperextensibility in, 260
  hypermobility in, 259
African Americans
  anterior fontanelles, 119
  blue nevus in, 315
  body hair, pubertal changes, 290
  ossification centers, 349
  palpebral fissure length, 134–136
Age-appropriate psychometric testing, 370
Aglossia (absence of tongue), 179
Amelogenesis imperfecta, 181
Anagen stage (of hair), 322
Anal stenosis, 303
Angel's kiss, 316
Anocutaneous anal fistula, 303
Anovulvar fistula, 303
Anterior fontanelle, 115–119
Anthropometric measurement, 106
Anthropometry
  defined, 6
  instruments used in, 7, 8
  photogrametric, 8
Anus
  anomalies, 302, 303
  development of, 286
  diameter of, 302
  placement of, 301
  stenosis of, 302
Anus-to-fourchette (AF) distance, 301–302
Apgar score, 366
Apocrine sweat glands, 286–287, 314, 319
Areola, 306–307, 367

Arm. *See also* Forearm; Hand
forearm length, 207–211
lower arm length, 6
sweat pores in, 321
total upper limb length, 6, 201–203
upper arm length, 6, 204–207
Array-based comparative genomic hybridization (aCGH), 394
Asians
blue nevus in, 315
epicanthal folds, 124
height, in Prader-Willis syndrome, 496–497
Ataxia-telangiectasia syndrome, 317
Auditory canal, 16, 18, 148
Auricle (ear), 141–145, 154

Babinski reflex, 366
Back. *See also* Spine; Vertebrae; Vertebral column
abnormalities, 263
lanugo hair whorls, 343
Barth syndrome
height, 418
weight, 419
Bathrocephaly, 95
Bayley Scales of infant development, 370
Beery-Buktenica test of visual-motor integration, 370
Biacromial diameter, 6
Biacromial distance, 278–279
Bi-iliac distance, 280–281
Biparietal diameter (BPD)
fetal biometric data measures, 378
fetal monitoring, 10
gestational age and, 381
head width and, 98
head-to-trunk ratio, 379
orbit size and, 388
Birth. *See also* Newborn
body mass index, 64, 66
body proportions, 14–15
crown-rump length at, 36, 37, 38
growth velocity, post-birth, 11
height velocity, 44, 47
length at, 16, 21, 25, 29, 30
parameters, landmarks, 10
recumbent length at, 27, 32
weight, 53–56, 58, 60
weight, by gestational age, 52
Birthmarks, 315–318
Birthweight by gestational age
in Down syndrome, 439
in Trisomy 13, 508
in Trisomy 18, 510
Bizygomatic distance (facial width), 109–110
Blaschko lines, 312
Blepharochalasis, 169
Blepharophimosis, 134
Blue nevus, 315
Body landmarks, 6
Body mass index (BMI)
at birth, 64, 66
calculation, 63
females, for age, 66
females, North American, 2-20 years, 65
males, for age, 64
males, North American, 2-20 years, 63
Body proportions, 14–15
Bone age. *See also* Ossification centers
in children, 547
definition, 345
dental analysis determination, 352–355
description, 11–12
height prediction and, 41
radiographic determination, 11
testicular volume from, 296–297
Bony interorbital distance, 122–123
Bony syndactyly, 199
BRAF mutation
length and height, 487
weight, 488
Brain
fetal abnormalities, 391
fontanelles/growth of, 114
head circumference and, 10
head shape and, 92

hindbrain malformation, 325
postmortem weight, 399, 400–401, 403–404
prenatal measurement, 391
scalp hair patterning and, 121–122, 341–342
skull development and, 92
Branchial arch abnormality, 109
Branchial cysts, 87, 192
Breasts
areola, 306–307, 367
development of, 265, 286–290, 304, 306–307, 367
internipple distance, 269–270
nipple. *See* nipple
ptosis of, 306
shape and size, 304–305
sweat pores in, 321
volume, 305–306

Café au lait macule, 315
Calf. *See* Lower leg
Calvaria sutures, 92–93, 112
Capillary hemangioma, 316–318, 317
Capillary malformation syndromes, 316
Capillary malformation-arteriovenous malformation syndrome, 316
Carpal angle, 362–363
Carrying angle, forearm, 211–212
Catagen stage (of hair), 322
Caucasian American
anterior fontanelles, 119
blue nevus in, 315
body hair, pubertal changes, 290
dentinogenesis imperfecta, 181
epicanthal folds, 124
mouth size variation, 168–169
ossification centers, 349
Cavernous hemangioma, 317
Cephalic index, 100
Cephalometry
effective mandibular length, 187
effective midfacial length, 183
lower facial height, 105, 106
palate length, 173
radiography employed by, 90
Cervical vertebrae, 192
CHARGE syndrome (ears), 146
Chest. *See also* Breasts; Ribs; Trunk
biacromial distance, 276–277
circumference, 10, 14, 266–268
inspection of, 265–266
sternal length, 273–275
thoracic index, 271–273
torso length, 276–277
Chest circumference
in Achondroplasia, 417
description, 266–268
fetal chest circumference, 10
gestational age and, 268
head circumference comparison, 14
in infants, 14
nipples and, 266
Children
head circumference (OFC), 10
height prediction, 41
measurement standards, 16
nasal root in, 158
total body length measurement, 17
weight position, 50
Circumference
abdomen, 378, 389
chest. *See* chest circumference
head. *See* head circumference
head-to-abdomen, 380
limbs, 250–252
lower leg (calf), 235
neck, 193–194
upper leg (thigh), 233, 252
Clavicle
development of, 263
length, 386
prenatal measurement, 377
radiograph measurement, 351
Cleft abnormality, 105
Cleft lip, with/without cleft palate, 113, 157, 167, 187
Cleft sternum, 263
Cleidocranial dysplasia (cleidocranial dysostosis), 112
Clitoris, 285–286, 302, 367
Cloverleaf skull, 96

Colon, 406
Columella length (nose), 161–162
Combination curve
  directions for use of, 41
  males/females, mid-parental height, 40
Compound nevus, 316
Congenital alopecia, 319
Congenital heart disease, 327
Congenital hip dislocation, 192
Connective tissue disorders, 255
Contractures
  crown-rump length and, 36
  foot, 235, 239
  hand/wrist, 214
  legs, 24, 229
  limbs, 198, 201, 203
  middle finger length, 217
Cornea
  dimensions, transverse diameter, 140–141
  megalocornea, 126
  microcornea, 126
  size/shape variance, 126
Cornelia de Lange syndrome
  head circumference, females, 429
  head circumference, males, 428
  height, females, 422–423
  height, males, 125, 420–421, 420–429
  weight, females, 426–427
  weight, males, 424–425
Costello syndrome, 124
  head circumference, males, females, 432
  height, males and females, 430
  weight, males and females, 431
Craniofacial dysostosis, 112
Craniofacies, 86–194
  age-related reductions, 91
  cephalometry method, 90
  craniofacial pattern profile analysis, 90
  dysmorphic features, 86
  ears, 141–156
  eyes, 122–141
  face. *See* face
  fontanelles, 93, 112–121
  Frankfort horizontal head orientation, 88
  head. *See* head
  mandible, 89, 105, 186–191
  maxilla, 86–87, 89, 92, 145, 169, 176, 180, 182–186
  mouth, 168–171
  neck, 192–194
  nose, 103–104, 156–165
  palate, 172–177
  palpable landmarks, 89
  philtrum, 87, 166–168, 169
  scalp/facial hair patterning, 121–122
  skull. *See* skull
  teeth, 87, 172, 180–182
Cranio-fronto-nasal syndrome, 326
Craniosynostosis, 83
Cri-du-chat syndrome
  head circumference, 438
  height, 432–435
  weight, 436–437
Crown-rump length (CRL)
  at birth, 36, 37, 38
  defined, 35
  fetal biometric data, 378
  fetal monitoring, 10
  instruments, 35
  landmarks, 35
  position, 35
  and sitting height, 37, 38
Cutaneous syndactyly, 199
Cutis aplasia, 318
Cutis aplasia, 318
Cyanotic congenital heart disease, 327
Cyclopia, 183
Cystic fibrosis, 327
Cystic hygroma, 318

Darwinian tubercle, 144
Deciduous teeth, 87, 180–182, 352
Deformational posterior plagiocephaly, 94
Dental age, 352–355
Dentinogenesis imperfecta, 181
Denver Development Screening Test (DDST), 370, 372

Denver Development Screening Test II (DDST II), 372–374
Depigmentation (birthmark), 316
Dermal ridges
  count of, 334
  pattern alteration, 337
  patterns, 332
Dermatoglyphics
  analysis/recording methods, 332–334
  definition, 330
  dermal ridge count, 334
  Down syndrome patterns, 338
  epidermal ridge pattern, 309, 319, 331–332
  fingerprint patterns, 335–337
  flexion creases analysis, 338–340
  hallucal patterns, 335
  hypothenar patterns, 335
  ridge pattern analysis, 332–337
  thenar patterns, 335
  triradii (deltas), 335
Dermis
  description, 309–310
  development of, 309
  pigmentation variation, 315, 317
  skin color and, 314
  sweat glands in, 320
Developmental assessment
  behavioral, 365
  gestational age estimates, 367–368
  growth and movement, 365
  intelligence, 369–371
  neonatal reflexes, 366
  neurodevelopment, 366
  reflex patterns, 365–366
Developmental screening, 371–375
Dimple, 318
Distichiasis, 124
Dolichocephaly, 93–95
Dolichocilia, 124
Doll's eyes reflex, 366
Double lip, 169
Down syndrome
  aberrant scalp patterns in, 122, 341
  birthweight, by gestational age, 439
  fetal phenotype manifestation, 12
  fontanelles in, 112–113, 120
  foot patterns in, 337–338
  hand patterns in, 337–338, 340
  head circumference, 440, 449–450, 459–460
  height, 442, 444, 451–454, 461–464
  iris hypoplasia in, 125
  keratoconus in, 126
  length, 441, 443, 455–456, 462–463
  macroglossia (large tongue) in, 179
  open hallucal fields in, 335
  small ears in, 146
  weight, 445–448, 457–458
Dubowitz syndrome, 124
Duodenum, 406
Dysmorphic features, 1, 4–7, 12–13, 544–547

Ears, 141–156
  abnormalities, 146
  anatomy of, 141–144
  angulation, 154–156
  auricle, 141–145, 154
  auricular hillocks, 144–145
  congenital malformation, 87
  cryptotia of, 143–144
  cupped/protuberance of, 148
  evaluation/assessment of, 142
  length, 145–147
  microtia, types I-IV, 143
  position, 152–154
  posterior angulation of, 147
  protrusion of, 149–151
  shape variation, 144
  width, 148–149
Eccrine sweat glands, 319
Ectodermal dysplasia, 182, 307, 321
Ectopic anus, 303
Ectopic thyroid gland, 192
Effective mandibular length, 187–188
Effective midfacial length, 183
Elbow joint
  development of, 351
  ossification centers, 351
  range of movement, 256
  sweat pores in, 321

Elevated vascular nevus, 317
Ellis-van Creveld syndrome, 465
Embryo and fetal pathology, 394–406
Enamel, 180–182, 314, 352
Encephalocele, 121
Endochondral ossification, 92
Epidermis
  birthmarks, 315
  description, 309–310, 312, 314
  development of, 197
  nail folds surrounded by, 325
  organoid nevus of, 318
  sweat glands in, 320
Epispadias, 293
Erythema nuchae, 316
Erythroblastosis/hydrops, 395
Esophagus, 406
Exophthalmos, 139
Expanded Interview of the Vineland Adaptive Behavior Scales II, 371
Extensibility of skin, 310–311
Eyes, 122–141
  bony interorbital distance, 122–123
  canthal distance, inner, 127–128
  canthal distance, outer, 129–130
  conjunctiva abnormalities, 126–127
  cornea size, shape variation, 126
  corneal dimensions, transverse diameter, 140–141
  developmental stages, 122–123
  epicanthal folds, 124–125
  eyelid assessment, 123–124
  interpupillary distance, 131–133
  iris color anomalies, 125–126
  orbital protrusion, 139
  palpebral fissure, inclination, 137–138
  palpebral fissure, length, 134–136
  periorbital edema, 122
  periorbital structures, 122
  related syndromes, 124–125
  supraorbital brows, 122

Face
  age-related growth, 90–91
  branchial arch abnormality, 109
  development of, 86–87
  epicanthal fold, 124
  evaluation positioning, 88
  facial height, 107–108, 110
  lower facial height, 105–106
  radiographic measurements, 90
  reconstructive surgery instruments, 7
  surface, photography, 8, 90
  uniqueness of, 86
  upper facial height, 103–104
  width (bizygomatic distance), 109–110
Facial cleft, 169, 187
Facial hair patterning, 121–122
Facial index, 110–111
Feet. *See* Foot
Female baldness, 324
Female genitalia
  clitoris, 285–286, 302, 367
  development of, 285–288
  labia minora, majora, 285–286, 367
  pubertal changes, 286–290
  racial differences, 290
  Tanner development stages, 288–289
  vagina, 285–286, 301
Fetal alcohol spectrum disorder, 124, 166
Fetal and embryo pathology, 394–406
Fetal organ weights
  by body weight, 400
  by ovulation age, 399
Fetal tissue weights, 401–402
Fetus
  biometric data, 378
  biparietal diameter (BPD), 10
  body proportion changes, 14
  chest circumference, 10
  clitoral development, 285
  crown-rump length, 10, 36, 378
  Down syndrome phenotype, 12
  epidermal layers, 309
  external genitalia differentiation, 286
  eyes, developmental stages, 122–123
  femur length, 10
  finger pads, whorl pattern, 330, 337
  hair follicle development, 323
  hand biometric data, 378
  head circumference biometric data, 378

intrauterine fetal death, 394–395
mouth development, 86
movement during gestation, 392
neonatal reflexes, 366
normal activity, during gestation, 392
ossification centers, 348, 350
palate development, 87
palm, flexion creases, 338
penile development, 291
reflex behavior, 365
reflex movements, 365
skin, blood vessel formation, 309
skull development, 92
supraorbital ridge shape, 342
thumb sucking, 392
tongue development, 87
ultrasound examination, 10, 376–392
umbilical cord length correlates, 264–265
Fingernails, 199, 325–327
Finger(s). *See also* Hand; Nails; Thumb
bone measurement, 356
clubbing, 327
development of, 331, 338, 340
epidermal ridge pattern, 309, 319, 331–332
family pattern profile, 357
flexion crease, 331, 338
middle finger length, 217–219, 222
nails. *See* nails
norms, finger bone length, 358–361
pad development, 330–331
polydactyly, 199
syndactyly, 199
thumb-finger grasp, 373
webbing, 198
Fingertips, 330, 335, 337
Flexion creases (of fingers)
evaluation, 338–339
five-finger crease, 339
three-finger crease, 340
thumb crease, 340
Flexion creases, of fingers, 338
Fontanelles, 93, 112–121
age-related changes, 113–114, 115
anterior fontanelle size, 115–119
at birth, 112–113
metopic fontanelle, 112
posterior fontanelle size, 120–121
of the skull, 93
Foot
contractures of, 235
development of, 351
in Down syndrome, 338
length, 6, 238–242
ossification centers, 350, 351
range of movement, 258
supernumerary digits, 199
in total lower limb length, 228–232
width, 6, 242–244
Forearm
carrying angle, 211–212
length, 207–211
Forehead
bulging/cloverleaf skull, 96
chin, relation to, 187
in craniosynostosis, 83
development of, 87
hair growth patterns, 341–342
height, 101–102
in newborns, 318
sweat pores in, 321
Frankfort horizontal plane, 18
Freeman-Sheldon syndrome, 124, 187
Frontonasal processes, 183
Fused dichorionic diamniotic placenta, 398

Gastrointestinal tract, 406
Gastroschisis, 264
Genitalia, 285–307
anus. *See* anus
breasts. *See* breasts
development of, 285–288
female. *See* female genitalia
male. *See* male genitalia
pubertal changes, 286–290
Gestational age
birth weight, 52–55
canthal distance, 128, 130

Gestational age (*Cont.*)
chest circumference, 268
clinical estimation of, 367
crown-rump length, 36
dental age, 352
developmental assessment, 367–368
Down syndrome, birth weight, 439
ear length, 146
foot length, 236
forearm length, 209
hand length, 214
head circumference, 78–79, 84
head length, 97
head width, 99
height standards, 16
intercommissural distance, 171
internipple distance, 270
interpupillary distance, 132
leg length, at birth, 230
length standards, 16, 18–21, 19
lower leg length, 236
middle finger length, 218
palm length, 221
palpebral fissure length, 135
penile length, 292
philtrum length, 167
skinfolds, 72
small for, 18
sternal length, 275
time of hair patterning, 341
torso length, 277
total upper limb length, 202
twin length, at birth, 21
ultrasound measurements in relation to, 376–391
umbilical cord length, 283
upper arm length, 205
weight and, 18
Glandular hypospadias, 293
Growth
brain, 10
defined, 4
parameters, landmarks, 10–11
patterns, 5
serial measurements, 2
tools for measuring, 7
Growth hormone deficiency, 11
Growth velocity, 5, 11
birth-4 years, 44
defined, 44
females, 46
males, 45

Hair
alopecia, 319, 325
balding, 324
body hair, pubertal changes, 286, 287–290
color, 312, 314, 323
daily growth of, 322
embryology, types of, 323
facial hair patterning, 121–122
follicle development, 121, 319, 320
growth on trunk, 322
lanugo hair pattern, 340–341, 343, 367
life cycle of, 322
lower spine, hair whorl, 343
parietal whorl, 121, 341
texture, 323–324
Hair follicle patterning (trichoglyphics), 340–342
Hair patterning
development of, 341–342
face, 121–122
hair whorl, 121, 341–343
lanugo hair pattern, 340–341, 343, 367
normal/abnormal patterns, 342–343
scalp, 121–122, 341
Hair whorl, 121, 341–343
Hand. *See also* Finger(s)
bone age determination, 11, 346–347
development of, 197–198, 330, 332
in Down syndrome, 338
fetal biometric data, 378
flexion creases, 332, 338, 339
gestational age determination, 368
length, 213–216
middle finger length, 217–219, 222
ossification centers, 350
palm length, 220–221

palm width, 222–225
palm width to length ratio, 225
pattern profile of, 356–357
supernumerary digits, 199
sweat pores in, 321
total upper limb length, 201–203
tubular bones, 357
Head
cephalic index, 100
cloverleaf skull, 96
fontanelles at birth, 112–113
head-to-trunk ratio, 379
length, 95–97
width, 98–100
Head circumference (occipito-frontal circumference), 10, 14–15
in Achondroplasia, 415–416
in Cornelia de Lange syndrome, 428–429
in Costello syndrome, 432
craniosynostosis variance, 83
in Cri-du-chat syndrome, 438
definition, 77
in Down syndrome, 440, 449–450, 459–460
females, 82, 83
fetal biometric data, 378
by gestational age, 79
infants, 80
instruments, 77
landmarks, 77
males, 80–81
in MOPD II, 476
in Neurofibromatosis, type I, 483–484
position, 77, 78
in Prader-Willi syndrome, 491
in Rubinstein-Taybi syndrome, 501
in Smith-Lemli-Opitz syndrome, 506
in Trisomy 13, 509
in Trisomy 18, 511
in Turner syndrome, 515
in 22q11.2 microdeletion syndrome, 533, 538–539
velocity, 84
in Williams syndrome, 520–521
in Wolf-Hirschhorn syndrome, 526
Head-to-abdomen circumference ratio, 380
Head-to-trunk ratio, 380
Heart
cyanotic congenital disease, 327
normal weight, 403–404
postmortem fetal weight, 399–401
Height. *See also* Standing height
in Achondroplasia, 409–410
for age, in males, 29
age group standards, 16
in *BRAF* mutation, 487
in Costello syndrome, 430
in Cri-du-chat syndrome, 432–435
in Down syndrome, 442, 444, 451–454, 461–464
in Ellis-van Creveld syndrome, 465
expected increments, both sexes, 47
for females, 33
in *KRAS* mutation, 487
in Marfan syndrome, 466–469
in MOPD II, 474
in Morquio A syndrome, 477–478
in Neurofibromatosis, type I, 481–482
in Prader-Willi syndrome, 489, 492, 496–497
prediction of, 41–42, 41–43
prospective, 42
in Pseudoachondroplasia, 498
in *PTPN11* mutation, 487
in *RAF1* mutation, 487
in Rubinstein-Taybi syndrome, 499–500
in Russell-Silver syndrome, 502–503
in *SHOC2* mutation, 487
sitting height, 6, 39
in Smith-Lemli-Opitz syndrome, 504
in *SOS1* mutation, 487
in spondyloepiphysial dysplasia congenita, 507
standing, 22–34
in Trisomy 13, 508
in Trisomy 18, 510
in Turner syndrome, 512–513
in 22q11.2 microdeletion syndrome, 527, 529–530, 534–535

Height (*Cont.*)
velocity, birth-4 years, 44
velocity, females, 46
velocity, males, 45
in Williams syndrome, 516–519
in Wolf-Hirschhorn syndrome, 522–523
Hemifacial microsomia, 146
Hemihyperplasia, 198
Hemihypertrophy, 198
Hemihypoplasia, 198
Hereditary hemorrhagic telangiectasia, 317
Hernia, umbilical, 264
Heterochromia iridis, 125
Hip joint
development of, 351
ossification centers, 351
range of movement, 254, 257
Humeral length, 383
Hydrops, 395
Hyperextensibility of limbs, 255, 259–260
Hypospadias, 293
Hypothenar patterns, 330–332, 335
Hypothyroidism, 125
Hypotonia, 272

Iliac crest, 265, 280
Imperforate anus, 303
Imperial measurement system, 8–9
Increased pupillary distance (IPD), 122
Infant scale, 7, 51
Infants. *See also* Newborn; Premature infants
gestational age, 18
head circumference, 10
nasal root in, 158
recumbent position measurement, 16
small for gestational age, 18
weight measurement, 50, 51
WHO growth chart development, 23
Ink staining, in dermatoglyphics, 332–333
Inner canthal distance, 127–128
Intelligence, developmental assessment, 369–371
adaptive functioning, 369–371
age-appropriate psychometric testing, 370
disability classification, 371
intelligence quotient (IQ), 369–370
Intelligence quotient (IQ), 369–370
Intervertebral disc, 263
Intrauterine fetal death, 394–395

Jadassohn nevus, 318

Karyotyping, 394–395
Kayser-Fleischer rings, 126
Keratoconus, 126
Kidney
age-based weight, 403–404
length, 386
postmortem fetal weight, 399–401
prenatal measure, 391
width, 387
Knee joint
development of, 351
ossification centers, 351
range of movement, 258
KRAS mutation
length and height, 487
weight, 488
Kyphosis, 263, 276

Labia minora, majora, 285–286, 367
Labioscrotal swelling, 285
Lacrimal punctae (primary telecanthus), 122–123, 131
Lambdoidal suture, 93, 114
Lanugo hair pattern, 340–341, 343, 367
"Late bloomers," 11
Leg. *See also* Foot
lower leg contracture, 24
lower leg length, 235–238
total limb length, 228–232
upper leg circumference, 252
upper leg length, 233–234
upper leg width, 251

Length
for age, in males, 29
age group standards, 16
in *BRAF* mutation, 487
in Down syndrome, 441, 443, 455–456, 462–463
for females, 33
gestational age, females, 20
gestational age, males, 19
in *KRAS* mutation, 487
in Marfan syndrome, 466, 468
in MOPD II, 474
in Morquio A syndrome, 477–478
North American females, birth-3 years, 30
North American males, birth-3 years, 25
in Prader-Willi syndrome, 489
in *PTPN11* mutation, 487
in *RAF1* mutation, 487
recumbent, 27
in *SHOC2* mutation, 487
in *SOS1* mutation, 487
total body, 11, 16–22
in 22q11.2 microdeletion syndrome, 527, 529–530, 534–535
twins, at birth, 21
Lentigo, 316
Limb(s), 197–260. *See also* Arm; Leg
absence of, 51
at birth, trunk comparison, 15
circumference, 250–252
congenital anomalies, 197–199
embryologic development, 198
hyperextensibility, 259–260
inspection questions, 198–199
range of movement, 253–258
span, 199–201
total lower limb length, 228–232
total upper limb length, 201–203
upper-to-lower segment ratio, 244–248
Lips
cleft lip, 113, 157, 167, 187
deformities of, 113, 157, 167, 169
ear position and, 152
lower lip cleft, 187
maxilla and, 87, 182
nasal height and, 159
philtrum and, 166, 167
Lordosis, 263
Lower leg. *See also* Leg
embryologic development, 198
total lower limb length, 228–232
Luedde exophthalmometer, 139
Lung
age-based weight, 403–404
fetal weight, 399–401
volume, 267
Lymphangioma, 318

Macrocephaly, 81
Macrocranium, 81
Macrodontia, 182
Macroglossia (large tongue), 179
Macrognathia (large jaw), 186
Macrostomia, unilateral congenital, 186
Majewski osteodysplastic primordial dwarfism II (MOPD II)
head circumference, 476
height, 474
length, 474
weight, 475
Male genitalia
penis. *See* penis
scrotum. *See* scrotum
Tanner development stages, 287, 289
testes. *See* testes
Male-pattern baldness, 322, 324
Mandible
absence of, 186
body, 89
cleft abnormality, 105
development of, 186
effective mandibular length, 187–188
lower lip cleft, 187
maxillomandibular differential, 189
median cleft of, 187
overdevelopment of, 186–187
temporomandibular joint, 187
underdevelopment of, 186
width of, 89, 190–191

Mandibular prominences, 86–87, 92, 169, 182, 186–187
Mandibular teeth, 180
Marfan syndrome
  height, 466–469
  length, 466, 468
  weight, 470–473
Maxilla
  absence of, 182–183
  development of, 182–183
  effective midfacial length, 183–184
  lips and, 87, 182
  outer canthal, nasal, outer canthal angle, 184–186
Maxillomandibular differential, 189
Measurements
  body landmarks, 6
  dual systems of, 8–9
  in dysmorphology, clinical genetics, 12–13
  metric-to-imperial conversions, 9
  parameters, landmarks, 10–11
  usefulness of, 1–2, 4–7
Megalencephaly-capillary malformation syndrome, 316
Megalocornea, 126
Melanin, 311–312, 314–315, 322
Menarche, and height prediction, 43
Meningomyelocoele, 112
Mental spurs, 187
Metatarsophalangeal (MTP) joint, 242
Metopic suture, 94, 112–113, 115, 119
Metric system, 8–9
Microcephaly
  brain growth and, 114
  central nervous system and, 341
  description, 78
  scalp hair patterning and, 121–122
Microcranium, 78, 81
Microdeletion syndrome (ears), 146
Microdontia, 182
Micrognathia, 107, 186
Microtia (of ears), types I-IV, 143
Middle finger
  length, 217–219
  ratio of, to total hand, 222
Midfacial length, effective, 183–184, 189
Mid-parental height
  definition, 39
  males/females, combination curve, 40
Milk line, 265, 307
Mole, 316
Monochorionic, diamniotic placenta, 398
Monochorionic, monoamniotic placenta, 398
MOPD II. *See* Majewski osteodysplastic primordial dwarfism II
Moro reflex, 366
Morquio A syndrome
  height, 477–478
  length, 477–478
  weight, 479–480
Mouth, 168–171. *See also* Lips; Palate; Tongue
  in facial height measure, 105, 107
  fetal development of, 86
  frenulae, 169–170
  size variations, 168–169
  width (intercommissural distance), 169, 170–172
Myotactic reflexes, 365

Nail-patella syndrome, 326
Nails
  color, 314, 326
  development of, 325, 326
  fingernails, 199, 325–327
  growth estimate method, 328
  in limb evaluation, 199
  quality, 326
  shape, 326
  structure, 325
  syndromes, 326
  toenails, 199, 325–326
Nail bed, 326
Nail dystrophy, 326
Nail field, 326
Nail fold, 326
Nail plate, 326
Nasal bridge prominence, 103
Nasal height, 103–104

Nasal root prominence, 101
Nasal tip, 103, 156, 158–159, 163
Neck
  circumference, 193–194
  congenital malformations, 192
  length, 192–193
  torticollis (wry neck), 192
  vertebrae, 192
  width, 192–193
Neonatal death, 394–395
Neonatal reflex assessment, 366
Neurocranium, 92
Neurofibromatosis, type I, 315
  head circumference, 483–484
  height, 481–482
Nevus
  blue nevus, 315
  compound nevus, 316
  elevated vascular nevus, 317
  Jadassohn nevus, 318
  nevus flammeus, 317
  nevus sebaceous, 318
  nevus simplex, 316
  Port wine nevus, 317
  strawberry nevus, 317
Newborn. *See also* Birth; Infant
  body proportions, 14
  small for gestational age, 18
  suprascapular skin thickness, 72
  total body length, 18, 22
  weight measurement, 50
Nipple
  areola measurement, 306–307
  in chest circumference, 266
  development of, 367
  in female breast, 304–306
  internipple distance, 269–270
  Noonan syndrome position, 267
  skin, post-pregnancy, 314
  in thoracic index, 271
Noonan syndrome
  eyebrow configuration, 124–125
  fingerprint whorl patterns, 337
  hairline placement, 343
  height, 485–487
  length, 487
  nipple position in, 267
  ptosis in, 124
  weight, 487
Nose
  assessment of, 156–157
  columella length, 161–162
  nasal bridge prominence, 103
  nasal height, 103–104, 159–160
  nasal root prominence, 101
  nasal tip, 103, 156, 158–159, 163
  nostrils, Topinard classification, 157–158
  protrusion, 162–163
  shape variations, 158
  width, 164–165

Obliquity of palpebral fissures, 124, 137–138
Occipito-frontal circumference (OFC). *See* Head circumference
Ocular hypertelorism, 122–123, 343, 545
Oligohydramnios, 192
Omphalocele, 264
Opisthocranion, 77, 89, 95
Orbital protrusion, 139
Organs
  fetal weights, by body weight, 400
  fetal weights, by ovulation age, 399
  miscellaneous sizes, 406
  normal mean weight, by age, 403–405
Ossification centers, 346–351
  of chest and trunk, 262–263
  in feet, 350
  fetal centers, 348
  in hand, 350
  in limbs, 197, 350
  in newborns, 348–349
  of skull, 92, 112
  standards comparison, 346
Osteogenesis imperfecta, 114, 127
Outer canthal, nasal, outer canthal angle, 184–186
Ovaries (combined), size by age, weight, 406
Oxycephaly, 95

Pachyonychia congenita, 326
Palate, 172–177
  congenital malformation of, 87, 113
  height, 175–176
  lateral palatine ridges, 172–173
  length, 172, 173–175
  width, 176–177
Palm
  creases, 331–332
  creases, in Down syndrome, 340
  in Down syndrome, 340
  length, 220–221
  pad development, 330
  sweat pores in, 321
  width, 222–224
  width to length ratio, 225
Palmer grasp reflex, 366
Palpebral fissure
  inclination of, 137–138
  length, 134–136
  obliquity of, 137–138
Pancreas
  age-based weight, 402–403
  fetal weight, 399–400
Panniculus adiposus, 310
Parathyroid glands, 406
Parietal (sagittal) fontanelle, 112
Peabody picture vocabulary test, 370
Pectus deformity, 272, 274
Penis
  development of, 286
  hypospadias, 293
  innervation of, 31
  length, 291–292
  pubertal changes, 286, 289
  scrotum. *See* scrotum
Perineal hypospadias, 293
Perioral fibrosis, 169
Petrosquamosal suture, 112
Philtrum
  congenital pits and, 169
  development of, 87
  length, 166–168
Photoanthropometric measurement, 89–90
Photogrametric anthropometry, 8
Pierre-Robin sequence, 186
Pituitary gland, size by age, weight, 406
Placenta
  abnormalities, 394–395
  cord insertion, 397
  fused dichorionic diamniotic, 398
  monochorionic, diamniotic, 398
  monochorionic, monoamniotic, 398
  separate dichorionic diamniotic, 398
  weight at term, 396
Plagiocephaly, 94
Polydactyly, 199
Port wine nevus, 317
Posterior fontanelle, 113, 115
  closure of, 113, 115
  hair whorl location and, 342
  location, 112, 113
  size, 120–121
Posterior parietal hair whorl, 121
Posterolateral fontanelle, 113, 115
Postmortem organ weights, 394–406. *See also* Placenta
  fetal organ weights, by body weight, 400
  fetal organ weights, by ovulation age, 399
  fetal tissue weights, 401–402
  miscellaneous organ sizes, 406
  normal mean weight, by age, 403–405
Postmortem photography, 394
Prader beads, 294
Prader-Willi syndrome, 489–497
  head circumference, 491
  height, 489, 492, 496–497
  length, 489
  weight, 490, 494–495
Precocious puberty, 41
Premature infants, 18, 78
  head circumference, 78
  measurement adjustments, 18
Prenatal ultrasound measurement, 376–392
Prognathism, 107

Proportional growth, and normal variants, 14–15
arm span with height comparison, ratio, 15
occipito-frontal circumference, 14
upper/lower segment ratio, 15
Prospective height, 42
Prostate gland, 406
Proteus syndrome, 318
Pseudoachondroplasia, 498
Ptosis, 139
of breasts, 306
of eyelid, 124
in Noonan syndrome, 124
in Smith-Lemli-Opitz syndrome, 124
PTPN11 mutation
length and height, 487
weight, 488
Puberty
genitalia development, 286
precocious puberty, 41
racial differences, 290
Tanner stages of, 287–289
timing of stages, 290
velocity of, 11, 41
Pubic hair, 287–290
Pulmonary disease, 327

Radiographic measurements, 345–363
adult height prediction, 352
bone age, 11, 345–351
carpal angle, 362–363
craniofacial, 83, 90, 101, 105, 174, 183, 187
dental age, 352–355
forearm length, 208
hand, pattern profile, 356–361
leg length, 229, 233, 235
upper arm length, 204
RAF1 mutation
length and height, 487
weight, 488
Range of movement (ROM), 253–258
ankle joint, 258
arm stretch position, 255
description, 253
elbow joint, 256
foot, 258
hip joint, 257
hip stretch position, 254
knee joint, 258
neutral screening positions, 253
shoulder joint, 256
shoulder stretch position, 254
squatting screening positions, 254
thumb, 226
wrist joint, 257
Recumbent length, 24, 27, 32
Reflex patterns assessment, 365–366
Rhombencephalosynapsis, 325
Ribs, 262–263, 274
Ridge pattern analysis
dermal ridge count, 334
graphite method, 333
hallucal patterns, 335
hypothenar patterns, 335
ink staining method, 332–333
pattern distribution, 335–337
photocopying method, 334
photographic emulsion method, 333
scanning method, 334
thenar patterns, 335
triradii (deltas), 335
Rubinstein-Taybi syndrome
head circumference, 501
height, 499–500
Russell-Silver syndrome, 502–503

Salmon patch, 316
Scalp
hair follicle formation, 341
hair patterning, 121–122
Scaphocephaly, 93, 95
Scapula, 70, 265–266, 278
Scoliosis, 263, 276
Scrotal hypospadias, 293
Scrotum
hypospadias, 293
labioscrotal swellings, 285–286
pubertal changes, 286
testicular descent and, 299

Sebaceous glands
  development of, 319, 320
  number variability of, 310
  skin anomalies and, 318
Sensory innervation of skin, 313
Separate dichorionic diamniotic placenta, 398
Serratus anterior muscle abnormalities, 278
SHOC2 mutation
  length and height, 487
  weight, 488
Shoulder joint
  development of, 351
  ossification centers, 351
  range of movement, 256
  stretch position, 254
  sweat pores in, 321
Sitting height, 6, 35, 37–39, 229, 245
Skeletal dysplasias, 198, 280, 345, 356
Skin. *See also* Dermis; Epidermis
  anomalies of, 318–319
  birthmarks, 315–318
  color, 312, 314
  dermatoglyphic studies, 331–332
  development of, 309, 320
  extensibility of, 310–311
  glands of, 319–321
  layers, 309–310
  patterns reflected by, 311
  sensory innervation of, 313
  surface, 310
  sweat glands. *See* sweat glands
  texture, 310
Skinfold thickness
  definition, 70
  instruments, 70
  landmarks, 70
  in nutritional problems, 11
  position, 70
  subscapular folds, 71–75
  suprailiac, 72
  triceps, 71–73
Skull
  abnormal suture fusion patterns, 94
  deformity/asymmetry, 98
  development of, 92–93
  facial width, 89
  fontanelles, suture landmarks, 93, 112–121
  head length, 89, 95–97
  head width, 89
  height (forehead), 101–102
  lower edge, bony orbit, 18
  lower facial height, 89
  mandibular width, 89
  upper facial height, 89
Small intestine, 406
Smith-Lemli-Opitz syndrome
  head circumference, 506
  height, 504
  ptosis in, 124
  weight, 505
SOS1 mutation
  length and height, 487
  weight, 488
Spina bifida occulta, 112
Spinal cord, 406
Spine
  abnormalities of, 263, 343
  in chest inspection, 266
  lower spine, hair whorl, 343
Stadiometer, 39
Standing height, 22–24
  North American females, 31
  North American males, 26
  North European females, 32, 34
  North European males, 27–28
Standing scale, 50, 51
Stanford Binet test, 369, 371
Sternal notch, 265
Sternum
  cleft sternum, 263
  development of, 262
  length, 273–275
  sternocostal relationship, 262
  in torso length, 276
Stillbirth, 394–395
Stork bite, 316
Strawberry nevus, 317
Sturge-Weber syndrome, 317
Subscapular skinfold thickness, 71–75

Subtle hypoplasia, 183
Subungual fibromas, 326
Supernumerary digits or toes (polydactyly), 199
Supine body length, 16
Suprailiac skinfold thickness, 72
Sutures of the skull
  abnormal fusion patterns, 94
  calvaria, 92–93, 112
  lambdoidal suture, 93, 114
  landmarks, 93
  metopic suture, 94, 112–113, 115, 119
  petrosquamosal suture, 112
Sweat glands
  apocrine, 286–287, 314, 319
  development of, 320
  eccrine, 319
  pore number, 321
  pubertal changes, 286
  quantification of number of, 319, 321
  skin texture and, 310
Syndactyly, 199
Syndromes
  Achondroplasia, 409–417
  Adams-Oliver, 318
  ataxia-telangiectasia, 317
  Barth, 418–419
  BRAF mutation, 487–488
  capillary malformation, 316
  capillary malformation-arteriovenous malformation, 316
  CHARGE, 146
  Cornelia de Lange, 125, 420–429
  Costello, 124, 430–432
  cranio-fronto-nasal, 326
  Cri-du-chat, 432–438
  Cushing, 11
  Down syndrome. *See* Down syndrome
  Dubowitz, 124
  Ellis-van Creveld, 465
  Freeman-Sheldon, 124, 187
  KRAS mutation, 487–488
  Marfan, 466–473
  megalencephaly-capillary malformation, 316
  MOPD II, 474–475
  Morquio A, 477–480
  nail-patella syndrome, 326
  Neurofibromatosis, type I, 481–484
  Noonan, 124–125, 267, 485–488
  Prader-Willi, 489–497
  Proteus, 318
  Pseudoachondroplasia, 498
  PTPN11 mutation, 487–488
  RAF1 mutation, 487–488
  Rubinstein-Taybi, 499–501
  Russell-Silver, 502–503
  SHOC2 mutation, 487–488
  Smith-Lemli-Opitz, 124, 504–506
  SOS1 mutation, 487–488
  spondyloepiphysial dysplasia congenita, 507
  Sturge-Weber, 317
  Treacher Collins, 146, 183
  Trisomy 13, 508–509
  Trisomy 18, 510–511
  Turner, 395, 512–515
  22q11.2 microdeletion, 146, 527–539
  Williams, 125, 516–521
  Wilms tumor–aniridia–genitourinary malformation, 126
  Wolf-Hirschhorn, 522–526
Synophrys, 125
Synostotic anterior plagiocephaly, 94
Synostotic brachycephaly, 94
Synostotic posterior plagiocephaly, 94
Synostotic scaphocephaly, 94
Synostotic trigonocephaly, 94

Tanner stages of puberty, 287–289
Taurodontia, 182
Teeth, 87, 172, 180–182
  abnormalities, 181, 182
  deciduous, 87, 180–182, 352
  enamel, 180–182, 314, 352
  macro-/microdontia, 182
  permanent, 180, 182
  shape variation, 182
  taurodontia, 182
Telangiectasia, 317
Telecanthus, 122–123, 131
Telogen stage (of hair), 322

Temporomandibular joint, 187
Testes
  descent of, 285, 299–300
  development of, 285, 367
  pubertal changes, 286
  size, by age and weight, 406
  volume, 294–298
Thigh. *See* Upper leg
Thoracic index, 271–273
Thoracic vertebrae, 262
Thumb. *See also* Finger(s)
  angle of attachment, 227–228
  crease, 339, 340
  fetal activity, sucking, 392
  hyperextensibility, 259
  nail dystrophy, 326
  nail size, shape, color, 326
  placement index, 226–227
  range of movement, 226
  wiggle, 373
Thumb-finger grasp, 373
Thyroglossal duct cysts, 192
Thyroid gland, size by age, weight, 406
Thyrotoxicosis, 327
Toenails, 199, 325–326
Tongue, 177–178
  anatomy of, 179
  atrophy of, 179
  congenital malformations of, 178
  fetal development of, 87
  lateral palatine ridges and, 172–173
  size variations, 178–179
Tonic-neck reflex, 366
Topinard classification, of nostrils, 157–158
Torso length, 276–277
Torticollis (wry neck), 192
Tower skull, 95
Treacher Collins syndrome, 146, 183
Trichoglyphics (hair follicle patterning), 340–342
Trigonocephaly, 94
Triradii (deltas), of ridge patterns, 335, 338
Trisomy 13, 508–509
Trisomy 13, 318
Trisomy 18, 510–511
Trunk. *See also* Breasts; Chest
  biacromial distance, 276–277
  bi-iliac distance, 280
  in breast measurement, 304
  development of, 365, 366, 377
  hair grown on, 322
  head-to-trunk ratio, 379
  landmarks, 265
  limb-to-trunk ratio, 197, 198
  in ROM inspection, 253, 259
  umbilical cord length and, 282
Tuberous sclerosis, 326
Turner syndrome, 395, 512–515
  fingerprint whorl patterns, 337
  hairline placement, 343
  head circumference, 515
  height, 512–513
  weight, 514
Turricephaly, 95, 101
22q11.2 microdeletion syndrome, 527–539
  external ear abnormalities, 146
  head circumference, 533, 538–539
  height, 527, 529–530, 534–535
  length, 527, 529–530, 534–535
  weight, 528, 531–532, 536–537

Ultrasound measurements, in relation to gestational age, 376–391
  abdominal circumference, 389
  biparietal diameter, 381
  clavicle length growth, 386
  crown-rump length, 380
  femur growth, 383
  fetal biometric data, 378
  fibula length growth, 385
  hand-to-abdomen circumference ratio, 380
  hand-to-trunk ratio, 379
  humerus length growth, 383
  kidney length growth, 386
  kidney width growth, 387
  lateral ventricle width, 390
  occipital-frontal diameter, 382
  ocular diameter growth, 389

orbit size growth, 388
radius length growth, 384
splenic length, 387
tibial length growth, 385
transverse cardiac diameter, 390
ulna length growth, 384
Ultrasound measurements, prenatal measurements, 391
Umbilical cord
abnormalities, 264–265
attachment location, 264, 397
development of, 264–265
length, 264–265, 282–283, 397
Umbilical hernia, 264
Unilateral congenital macrostomia, 186
Unilateral maxillary absence, 182–183
Upper arm length, 6
Upper body-to-lower body segment ratio, 244–248
Upper facial height, 103–104
Upper leg (thigh)
circumference, 252
length, 233–234
width, 251
Upper limb length, 201–203
Upper lip
development of, 87, 323
ear position and, 132
maxilla and, 182
nasal height and, 159
philtrum and, 166–167, 169
telangiectasia and, 317
Urethrolabial fold, 286
Uterine fibroid, 192
Uterus, 406

Vagina, 285–286, 301
Vascular nevus, elevated, 317
Velocity
growth velocity, 5, 11, 44–46
head circumference, 84
height, 44–48
of puberty, 11, 41
weight, 67–69
Vertebrae, 192, 262–263, 271
Vertebral arch, 263
Vertebral column, 262–263
Vesicourethral canal, 285
Vineland Adaptive Behavior Scales II, 371
Viscerocranium, 92

Wechsler Intelligence Scale for Children (WISC), 369
Weight
in Achondroplasia, 411–414
adult measurement, 11
at birth, gestational age, 52
in *BRAF* mutation, 488
in Costello syndrome, 431
in Cri-du-chat syndrome, 436–437
definition, 50
in Down syndrome, 445–448, 457–458
females, 2-20 years, 59
females, birth-3 years, 58
females, for age, 60
females, N. European, 7-19 years, 62
females, N. European, at birth, 55
gestational age and, 18
instruments, 50, 51
in *KRAS* mutation, 488
males, 2-20 years, 57
males, at birth, N. European, 54
males, birth-3 years, 56
males, for age, 58
males, N. European, 7-19 years, 61
in Marfan syndrome, 470–473
metric to imperial conversion, 9
in MOPD II, 475
in Morquio A syndrome, 479–480
normal standards curves, 10–11
in nutritional problems, 11
position, 50
in Prader-Willi syndrome, 490, 494–495
in *PTPN11* mutation, 488
in *RAF1* mutation, 488
in *SHOC2* mutation, 488
in Smith-Lemli-Opitz syndrome, 505
in *SOS1* mutation, 488
in Trisomy 13, 509

in Trisomy 18, 511
in Turner syndrome, 514
in 22q11.2 microdeletion syndrome, 528, 531–532, 536–537
twins, both sexes, at birth, 53
in wheelchair measure, 50
in Williams syndrome, 519–520
in Wolf-Hirschhorn syndrome, 524–525
Weight velocity, 67–69
Wharton's jelly, 264
Widow's peak, 342–343
Width
ears, 148–149
face, 89, 109–110
foot, 6, 242–244
hand, palm width, 222–225
head, 98–100
kidney, 387
mandible, 89, 190–191
mouth, 169, 170–172
neck, 192–193
nose, 164–165
palate, 176–177
palm, 222–224
upper leg, 251
Williams syndrome
eyebrow configuration, 124–125
head circumference, 520–521
height, 516–519
weight, 519–520
Wilms tumor–aniridia–genitourinary malformation, 126
Winged scapula, 278
Wolf-Hirschhorn syndrome
head circumference, 526
height, 522–523
weight, 524–525
Wrist joint
carpal angle, 362–363
development of, 351
ossification centers, 351
range of movement, 257

Xiphoid process, 265

Yale Developmental Schedule, 372